D1403813

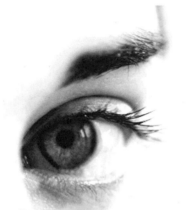

The
Ophthalm✺logy
Examinations Review

Second Edition

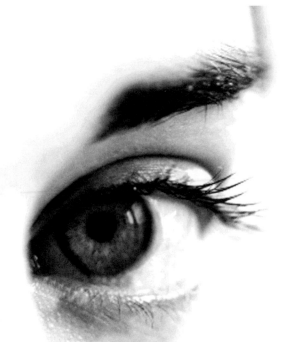

The Ophthalmology Examinations Review

Second Edition

Tien Yin WONG

*National University of Singapore, Singapore
& University of Melbourne, Australia*

With Contributions From

Chelvin SNG
National University Health System, Singapore

Laurence LIM
Singapore National Eye Centre, Singapore

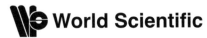 **World Scientific**

NEW JERSEY · LONDON · SINGAPORE · BEIJING · SHANGHAI · HONG KONG · TAIPEI · CHENNAI

Published by

World Scientific Publishing Co. Pte. Ltd.

5 Toh Tuck Link, Singapore 596224

USA office: 27 Warren Street, Suite 401-402, Hackensack, NJ 07601

UK office: 57 Shelton Street, Covent Garden, London WC2H 9HE

British Library Cataloguing-in-Publication Data
A catalogue record for this book is available from the British Library.

THE OPHTHALMOLOGY EXAMINATIONS REVIEW (2nd Edition)
Copyright © 2011 by World Scientific Publishing Co. Pte. Ltd.

ISBN-13 978-981-4304-40-5
ISBN-10 981-4304-40-9
ISBN-13 978-981-4304-41-2 (pbk)
ISBN-10 981-4304-41-7 (pbk)

Typeset by Stallion Press
Email: enquiries@stallionpress.com

Printed in Singapore by World Scientific Printers.

INTRODUCTION TO SECOND EDITION

In the past decade, there have been many discoveries made in understanding the pathogenesis of, and risk factors for, eye diseases. There have been developments in new diagnostic procedures including advances in ocular imaging, and in new treatments, particularly of retinal diseases such as age-related macular degeneration and diabetic retinopathy.

We therefore felt a revised edition of this book reflecting updated knowledge is warranted. In this new edition, we have specifically included topics covering new investigations (e.g. OCT), procedures and treatments (e.g. use of anti-vascular endothelial growth factors and new refractive surgical techniques).

The scope and aim of the book remains consistent with the first edition in that it will provide a broad review for the final year ophthalmology residents and trainees taking the specialist ophthalmology examinations. We have made sure the book deals primarily with *key facts and topics* that are important from an examination perspective. We have tried to ensure that only information that is considered relevant to the examinations is covered, with topics that may be of broader scientific interest, but which are not commonly assessed in the examinations, specifically left out.

We have received extremely good feedback from the first edition and feel this book will still fill a gap in helping the residents organize and synthesize knowledge acquired from various other sources or textbooks.

We emphasize once again it is not meant to replace standard textbooks, although we know now that many residents/trainees believe there is sufficient information contained in our book to serve as the main revision text nearer the exams. **"Caveat emptor"!**

Professor Tien Y Wong
MBBS, MMED (Ophth), MPH, PhD (Johns Hopkins), FRCS (Edin), FRANZCO, FAMS
Director, Singapore Eye Research Institute
Professor, Department of Ophthalmology, National University of Singapore
Senior Consultant Ophthalmologist, Singapore National Eye Centre and National University Hospital
Professor, Centre for Eye Research Australia, University of Melbourne, Australia

Dr Chelvin Sng
BA, MB BChir, MA (Cambridge), MMED (Ophth), MRCS (Edin)
Registrar, National University Health System, Singapore

Dr Laurence Lim
MBBS, MMED, MRCS
Registrar, Singapore National Eye Centre

ABOUT THE AUTHORS

Tien Y Wong is currently Professor and Director of the Singapore Eye Research Institute and Senior Consultant Ophthalmologist at the Singapore National Eye Centre and National University Health System. Professor Wong balances clinical practice as a retinal specialist with a broad-based research program focused on diabetic retinopathy, age-related macular degeneration and the use of retinal imaging to predict cardiovascular risk. He has published more than 500 papers, including papers in the *New England Journal of Medicine* and *The Lancet*. Prof Wong was previously Chairman of the Department of Ophthalmology at the University of Melbourne.

For his clinical service, academic leadership and research, Professor Wong has been recognized internationally with numerous awards, including the Ten Outstanding Young Persons of the World for "academic leadership in people younger than 40 years of age" (1999), the Sandra Doherty Award from the American Heart Association (2004), the Woodward Medal from the University of Melbourne (2005), the Alcon Research Institute Award (2006), the Novartis Prize in Diabetes (2006), the Australian Commonwealth Health Minister's Award for Excellence in Health and Medical Research (2006), and the Australian Society of Medical Research Medical Research of the Year Award (2006). In 2008, Prof Wong was the recipient of the inaugural Singapore Translational Researcher Award (STaR), in 2009, the Outstanding Researcher Award from National University of Singapore, and in 2010, the National Clinician Scientist Award. He is the recipient of the 2010 President's Science Award in Singapore.

He is married to a very supportive family physician wife and have two boys, aged 9 and 13, who do not see a lot of him (although he is trying to change this). He enjoys movies, reading, jogging and squash.

Chelvin Sng is a typical struggling Ophthalmology resident with "too much to do" and "too little time." To compound matters, there is "too much to learn" and "too little cerebral capacity." Hence, she is forever indebted to the first edition of "Ophthalmology Examinations Review," without which she would not have passed her postgraduate assessments. Dr Sng is currently a registrar at the National University Health System in Singapore, where she has developed a healthy interest in glaucoma, myopia and epidemiology. She has a few publications under her belt, but certainly hopes to acquire many more. She has ambitions of traveling the world and owning a dog, but is soon coming to the realization that both may not be compatible with the lifestyle of an Ophthalmology resident.

Dr Sng graduated from Gonville and Caius College in Cambridge University with First Class Honours, and distinctions in Medicine, Pathology and Obstetrics and Gynecology. For her academic achievements, she was the elected senior scholar at Gonville and Caius College (2001), and also received the Max A. Barrett Prize (2002), William Harvey Studentship (2002–2004) and the Charles and Iris Brook Prize (2004). After graduation, she was awarded the Singhealth House Officer Award (2006), the International Travel Grant from the Association for Research in Vision and Ophthalmology (2008), and the Australian and New Zealand Glaucoma Interest Group Scholarship (2010).

Laurence S Lim is currently a registrar at the Singapore National Eye Centre. He hopes to complete his Advanced Specialty Training in Ophthalmology soon and thereafter pursue sub-specialty training in vitreo-retinal diseases. Dr Lim is privileged to have worked under the mentorship of Prof Wong, and the opportunity of participating in this latest edition of the Ophthalmology Examinations Review.

Dr Lim pursued medical studies at the National University of Singapore, in the course of which he earned several medals and prizes for best performance in various subjects. He was recognized on the Dean's List every year and was also a University Scholar. Graduating in 2002 as the best student throughout the entire course of study, he was awarded the Lee Kuan Yew Gold Medal. He has a strong interest in research and published his first paper as an undergraduate. He has continued to do research and, to date, has published 25 papers in international journals including the *Lancet, Ophthalmology, Investigative Ophthalmology and Visual Sciences*, and the *Archives of Ophthalmology*. He also serves frequently as a peer reviewer for several ophthalmic publications. He has attended many international, regional and local scientific meetings at which he has participated as an invited speaker, a course instructor, session moderator, judge and presenter.

He is married to a fellow ophthalmologist in training, and their preferred distractions include running, painting, and spending time in the kitchen.

CONTENTS

Section 3: Corneal and External Eye Diseases 107

Section 4: Surgical Retina 171

Section 5: Medical Retina 195

Section 6: Neuroophthalmology 267

Section 7: Oculoplastic and Orbital Diseases 345

Section 8: Uveitis, Systemic Diseases and Tumors 389

Cataract and Cataract Surgery

TOPIC 1

THE LENS

Overall yield: ✹✹   **Clinical exam:**   **Viva:** ✹✹   **Essay:** ✹   **MCQ:** ✹✹✹

Q Opening Question: What is the Anatomy of the Lens?

"The lens is located between the anterior and posterior segments of the eye."

Anatomy of the Lens

1. **Gross anatomy**
   - Biconvex, transparent structure that divides eye into anterior and posterior segment
   - General dimensions: 10 mm diameter, 4 mm thickness, 10 mm anterior surface radius, 6 mm posterior surface radius

2. **Microscopic anatomy**
   - Capsule
     - **Acellular** elastic structure
     - Similar to basement membrane (type 4 collagen)
     - Zonules run from ciliary processes and fuse onto outer layer of capsule
     - Main function is to mould the shape of lens in response to tension on zonules
     - Important barrier to forward migration of the vitreous during/after lens extraction
   - Anterior epithelium
     - Functionally divided into 2 zones:
       - Equatorial zone
         - Actively dividing and differentiating into lens **cell fibers**
       - Non-equatorial zone
         - **Transports** solutes between lens and aqueous humor
         - Secretes **capsular material**
     - All epithelial cells are nucleated
     - Cytoplasm contains organelles (ribosomes, sER, rER, GA, mitochondria)
   - Lens fibers
     - Divided into cortex and nucleus
     - Cortex
       - **Suture lines** (anterior Y shape, posterior inverted Y)
       - Only the young lens fibers have normal cellular organelles which subsequently disintegrates with aging
       - Newly formed cortical fibers elongate, with one end of the cell moving anteriorly and the other end posteriorly
     - Nucleus
       - Consists of cells that have been retained throughout life
       - Metabolism of cells in the nuclear region is minimal

Exam tips:
- **Not a very common question, but considered "basic" anatomical knowledge.**
- **In general, anatomy questions like "What is the anatomy of...." can be answered by first dividing the structure into gross and microscopic anatomy.**

Q What is the Function of the Lens? Why is it Transparent?

"The main functions of the lens are..."

Functions of Lens

1. **Function of lens**
   - Refraction
     - Accounts for **35%** of total refractive power of eye (15D out of total of 58D)
   - Light transmission
2. **Maintenance of transparency**
   - Regular arrangement of lens fibers
   - Small differences in refractive index between components
   - Little cellular organelles
   - Little extracellular space (tight 'ball and socket' junctions)

Q What is the Embryology of the Lens?

Embryology

1. **Formation of lens vesicle**
   - 4 mm stage (4 weeks)
   - Optic vesicle induces lens **placode** from ectoderm
   - Lens placode invaginates and becomes lens **pit**
   - Optic vesicle also invaginates and becomes the optic cup
   - Lens pit separates from ectoderm to become lens **vesicle**
2. **Formation of lens fibers and zonules**
   - Primary lens fibers
     - Cells in **posterior** portion of lens vesicle elongate to fill vesicle
   - Secondary lens fibers
     - Cells in **anterior** portion of vesicle divide actively and elongate
   - Tertiary lens fibers
     - Cells in **equatorial** zone of lens epithelium divide and differentiate into long lens fibers
   - Lens zonules
     - Develop from neuroepithelium running from inner surface of ciliary body to fuse with lens capsule

Q How is Glucose Metabolized in the Lens?

Carbohydrate and Energy Metabolism

1. **Energy production entirely dependent on glucose metabolism**
   - Glucose enters lens by simple diffusion and facilitated diffusion
   - Glucose is rapidly metabolized via glycolysis so that level of free glucose in lens < 1/10 glucose in aqueous
2. **4 pathways**
   - **Anaerobic glycolysis**
     - Accounts for **85%** of glucose metabolism by lens
     - Provides **> 70%** of energy for lens
     - 1 mole of glucose gives 2 moles of ATP
     - Lactate generated undergoes 2 pathways of metabolism:
       - Further metabolism via Kreb's cycle
       - Diffusion from lens into aqueous
   - **Aerobic metabolism (Kreb's cycle)**
     - Limited to **epithelium**
     - 1 mole of glucose gives 38 moles of ATP
     - Only **3%** of lens glucose metabolized by this pathway
     - But generates up to **20%** of total ATP needs of lens
   - **Hexosemonophosphate shunt**
     - Accounts for 5% of glucose metabolism by lens
     - Important source of **NADPH** required for other metabolic pathways e.g. sorbitol pathway and glutathione reductase
   - **Sorbitol pathway**
     - Glucose → **sorbitol** via aldose reductase → **fructose** via polyol dehydrogenase
     - Accounts for 5% of glucose metabolism by lens
     - When sorbitol accumulates within cells of lens, it sets up an osmotic gradient that induces influx of water and lens swelling and ultimately loss of lens transparency

Q What is the Biochemical Structure of Lens Proteins?

"There are 2 types of lens proteins...."

Biochemical Structure of Lens Proteins

1. **Water soluble lens crystallins**
   - **90%** of total lens protein
   - Alpha crystallin
     - Largest crystallin
     - Accounts for 35% of total lens protein
   - Beta crystallin
     - Most abundant crystalline; accounts for 55% of total lens protein
     - Most heterogenous group; 4 distinct subgroups
   - Gamma crystallin
     - Smallest crystallin
     - Least abundant

2. **Water insoluble proteins – includes:**
   - Membrane proteins – urea insoluble
   - Cytoskeletal proteins and crystallin aggregates – urea soluble

TOPIC 2

CATARACTS

Overall yield: ✸✸✸   **Clinical exam:** ✸✸   **Viva:** ✸✸✸   **Essay:** ✸✸   **MCQ:** ✸✸✸

Q **Opening Question:** What are the Causes of Cataracts?

"By far the most common cause of cataract is aging."
"Other causes can be classified into 2 types: congenital and acquired...."

Etiology of Cataracts

1. **Congenital**
   - Genetic and metabolic diseases
     - Down's syndrome, galactosemia, Lowe's syndrome
   - Intrauterine infection
     - Rubella
   - Ocular anomalies
     - Aniridia
   - Hereditary cataract

2. **Acquired**
   - Age-related cataract
   - Traumatic cataract
   - Metabolic diseases
     - DM
   - Toxic
     - Steroid use, chlorpromazine
   - Secondary to ocular disease
     - Uveitis
     - Angle closure glaucoma (glaukomflecken)

Exam tips:
- In general, etiology questions like "What are the causes of...?" can be answered in a common opening statement: "The causes can be classified into congenital or acquired. Congenital causes include...."
- In other situations, it may be best to answer directly the most common cause first (which gives the impression that you're not memorizing from the book!).
- Do not list the rare conditions. For example, under metabolic diseases, say "diabetes," and avoid "hyperparathyroidism."

Q What is the Pathophysiology of Age-related Cataracts?

Pathophysiology of Age-related Cataracts

1. **General risk factors**
   - Age
   - Smoking
   - Ultraviolet light exposure
   - Medications and other environmental exposures (controversial)

2. **Cortical cataract**
   - Usually results from derangement of **electrolyte and water balance**
     - Increased levels of sodium, chloride and calcium
     - Decreased levels of potassium

- Associated with marked increase in lens membrane permeability
- Associated with liquefaction of lens material and osmotic phenomena (lens intumescence)

3. **Nuclear cataract**
   - Associated with **protein modification** and increased coloration (urochrome pigment)

- Other lens metabolism changes
  - Increase in proteolysis
  - Decrease in ATP production
  - Decrease in glutathione levels
    - Inability to withstand oxidative stress

Q **What is the Pathophysiology of Diabetic Cataracts?**

"There are two pathogenic mechanisms in diabetic cataracts...."

Pathophysiology of Diabetic Cataracts

1. **Osmotic effect**
   - Glucose → **sorbitol** via aldose reductase (rapid) → **fructose** via polyol dehydrogenase (slow)
   - Sorbitol cannot diffuse out of intracellular compartment → accumulates in lens → creates an osmotic gradient and movement of water

into cells → swelling and rupture of cells → results in opacification and cataract formation

2. **Direct damage**
   - Glucose may directly interact with lens proteins via glycosylation, leading to protein aggregation and cataract formation

Q **Tell me about Galactosemia.**

"Galactosemia is an inborn error in metabolism." "The inheritance is AR and there are 2 types."

Galactosemia

1. **Galactosemia (type II or classic galactosemia)**
   - Pathophysiology
     - Deficiency of **galactose-1-phosphate uridyl transferase (GPUT)**
     - Galactose → dulcitol/galactitol via aldose reductase (no further metabolism)
     - Accumulation of dulcitol results in osmotic disturbance in lens, leading to cataract formation
   - Clinical features
     - Central **oil droplet** cataract
     - Nonglucose reducing substance present in urine
     - Generally **sick** (failure to thrive, hepatosplenomegaly, CNS disease, renal disease)

2. **Galactokinase deficiency (type I)**
   - Pathophysiology
     - Deficiency of **galactokinase**
     - Galactose → dulcitol/galactitol via aldose reductase (no further metabolism)
     - Accumulation of dulcitol results in similar pathway as in Galactosemia type II
   - Clinical features
     - **Lamellar cataract** (early cataract formation that sinks into lens substance with subsequent growth following institution of dietary control)
     - Generally **healthy**

Exam tips:
- Note that aldose reductase is important in the pathogenesis of both diabetic and galactosemic cataracts.

Q **What are the Ocular Signs in Down's Syndrome?**

"The ocular features of Down's syndrome can be divided into anterior segment and posterior segment signs."

Down's Syndrome

1. **Inheritance**
   - **Nondisjunction** (95%)
     - 47 chromosomes (3 chromosome 21)
     - Nonhereditary
     - Risk to siblings 1%
   - **Translocation** (4%)
     - 46 chromosomes (segment of chromosome 14 translocates to chromosome 21)
     - Hereditary
     - Risk to siblings 10% (with high rates of spontaneous abortion)
   - **Mosaic** (1%)
     - 47 chromosomes in some cells, 46 in others
     - Nonhereditary
2. **Systemic features**
   - Mental retardation
   - Stunted growth
   - Mongoloid facies
   - Congenital heart defects
3. **Ocular features**
   - Anterior segment
     - Lid (**blepharitis**, epicanthal fold, mongoloid slant)
     - Nasolacrimal duct obstruction
     - Cornea (**keratoconus**)
     - Iris (**brushfield spots**, iris atrophy)
     - Cataract
   - Posterior segment
     - Increased retinal vessels across optic disc
   - Others
     - High myopia
     - Strabismus, nystagmus and amblyopia
     - Macular hypoplasia

Exam tips:
- Questions like "What are the ocular signs of...?" can be answered with a common opening statement, "The ocular signs can be divided into anterior segment or posterior segment signs. Anterior segment signs include...."
- You may consider either answering directly the commonest eye sign first, "The commonest ocular feature is...."
- Or answering the most important eye sign first: "The most important eye sign is...."

CONGENITAL CATARACTS

Overall yield: ✪✪✪ **Clinical exam:** **Viva:** ✪✪✪ **Essay:** ✪✪✪✪ **MCQ:** ✪✪✪

Q **Opening Question No. 1:** What are the Causes of Congenital Cataracts?

"Congenital cataracts can be classified into 2 types: primary and secondary."
"Secondary causes include…."

Classification of Congenital Cataract

1. **Primary**
   - Idiopathic (50% of all congenital cataracts)
   - Hereditary (30%, usually AD)

2. **Secondary**
   - Systemic disorders
     - Chromosomal disorders (Down's syndrome)
     - Metabolic disorders (galactosemia, Lowe's syndrome)
   - Maternal infections (toxoplasmosis)
   - Ocular developmental disorders
     - Persistent hyperplastic primary vitreous
     - Anterior segment dysgenesis, aniridia
     - Congenital ectropian uvea, nanophthalmos
   - Ocular diseases
     - Trauma, uveitis, retinoblastoma

Exam tips:
- Do not list the rare causes of congenital cataract. For example, remember "galactosemia" but avoid "Alport's syndrome" (unless you know it well!)
- The classification is identical to that of congenital glaucoma (see page 57) and subluxed lens (see page 35).

Q **Opening Question No. 2:** How do You Manage Congenital Cataracts?

"The management of congenital cataract is **difficult.**"
"And involves a **multidisciplinary team** approach."
"The important **issues** are…."
"And **factors** that will influence the decisions include…."
"The management consists of a thorough history…."

Management of Congenital Cataracts

1. **Important issues (see below for detailed discussion)**
   - **Indications** for cataract extraction
   - **Timing** of surgery
   - **Type** of surgery
   - **Aphakic** correction

2. **Factors that influence the decisions**
   - **Cataract** factors (type of cataract, location of cataract, severity of cataract, unilateral or bilateral cataract)
   - **Child** factors (age of onset, associated systemic diseases)

- **Parent** factors (motivation of amblyopia correction)

3. **History**
   - Age of presentation
   - Unilateral/bilateral
   - Family history (AD, AR, etc), consanguinity
   - Birth history – Low birth weight (ROP), trauma at birth (cataract)?
   - Maternal infection?
   - Drug exposure?
     - Naphthalene, phenothiazines, steroids, sulphonamides
   - Radiation exposure?

4. **Clinical examination**
   - Visual acuity
     - Forced preferential looking charts (hundreds and thousands), Catford drum, optokinetic drum
     - Kay picture chart, Sheridan Gardiner, Illiterate "E"
   - Lens opacity
     - Location
       - Polar, subcortical, cortical, lamellar, total
     - Type
       - Spoke-like (Fabry's disease, mannosidosis)
       - Vacuoles (DM, hyperalimentation, ROP)
       - Multi-color flecks (hypoparathyroidism, myotonic dystrophy)
       - Oil droplet (galactosemia, Alport's syndrome)
       - Thin, wafer-shaped (Lowe's syndrome)
       - Green sunflower (Wilson's disease)
   - Associated ocular anomalies
     - Anterior segment
       - Microophthalmos (rubella)
       - Megalocornea, sclerocornea, keratoconus
       - Cloudy cornea (Peter's plus syndrome, Lowe's syndrome, Fabry's disease, glaucoma)
       - Uveitis (juvenile rheumatoid arthritis)
       - Aniridia, mesenchymal dysgenesis, coloboma
       - Glaucoma (aniridia, Peter's plus syndrome, Lowe's syndrome, rubella, trisomy 18)
     - Posterior segment
       - Vitreous strands (persistent fetal vasculature, Stickler's syndrome)
       - Retinal abnormalities
         - ROP, retinoblastoma,
         - Pigmentation (rubella, Bardet-Biedl syndrome, Refsum's disease)
         - Atrophy (Cockayne's syndrome)
         - White flecks (Alport's syndrome)
       - Optic nerve abnormalities
   - Associated systemic anomalies
     - Chromosomal (Down's syndrome and others)
     - Skin rash (atopic dermatitis)
     - Deafness (Alport's syndrome, Rubella, Refsum's disease)
     - Hepatic dysfunction (Wilson's disease, Zellweger's syndrome)
     - Renal disease (Lowe, Alport's, Zellweger's syndrome)
     - CNS disease (Zellweger's syndrome, Lowe)

5. **Investigations**
   - Serum
     - Complete blood count
     - Renal function tests, serum calcium (hypoparathyroidism)
     - Serology for virus (toxoplasmosis)
     - GPUT and galactokinase activity in red blood cells (galactosemia)
     - Arterial blood gas (Lowe's syndrome)
   - Urine
     - Reducing substance (galactosemia)
     - Amino acid (Lowe's syndrome)
     - Sediments (Fabry's disease)
     - Copper (Wilson's disease)
     - Blood (Alport's syndrome)
   - SXR for calcifications (toxoplasmosis, hypoparathyroidism)
   - Others
     - Karyotyping (chromosomal disorders)
     - Cultured fibroblasts with low mannosidase level (mannosidosis)
     - Conjunctival biopsy with birefringent cell inclusions (Fabry's disease)
     - Audiological evaluation

Important Issues in Cataract Management

1. **Indications for surgery**
   - "**Severe**" cataract
     - Frequent assessment of visual function needed
     - In general, operate when cataract is severe enough to affect visual function and development of the eye
     - Earlier surgery indicated when cataract is unilateral (more amblyogenic)
   - Common indications — cataract is associated with:
     - Compromised fixation (infants)
     - Snellen VA or equivalent VA < 6/24 (older baby)
     - Strabismus
     - Poor visualization of fundus
     - Opacity occupying central 3 mm

2. **Timing of surgery**
   - Depends on **laterality** and **severity**
   - Bilateral severe
     - < 2–3 months
     - Operate fellow eye within 1 week of first operation
   - Unilateral severe
     - < 4 months (best outcomes when performed < 16 weeks)
     - If persistent hyperplastic primary vitreous present, consider operating earlier
     - After 9 years of age, operate for cosmetic results only
   - Bilateral or unilateral mild
     - May consider waiting until child is older

3. **Type of surgery**
   - "What are the problems associated with congenital cataract surgery?"
     - Intraoperative problems
       - Risk of GA (prematurity, systemic diseases)
       - Small eye
       - Hard to dilate pupil
       - Low scleral rigidity
       - Solid vitreous
       - Elastic anterior capsule
     - Postoperative problems
       - Higher incidence of posterior capsule opacification
       - Increased inflammation
       - IOL decentration
       - Difficulty in refraction
       - Refractive correction and amblyopia treatment
   - Standard technique is usually combination of:
     - Lens aspiration/lensectomy

   - Primary posterior capsulotomy
   - Anterior vitrectomy: At least 1/3 of anterior vitreous must be removed
   - May be either corneal/transpupillary or pars plana approach
   - IOL material: Single piece PMMA lens has longest safety record, acrylic foldable lenses increasingly utilized
   - IOL frequently captured in posterior CCC to improve centration and block vitreous migration
   - Additional considerations
     - < 18 months (corneal 2-stab incision lensectomy, 1 for AC maintainer, 1 for ocutome/vitrector)
     - 18–24 months (scleral tunnel lensectomy, with phacotome)

4. **Aphakic correction**
   - Depends on **laterality** and **age**
   - IOL implantation
     - Indication: **unilateral aphakia** in children 6 months to 1 year or older (not indicated for children < 6 months)
     - Biometry done under GA prior to operation
     - "How do you choose the IOL power?"
       - Difficult to estimate because of the progressive myopic shift with age (axial length of 16.8 mm at birth, this space becomes 20 mm by 1 year)
       - 5 different approaches
         - Preferred approach: Undercorrecting eye by 1–4D from IOL power that is calculated for emmetropia based on age of child (aim for initial hypermetropia)
         - IOL based on emmetropia
         - IOL that matches refractive error of fellow eye
         - IOL based on axial length alone
         - IOL of 21–22D in all normal sized eyes in children more than 12 months old
   - Aphakic glasses
     - Indication: **Bilateral aphakia** in **older** child
   - Contact lens
     - Indication:
       - bilateral or unilateral aphakia in **infants**
       - frequently needed for correction of anisometropia after IOL implantation in very young children/infants
     - Family support/compliance essential
     - Extended wear soft lens
       - Keratometry under GA
       - Lens diameter of 13.5
       - Overcorrect by 2.5–3D (near vision more important to prevent amblyopia)
   - Infantile Aphakia Treatment Study (in progress)

- Background:
  - IOL use for correction of infantile apahakia still controversial due to problems with IOL power selection and safety concerns
  - Two-thirds of aphakic infants treated with contact lenses remain legally blind in the aphakic eye
- Aim: To compare the use of contact lenses and IOL implantation in the correction of unilateral aphakia
- Study groups: Infants up to 7 months of age with unilateral cataracts randomized to cataract surgery with IOL vs contact lens correction

TOPIC 4

CATARACT SURGERY

Overall yield: ✦✦✦   Clinical exam: Viva: ✦✦✦✦   Essay: ✦   MCQ: ✦✦

Q **Opening Question:** What are the Types of Cataract Surgery?

"There are 3 basic types of cataract surgery."

Cataract Surgery

1. **Intracapsular cataract extraction (ICCE)**
2. **Extracapsular cataract extraction (ECCE)**
3. **Phacoemulsification**

Exam tips:
- **In general, give short simple answers to straightforward questions.**

Q What are the Advantages of ECCE over ICCE?

Advantages of ECCE over ICCE

1. **Smaller wound size**
   - Faster healing time
   - Fewer wound problems (wound leak and iris prolapse)
   - Less astigmatism
   - Less risk of iris incarceration
2. **No vitreous in AC**
   - Lower risk of bullous keratopathy
   - Lower risk of cystoid macular edema
   - Lower risk of retinal detachment
   - Lower risk of glaucoma
3. **Intact posterior capsule**
   - PC IOL implantation possible
   - Eliminate complications associated with AC IOL

Q What are the Advantages (and Disadvantages) of Phacoemulsification over ECCE?

Phacoemulsification vs ECCE

1. **Advantages**
   - Smaller **wound** size
     - Faster healing time
     - Fewer wound problems (wound leak and iris prolapse)
     - Less astigmatism
   - Less risk of expulsive hemorrhage
   - Operation can be performed under **topical anesthesia**
   - **Conjunctival** sparing (important in patients with glaucoma)

2. **Disadvantages**
   - Machine dependent
   - Longer learning curve
   - Higher complication rate during learning curve

Q How do you Perform an Extracapsular Cataract Extraction?

"I would perform an extracapsular cataract extraction with IOL implantation as follows...."

ECCE with IOL

1. **Preparation**
   - Retrobulbar or peribulbar anesthesia
   - Superior rectus suture with 4/0 silk
2. **Conjunctival peritomy**
3. **Partial thickness limbal incision**
   - 2-plane technique (vertical and horizontal)
   - Vertical component made with Beaver blade to 2/3 of scleral thickness, from 10–2 o'clock
4. **Anterior capsulotomy**
   - Enter AC with 27 G needle
   - Fill AC with viscoelastic
   - Perform anterior capsutomy using "tin can" technique
5. **Nucleus expression**
   - Complete horizontal component of the limbal incision with scissors
   - Express nucleus with alternating superior and inferior pressure
6. **Soft lens aspiration**
   - Temporarily close the wound and reform the AC with adequate 10/0 nylon sutures
   - Aspirate soft lens with infusion-aspiration cannula
7. **IOL implantation**
   - Reform AC with viscoelastics
   - Insert IOL into PC capsular bag
8. **Wound closure**
   - 10/0 nylon sutures
   - Subconjunctival steroid/antibiotic injection

> **Exam tips:**
> - **When asked about a certain surgical technique, describe what you are familiar with and make your own notes.**
> - **Be prepared to answer further questions related to the procedure you choose.**
> - **Be concise but accurate with the steps, as if you had done the procedure a hundred times. Say, "I will make a 2-plane limbal incision from 10 to 2 o'clock with a beaver blade" rather than "I will make an incision at the limbus."**
> - **Avoid abbreviations. Say "extracapsular cataract extraction" instead of "ECCE."**

Q What are Some Potential Problems with Anterior Capsulotomy and Nucleus Expression During ECCE?

Anterior Capsulotomy and Nucleus Expression

1. **Problems with anterior capsulotomy**
   - Zonulolysis
   - Endothelium damage
   - Miosis
   - Loss of aqueous (AC shallowing)
2. **Problems with nucleus expression**
   - Wound too small (PCR)
   - Incomplete capsulotomy (PCR)
   - Difficult to express nucleus in soft eye
   - Sphincter rupture with small pupil
   - Tumbling of nucleus (endothelium damage)

Q How do you Perform an Intracapsular Cataract Extraction?

"Currently, the only common indication for planned ICCE is a subluxed lens."
"I would perform an intracapsular cataract extraction with IOL implantation as follows..."

ICCE with AC IOL

1. **Preparation**
   - Retrobulbar or peribulbar anesthesia
   - Superior rectus suture with 4/0 silk
2. **Conjunctival peritomy**
3. **Full thickness limbal incision with Beaver blade and complete incision with scissors, from 9–3 o'clock (larger than ECCE)**
4. **Peripheral iridectomy with Vanna scissors**
5. **Lens removal**
   - Dry lens with Weck sponge
   - Apply cryoprobe between iris and cornea onto lens
   - Alternatively, use vectis and forceps to remove lens
6. **AC IOL implantation**
   - Constrict pupil
   - Reform AC with viscoelastics
   - Insert AC IOL with help of lens glide
7. **Wound closure**
   - 10/0 nylon sutures
   - Subconjunctival steroid/antibiotic injection

Q How do You Perform Phacoemulsification?

"I would perform phacoemulsification as follows…."

Phacoemulsification

1. **Preparation**
   - Retrobulbar, peribulbar or topical anesthesia
2. **Clear corneal tunnel**
   - Stab incision with 2.5 mm keratome for main wound at 12 o'clock
   - Stab incision with Beaver blade for side port at 3 or 9 o'clock
3. **Capsulorrhexis**
   - Fill AC with viscoelastic
   - Perform continuous circular capsulorrhexis with 27 G bent needle
   - Perform hydrodissection (cleavage between cortex and capsule) and hydrodelineation (cleavage between nucleus and epinucleus)
4. **Phacoemulsification of nucleus**
   - The aim of phacodynamic control is to remove lens material in a stable chamber, thereby minimizing the risk of complications related to chamber instability
   - Main parameters:
     - Flow/aspiration
     - Vacuum
     - Power
     - Bottle height
   - Peristaltic systems: Flow and vacuum dissociated and can be controlled individually
   - Venturi systems: Only vacuum can be controlled, and serves to determine flow
   - 'Common' settings:
     - Sculpting:
       - Continuous power, 30%
       - Low vacuum: 30 mm Hg
       - Low flow: 20–30 cc/min
     - Nucleus disassembly:
       - Burst/pulse/hyperpulse power: 25–30%
       - High vacuum: 250–300 mm Hg
       - High flow: 30–40 cc/min
   - Dealing with chamber instability:
     - Proper wound construction to prevent leaks
     - Lower vacuum and flow/aspiration
     - Raise bottle height
     - Check inflow for kinks/interruptions in tubing or connections
     - Viscoelastic tamponade
   - Start with central sculpting
   - Remove rest of nucleus with various techniques
     - Divide and conquer
     - Chop techniques
5. **Soft lens aspiration**
   - Aspirate soft lens with automated infusion-aspiration cannula
6. **IOL implantation**
   - Reform AC with viscoelastics
   - Enlarge main wound to 3 mm (depending on lens insertion technique)
   - Insert foldable IOL into capsular bag
7. **Wound closure**
   - One 10/0 nylon suture if necessary
   - Subconjunctival steroid/antibiotic injection

ANESTHESIA AND VISCOELASTICS

Overall yield: ✪✪✪   **Clinical exam:**   **Viva:** ✪✪✪   **Essay:** ✪✪✪   **MCQ:** ✪✪✪

Q Opening Question: How do You Administer Regional Anesthesia...? What are the Possible Complications?

"I prefer to use the peribulbar anesthesia technique...."

Retrobulbar and Peribulbar Anesthesia

1. **Amount**
   - 5 ml of lignocaine 1% +
   - Wydase (1 ml diluted into 20 ml of lignocaine) +
   - Adrenaline (2/3 drops of 1:1000)

2. **Advantages of peribulbar over retrobulbar anesthesia**
   - Lower risk of optic nerve damage
   - Lower risk of systemic neurological effects of anesthesia
   - Lower risk of globe perforation (controversial)
   - No need for facial block

3. **Disadvantages of peribulbar over retrobulbar anesthesia**
   - Need more anesthetic
   - Less akinesia
   - Longer onset (30 min to attain maximum effect)
   - Higher intraorbital pressure
   - Greater degree of chemosis
   - May need additional superior oblique block (therefore ending up with 2 injections around the globe)

4. **Complications and management**
   - Retrobulbar hemorrhage
     - Most common complication
     - Proceed with surgery if hemorrhage is small
     - Abort surgery if hemorrhage is large
   - Apply intermittent pressure to compress eye
   - Lateral canthotomy if pressure is too high
   - Globe penetration
     - Abort surgery
     - Fundal examination
     - Usually no need to explore scleral wound (self-sealing)
     - B-scan if vitreous hemorrhage obscures view
     - Refer for retinal consult
       - Cryotherapy or laser photocoagulation for the retinal break
   - Optic nerve damage
     - Direct damage or ischemia
   - Extraocular muscle damage (post-operative motility problems)
   - Neurological effects of anesthetic agents
   - Ptosis (from compression/ocular massage)

5. **Alternatives to regional blocks**
   - Topical anesthesia
     - Advantages:
       - No complications of injection
       - No increase in orbital volume
       - Avoids periorbital bruising
     - Disadvantages:
       - No akinesia
       - Less anesthetic effect (intraocular structures till sensitive; e.g. iris)
   - Sub-Tenon's injection
   - Intracameral anesthesia
     - 1% preservative-free lignocaine

Exam tips:
- Be precise about the concentration of drugs and amount you give. Say "In my practice, I'll use 5 ml of 1% lignocaine...." rather than "I'll use lignocaine...."

Q How are the Irrigating Solutions Used During Cataract Surgery?

Irrigating Solutions

1. **Balance salt solution (BSS)**
   - Physiological balanced salt solution
   - Sterile
   - Isotonic
   - Preservative-free
   - Includes: Sodium chloride, potassium chloride, calcium chloride, magnesium chloride, acetate, citrate

- Epinephrine/antibiotics can be added as well
2. **BSS – Plus**
   - Enriched with bicarbonate, dextrose, glutathione
   - Less endothelial damage and better lens nutrition (not proven)

Q Tell me about Viscoelastics.

"Viscoelastics are substances with dual properties of a viscous liquid and elastic solid."
"They are used extensively in intraocular surgeries."
"They display various physical properties...."
"The ideal viscoelastic material has the following characteristics...."

Viscoelastics

1. **Physical properties**
   - Related to chain length and molecular interaction of substances
   - 4 characteristics:
     - Viscoelasticity
       - Refers to tendency to retain original shape and size → shock absorption and endothelial protection
     - Viscosity
       - Refers to resistance to flow → maintain anterior chamber and intraocular volume
     - Pseudoplasticity
       - Refers to ability to transform under pressure from gel to liquid → ease of insertion with increase in pressure
     - Surface tension
       - Refers to coating ability → endothelial protection and surface coating

Exam tips:
- Remember the properties of ideal viscoelastic and compare the advantages and disadvantages of cohesive vs dispersive viscoelastics in terms of these factors.

2. **Ideal viscoelastic**
   - Optically clear, nontoxic, noninflammatory
   - Chamber maintenance
   - Shock absorption
   - Endothelial protection
   - Surface coating
   - Ease of insertion
   - Ease of removal
   - No IOP rise

3. Example

	Cohesive	Dispersive
Examples	Healon • Sodium hyaluronate 1% • Derived from rooster combs • Generally better shock absorption, easier to insert and remove, better view	Viscoat • Hyaluronate 3% + Chondroitin sulfate 4% • Derived from shark cartilage • Generally better coating and endothelial protection, but poorer shock absorption, poorer view, difficult to insert and remove
Properties		
1. Optically clear	+++	+
2. Chamber maintenance	+++	+++
3. Shock absorption	+++	+
4. Endothelial protection	+	+++
5. Surface coating	+	+++
6. Ease of insertion	+++	+
7. Ease of removal	+++	+
8. IOP rise	++	++

4. Indications

- Cataract surgery — commonly used during:
  - Anterior capsulotomy
  - Prior to nuclear expression (for ECCE)
  - IOL insertion
  - Other scenarios in which it is used – pupil dilation, free soft lens matter during aspiration of soft lens, tamponade vitreous after PCR
- Penetrating keratoplasty
- Glaucoma surgery
- Corneal laceration
- Retinal detachment surgery (retinal incarceration during SRF drainage)

INTRAOCULAR LENS

Overall yield: ✸✸✸   Clinical exam: Viva: ✸✸✸   Essay: ✸   MCQ: ✸✸

Q Opening Question: What are the Types of Intraocular Lens?

"An intraocular lens (IOL) is a clear optical device."
"Implanted into the eye to replace the crystalline lens."
"Intraocular lens can be classified as follows…."

Intraocular Lens

1. **Rigid posterior chamber intraocular lens (PC IOL)**
   - Divided into: Optic and haptic components
   - Either one or three pieces
   - Overall length (12–14 mm)
   - Optic
     - Material (PMMA — Polymethylmethacrylate)
     - Diameter (4.5–7 mm)
     - Design (piano-convex, biconvex, meniscus)
   - Haptic
     - Material (PMMA, prolene — easily deformed, nylon — gradually hydrolyzed)
     - Configuration (closed loop, J or C loop)
     - Angulation of haptic to optic (flat, 10° posterior bowing)
   - Additional features
     - Positioning hole
       - Problem of postoperative diplopia
     - Laser ridges
       - Prevent PCO and decrease damage with Nd:YAG laser capsulotomy
       - Problem of postoperative diplopia
     - Multifocal
       - Central portion for near vision
       - Mechanisms – 3 types
         - Refractive, diffractive and aspherical
         - Problems of postoperative diplopia, haloes, glare and loss of VA
     - Heparin-coated
       - Surface more hydrophilic
       - Decrease inflammation, pigment dispersion and synechiae formation (not proven)

2. **Anterior chamber intraocular lens (AC IOL)**
   (see below)

3. **Foldable PC IOL**
   - For small incision cataract surgery
   - Materials:
     - Silicone
     - Acylic
       - Hydrophobic
       - Hydrophilic
     - Optic color/tints:
       - Clear
       - Yellow (blue-blocker)
       - Violet
     - Optic design
       - Convexity (Cornea has positive spherical aberration (SA), normal lens has negative SA)
         - Biconvex std IOL – Positive (SA)
         - Aspheric:
         - Tecnis: Prolate anterior surface = negative SA
         - Acrysof IQ: Negative SA on posterior surface
       - Sorport AO: Pos aspheric — SA free (even power from centre to periphery — not affected by centration/tilt)
     - Edge design:
       - Square
       - Round
       - OptiEdge (Tecnis)
     - Toricity
     - Multifocality
       - Refractive
       - Diffractive
   - Haptic design
     - Material:
       - PMMA (dyed)
       - Prolene – MA60

- Same as optic
- PVDF (Tecnis)
- Shape:
  - Plate
  - Loop
  - Four-point

4. **Injectable IOL**
5. **Scleral-fixated IOL**
6. **Phakic IOL**

Exam tips:
- **Remember that you are implanting this foreign object into a patient's eye. You are therefore expected to know quite a bit about it!**

Q **Tell me about AC IOL.**

"AC IOL is divided into 3 different types.
"It is usually indicated for…."

AC IOL

1. **Types**
   - Pupil plane – suture or clip
   - Iris supported – suture or clip
   - Angle supported – divided into:
     - Rigid angle supported
     - Flexible angle supported – further divided into:
       - Closed loop
       - Open loop "S/Z" shaped or 2/3/4 legs

2. **Indications (3 scenarios)**
   - Secondary IOL implant
   - During ECCE/phaco after PC rupture/zonulolysis

- During planned ICCE

3. **Complications with AC IOL**
   - Endothelial fallout (bullous keratopathy)
   - CME (most common cause of poor VA after AC IOL implant)
   - Chronic pain and ache (older AC IOL with rigid haptics)
   - Glaucoma (uveitis-glaucoma-hyphema (UGH) syndrome)

4. **Calculations of AC IOL power (see below)**

 Clinical approach to anterior chamber IOL

"This patient is pseudophakic with an AC IOL."
"There is a peripheral surgical iridectomy seen at 2 o'clock."

Look for
- *Bullous keratopathy*
- *AC activity (uveitis)*
- *Vitreous in AC/vitreoendothelial touch*
- *Outline of PCR/shape of pupil (round/peaked)*

I'll like to
- *Check IOP*
- *Check fundus (CME, RD)*

Q **What are the Indications and Complications with PC Scleral-Fixated IOL?**

1. **Indications**
   - Similar to AC IOL indications plus
   - Relative **contraindication** to AC IOL implant
     - Younger patient
     - Glaucoma
     - Peripheral anterior synechiae
     - Corneal/endothelial problems
2. **Complications of PC scleral-fixated IOL**
   - IOL tilt/dislocation

- Persistent iritis (IOL instability)
- CME
- Pupil distortion
- Hyphema
- Endophthalmitis
- Suture erosion over time

Q **Under What Situation During Cataract Surgery would You Consider NOT Implanting an IOL?**

"In certain scenarios, IOL is not routinely used...."

Patients With
- Congenital cataract (most common contraindication)
- Aphakia in fellow eye
- Recurrent uveitis
- Posterior segment problems (proliferative DR, RD) and IOL will interfere with treatment of such problems

- PCR with significant vitreous loss
- Severe glaucoma
- Corneal endothelial dystrophy

Q **What are the Different IOL Materials?**

"What are the different IOL materials?"
"There are many different types of IOL materials...."
"These include...."

IOL Materials

1. **Ideal material**
   - High optical quality
   - High refractive index (RI)
   - Lightweight
   - Durable
   - Nontoxic/inert (no inflammation, antigenicity, carcinogenicity)
   - Ease of manufacture and sterilization
2. **PMMA**
   - All the above properties except ease of sterilization (altered by heat, steam, gamma radiation)
3. **Glass**
   - Potential advantages
     - Good optical quality
     - Autoclavable
   - But
     - Heavy
     - Crack after Nd:YAG capsulotomy
4. **Silicone**
   - Potential advantages
     - Foldable, inserted into small wound

   - Similar optical quality as PMMA
   - Cast/injection molded (no polishing required)
   - Autoclavable
   - Minimal trauma to tissues
   - But (compared to PMMA)
     - Low RI (thicker)
     - Low tensile strength (tears easily)
     - Slippery (needs dry instruments)
     - Elastic (needs controlled release in anterior chamber)
     - Capsular phimosis
     - Discoloration
     - Contraindicated in patients who need silicon oil later (e.g. DM)
5. **Acrylic**
   - Potential advantages
     - More control over folding and release of IOL
     - Sticky (less PCO, less capsular phimosis)
     - Less inflammation
     - More resistant to Nd:YAG capsulotomy
   - But (compared to silicone)
     - Less compliant (longer time to compress and results in larger wound)
     - Low tensile strength (tears easily)
     - Higher cost

"There are 3 types of formulas available…."

IOL Power Calculation

1. **Theoretical formulas**
   - Based on optics/vergence equations
   - E.g. Holliday, Binkhorst

2. **Empirical formulas**
   - Based on regression analysis on refraction results from patients with cataract surgery and IOL
   - E.g. SRK (Sander-Retzlaif-Kraff)

3. **Combination formulas**
   - Theoretical formula with regression analysis added to optimize the equations
   - E.g. SRK-T

4. **Choice of formula**
   - Main factor is axial length of eye
   - Royal College of Ophthalmologists' recommendations:
     - AL <22.0 mm – Hoffer/SRK-T
     - AL 22.0–24.5 mm – SRK-T/Holladay, Haigis
     - AL >24.6mm: SRK-T

"The SRK is an IOL power calculation formula and stands for…."

SRK Formula

1. **Power = (A constant) – 2.5 (axial length) – 0.9 (keratometry)**

2. **Factors which affect the A constant**
   - Position of IOL in eye (closer the IOL to retina, higher the A constant, therefore AC IOL has lower A constant!)
   - Shape of IOL (convex, biconvex etc)
   - Haptic angulation

3. **Choosing power of AC IOL when PCR occurs**
   - Suppose a 20D PC IOL was chosen with an A constant of 118
   - The AC IOL has A constant of 114
   - Then the desired power of AC IOL is 20D – (118 – 114) = 16D

"Selection is based on the patient's refractive status in the eye due for cataract surgery, the patient's visual requirements and the state of the fellow eye."

IOL Power Selection

1. **Emmetropic eye (−0.5 to +0.5D)**
   - Active patient → aim for emmetropia
   - Sedentary, elderly → aim for slight myopia

2. **Slight hyperopia (+0.5 to 3.0D)**
   - Aim for emmetropia

3. **High hyperopia (> +3.0D)**
   - Fellow eye needs cataract operation → aim for emmetropia
   - Fellow eye does not need operation → aim for slight hyperopia

4. **Slight myopia (−1.0 to 3.0D)**
   - Active patient → aim for emmetropia
   - Sedentary, elderly → aim for slight myopia of −2.0 to 2.5D

5. **High myopes**
   - Many surgical issues involved must be explained (see page 27)
   - Fellow eye needs cataract operation → aim for slight myopia (then aim for emmetropia in fellow eye)
   - Fellow eye is as myopic but does not need cataract operation → aim for myopia with 2–3D difference compared with fellow eye (or aim for emmetropia and use contact lens for fellow eye)
   - Fellow eye is emmetropic → consider the possibility that operated eye may have amblyopia!

Ultrasound Biometry

1. **Principles**
   - Ultrasound = acoustic (sound) waves at frequency >20 kHz (20,000 cycles/sec)
   - Produced from an electric pulse in **piezoelectric crystal** (keyword)
   - Echoes
     - A-scan (time–amplitude)
     - B-scan (brightness modulated)
   - Frequency
     - Increase in frequency is associated with a decrease in penetration, but an increase resolution
     - Ophthalmic use (8–12 MHz) vs obstetric use (1 MHz)
   - Sound velocity
     - Faster through denser medium
     - Velocities
       - Cornea/lens (1,641 m/sec)
       - Aqueous/vitreous (1,532 m/sec)
       - PMMA (2,718 m/sec)
       - Silicone (980 m/sec)
   - Acoustic impedance
     - Impedance = density × sound velocity
   - Acoustic interface
     - Formed when sound travels between media of differing acoustic impedances

2. **Measurements**
   - A-scan ultrasound determines time required for sound to travel from cornea to retina and then back to probe
     - (Distance = velocity × time/2)
   - Gain
     - Increase in gain is associated with an increase in tissue penetration and sensitivity but decrease in resolution
   - Accuracy of axial length
     - 0.1 mm = error of 0.25D in an emmetropic eye, more in a short eye and less in a longer eye (see SRK formula)
   - Standard dimensions
     - Multiple measurements between two eyes should be within 0.2 mm and difference in length between two eyes should be within 0.3 mm
   - Mean values
     - Axial length = 23.5 mm
     - Corneal thickness = 0.55 mm
     - AC depth = 3.24 mm
     - Lens thickness = 4.63 mm

3. **Measurement errors and other issues**
   - Artificially too short
     - Corneal compression
     - Sound velocity too slow, improper gate settings or gain too high
     - Misalignment of sound beam
   - Artificially too long
     - Fluid between cornea and probe
     - Sound velocity too fast, improper gate settings or gain too low
     - Misalignment of beam
     - Staphyloma
     - Silicone oil
   - Pseudophakia
     - PMMA IOL – eye measure shorter
     - Silicone IOL – eye measure longer
     - Conversion factors (measure using aphakic sound velocity and add the above factors)
       - PMMA (+0.4)
       - Silicone (−0.8)
       - Acrylic (+0.2)

"Partial coherence biometry (e.g. IOL Master) is a new biometric tool that utilizes infrared light (wavelength 780 nm) instead of sound waves for biometric measurements."

Advantages Over Ultrasound Biometry:
- Non-contact
- Faster (<1 sec)
- Easier to perform
- Measures along fixation beam: More accurate for high myopia (almost mandatory in presence of staphyloma!)
- No correction needed for silicone oil filled eyes

"Ultrasound is used for diagnosis and treatment."

Diagnostic

1. **Anterior segment**
   - Pachymetry
   - Biometry
   - Biomicroscopy (AC angles)
   - Lens thickness

2. **Post segment**
   - Vitreous opacity (vitreous hemorrhage, posterior vitreous detachment)
   - Retina (RD, tumors)
   - Choroid (choroidal detachment, tumors)
   - IOFB

3. **Orbit**
   - Tumor, cyst, mucocoele, FB (superceded by CT scan)

4. **Doppler**
   - Carotid duplex
   - Blood flow to optic nerve head
   - Orbital color doppler imaging
   - Ophthalmic artery duplex

Therapeutic

1. **Phacoemulsification**
2. **Ciliary body destruction for end stage glaucoma**

Post-Keratorefractive Surgery Biometry

1. **Main challenges in post-refractive surgery biometry**
   - Keratometers only measure K in central zone which may not encompass entire treatment/ablation zone
   - Standard Keratometry index (1.3375) assumes constant relationship between anterior and posterior corneal surfaces – not true after corneal ablation

2. **Approaches to biometry:**
   - Methods which do not rely on current data (historical data methods)
     - Based on records of pre-refractive surgery K values, with adjustment based on amount of refractive correction
     - Various formulae
   - Methods based on current data
     - Contact lens overrefraction: Effective K = contact lens base curve – difference between refraction with and without contact lens

   Pentacam based formulae (direct measurement of posterior corneal curvature)

CATARACT SURGERY IN SPECIAL SITUATIONS

Overall yield: ✪✪✪✪✪ Clinical exam: ✪✪ Viva: ✪✪✪✪✪ Essay: ✪✪✪✪✪ MCQ: ✪✪

Q **Opening Question:** How do You Manage this Patient with Glaucoma and Cataract?

"In this patient, there are 2 clinical problems that have to be managed simultaneously."
"This would depend on the severity of each condition...."
"Factors to consider would include...."

Management of Glaucoma and Cataract

Severity of glaucoma	Severity of cataract	Possible options
+++	+	• Trabeculectomy first, cataract operation later • Alternatively, discuss with patient about advantages of combined cataract operation and trabeculectomy (triple procedure) (see below)
+	+++	• Cataract operation first, manage glaucoma conservatively • Alternatively, discuss with patient about advantages of triple procedure (see below)
+++	+++	• Consider triple procedure

Factors that Determine the Management of Glaucoma and Cataract

1. **Severity and progression of glaucoma**
   • IOP level (most important factor)
   • Optic nerve head changes
   • Visual field changes
   • Ocular risk factors (CRVO, Fuch's endothelial dystrophy, retinitis pigmentosa)

2. **Severity and progression of cataract**
   • VA and visual requirements

3. **Patient factors**
   • Age
   • Race (blacks higher rate of glaucoma progression)
   • Family history of blindness from glaucoma
   • Fellow eye blinded from glaucoma
   • Concomitant risk factors for glaucoma (DM, HPT, myopia, other vascular diseases)
   • Compliance to follow-up and medication use

Exam tips:
- Remember there are no RIGHT or WRONG answers. You must be able to come up with a position and defend it.
- Be as conservative as possible. Therefore give extremes of each scenario first (least controversial), then go on to the more difficult and controversial areas.
- Opening statement is similar in all situations in which there are 2 problems, "There are 2 clinical problems that must be managed simultaneously. Factors to consider in these patients include…."
- See factors that determine glaucoma management (page 63).

Q What are the Indications for a Combined Cataract Extraction and Trabeculectomy?

"In general, this procedure is indicated when there is SIMULTANEOUS need for trabeculectomy and cataract operation."

Combined Cataract Extraction and Trabeculectomy

1. **Indications**
   - General principle: Indications for trabeculectomy (when IOP is raised to a level that there is evidence of progressive VF or ON changes despite maximal medical treatment) **plus** indication for cataract surgery (visual impairment)

2. **Advantages**
   - One operation
   - Faster visual rehabilitation
   - Patient may be able to be taken off all glaucoma medications
   - Prevents post-op IOP spikes
   - HVF monitoring easier with clear media
   - No subsequent cataract operation needed (lower risk of bleb failure)

3. **Disadvantages**
   - **Strong** evidence that IOP control with trabeculectomy alone is better than combined surgery
   - More manipulation during the combined operation (higher risk of bleb failure)
   - Vitreous loss during cataract surgery (higher risk of bleb failure)
   - Larger wounds created (higher risk of wound leakage and shallow AC)

4. **Alternative ways to perform the combined operation**
   - Corneal section ECCE plus trabeculectomy
     - Advantages
       · More control
       · Less conjunctival manipulation
       · Smaller wound (lower risk of leakage and shallow AC)
     - Disadvantages
       · Longer
       · Higher corneal astigmatism
   - Limbal section ECCE plus trabeculectomy
     - Advantages
       · Faster
       · Less astigmatism
     - Disadvantages
       · Larger wound
       · More conjunctival manipulation
       · Increased risk of flat AC
   - Phacoemulsification plus trabeculectomy
     - Advantages
       · More control of AC
       · Less conjunctival manipulation (main reason)
       · Smallest wound of the 3 techniques
       · Less astigmatism
       · Faster
     - Disadvantage:
       · More difficult operation for the inexperienced surgeon

Exam tips:
- **Essentially identical to the indications for trabeculectomy (page 80).**

- "What are the common scenarios for trabeculectomy?"
  - Uncontrolled POAG with maximal medical treatment
    - **Failure** of medical treatment (IOP not controlled with progressive VF or ON damage)
    - **Side effects** of medical treatment
    - **Noncompliance** with medical treatment
    - Additional considerations
      - Young patient with good quality of vision
      - One-eyed patient (other eye blind from glaucoma)
      - Family history of blindness from glaucoma
      - Glaucoma risk factors (HPT, DM)
  - Uncontrolled PACG after laser PI and medical treatment
  - Secondary OAG or ACG

Q **What are the Potential Problems in Removing a Cataract in a Patient with High Myopia?**

"There are several potential problems, which can be divided into…."

High Myopia and Cataract Surgery

1. **Preoperative stage**
   - Need to assess visual potential (amblyopia, myopic macular degeneration)
   - Choose IOL power carefully (counseling for anisometropia)
   - Harder to do biometry (need special formulas to adjust for longer axial lengths)
   - IOL Master biometry in view of high prevalence of staphylomata

2. **Intraoperative stage**
   - Risk of perforation with retrobulbar anesthesia (consider topical anesthesia or GA)
   - Lower IOP (harder to express nucleus during ECCE)
   - Deeper AC (harder to aspirate soft lens material)
   - Increased risk of PCR (weak zonules)

3. **Postoperative stage**
   - Risk of RD

Q **What are the Potential Problems in Removing a Cataract in a Patient with Uveitis?**

Uveitis and Cataract Surgery

1. **Preoperative stage**
   - Need to control inflammation
     - Consider waiting 2 to 3 months until inflammation settles after an acute episode
     - Consider course of preoperative steroids
   - Assess visual potential (CME, optic disc edema)
   - Dilate pupil in advance (atropine, subconjunctival mydriacaine)
   - Perform gonioscopy (if synechiae is severe superiorly, consider corneal section)

2. **Intraoperative stage**
   - Problem of small pupil (see below)
   - Increased risk of PCR (weak zonules)
   - Increased inflammation (consider heparin coated IOL or leave aphakic)
   - Increased risk of bleeding

3. **Postoperative stage**
   - Higher risk of complications
     - Corneal edema
     - Flare up of inflammation
     - Glaucoma or hypotony
     - Choroidal effusion
     - CME
   - Consider prophylaxis for infectious etiologies (e.g. herpetic lesions)

Small Pupil During Cataract Surgery

1. **Preoperative stage**
   - High risk patients (uveitis, DM, pseudoexfoliation syndrome, Marfan's syndrome, glaucoma on pilocarpine treatment)
   - Prior to operation, prescribe mydriatics (3 days of homatropine 2% three times a day or atropine)
   - 2 hours before operation, intensive dilation with
     - Tropicamide 1%
     - Ocufen 0.03%
     - Phenylephrine 10%

2. **Intraoperative stage**
   - Infuse AC with balanced salt solution mixed with a few drops of 1:1000 Adrenaline

- Use viscoelastics to dilate pupil
- Remove pupillary membrane (previous inflammation)
- Stretch pupil gently (with Kuglen hooks)
- Perform sphincterotomy at 6-, 3-, 9- and 12 o'clock positions
- Perform broad iridectomy at 12 o'clock position
- Perform basal iridectomy and mid-peripheral iridotomy (better apposition than broad iridectomy)
- Iris hooks
- Pupil expansion devices (e.g. Morcher pupil expansion ring)

Exam tips:
- **Common follow-up question of pseudoexfoliation (page 18) and uveitis (see above).**
- **Give practical answers. Do not say "iris hooks" first or you will be asked in detail how to do it!**

Mature Cataract

1. **Need to assess visual potential**
   - Pupils (optic nerve function)
   - Light projection (gross retinal integrity), color perception
   - Potential acuity meter (macular function)
   - B-scan ultrasound (gross retinal anatomy)

2. **Poor view of capsulotomy/capsulorrhexis edge**
   - Consider endocapsular technique

- Consider using air instead of viscoelastics
- Use of capsular stains (vision blue/trypan blue): possibly toxic to endothelium, capsular fragility, teratogenic

3. **High intra-capsular pressure**
   - CCC runs out/splits easily

4. **Floppy capsule due to chronic bulky lens**
   - Viscoelastic tamponade

"The 2 main issues are…."

Diabetes and Cataract

1. **Issues**
   - Difficult cataract surgery
   - Progression of diabetic retinopathy after operation

2. **Preoperative stage**
   - Assess visual potential
     - Consider FFA

- Laser PRP if necessary prior to the surgery
- Medical consult
- List for first case in morning

3. **Intraoperative stage**
   - Protect corneal epithelium (risk of abrasion and poor healing)

- Problems with small pupil (see above)
- Consider stitching wound
- Selection of IOL
  - Large optics (7 mm)
  - Use acrylic IOL (avoid silicone IOL)
  - Avoid IOL if PDR (risk of neovascular glaucoma)
- Avoid AC IOL
- Consider heparin-coated IOL

4. **Postoperative stage**
   - Control inflammation (especially in eyes with PDR)
   - Risk of PDR/CSME
   - Risk of glaucoma
   - Risk of PCO

Notes
- "Why does diabetic retinopathy progress?"
  - Removal of anti-angiogenic factor in lens
  - Secretion of angiogenic factors from iris
  - Increased intraocular inflammation
  - Decreased anti-angiogenic factor from RPE
  - Migration of angiogenic factors into AC

TOPIC 8

CATARACT SURGERY COMPLICATIONS

Overall yield: ✵✵✵✵✵   **Clinical exam:** ✵   **Viva:** ✵✵✵✵✵   **Essay:** ✵✵✵   **MCQ:** ✵✵✵✵

Q **Opening Question:** What are the Issues in Cataract Extraction for Diabetic Patients?

"The complications can be classified into 3 categories: Preoperative, intraoperative and postoperative complications…."

Complications of Cataract Surgery

1. **Intraoperative**
   - Posterior capsule rupture (PCR) and vitreous loss
   - Suprachoroidal hemorrhage
   - Dropped nucleus

2. **Early postoperative**
   - Endophthalmitis
   - Wound leak
   - IOP related problems (raised IOP, low IOP and shallow AC)
   - Corneal edema (striate keratopathy)

   - Undetected intraoperative PCR with vitreous in AC
   - Cystoid macular edema (CME)

3. **Late postoperative**
   - Late endophthalmitis
   - Wound astigmatism
   - Glaucoma
   - Bullous keratopathy
   - Posterior capsule opacification
   - Retinal detachment

Exam tips:
- **Complications of all eye operations are extremely important, because you are expected to manage them.**
- **There are a few ways to answer these questions, choose one and be comfortable with it.**
- **The most common complication answer, "The commonest ocular complication is…."**
- **The most important complication answer, "The most important complication is endophthalmitis…."**
- **The clinical classification answer, "The complications can be classified into preoperative, intraoperative and postoperative complications…."**
- **The anatomical classification answer, "The complications can be divided into anterior or posterior segment…."**

Exam tips:
- **Notice an intentional grouping of early postoperative and late postoperative complications into similar groups (i.e. endophthalmitis, would problems, IOP problems, corneal problems, PC problems and retinal problems)!**

"The management depends on the **stage** of the operation, the **size** and extent of PCR and whether **vitreous loss** has occurred."
"The risk factors include…."

Management of PCR

1. **Management depends on**
   - **Stage** of operation at which PCR occurs, commonly during:
     - Nucleus expression
     - Aspiration of soft lens
     - IOL insertion
   - **Size** and extent of PCR
   - Presence or absence of **vitreous** loss

2. **Risk factors**
   - Ocular factors
     - Difficult cataracts (brunescent, morgagnian, pseudoexfoliation, posterior polar cataracts)
     - Glaucoma
     - High myopia
     - Increase in vitreous pressure observed after retrobulbar and peribulbar anesthesia
     - Small pupils
     - Small CCC
   - Patient factors
     - HPT
     - Chronic lung disease
     - Obese patient with short thick neck

3. **Clinical signs of PCR**
   - Presence of ring reflex in the posterior capsule
   - Inability to aspirate soft lens matter (vitreous stuck to port)
   - Outline of PCR seen
   - Peaked pupil
   - Vitreous seen in AC
   - Sudden deepening of AC
   - Fragments disappear form view
   - Pupil-snap sign: PC rupture during hydrodissection

4. **General principles of management**
   - Intraoperative stage
     - Stop surgery immediately and assess situation
     - Limit size of PCR (inject viscoelastic into AC)
     - Dealing with remaining lens matter
       - Small fragment
         - Enlarge wound and express with Vectis

   - Phaco over Sheets glide (reduce parameters)
   - Large fragment – convert to ECCE/posterior assisted techniques
   - Remove remaining soft lens matter with gentle and "dry" aspiration
   - Vitreous loss
     - Anterior vitrectomy (sponge vitrectomy or automated vitrectomy) settings
   - Consider IOL implantation
     - PC IOL (small PCR) – convert rupture to round posterior CCC
     - Sulcus IOL (moderate to large PCR with adequate PC support)
       - Avoid one-piece lenses: Chafing and instability
       - IOL power has to be adjusted (reduced) to account for more anterior position
     - AC IOL (large PCR with inadequate posterior capsule support)
     - Leave aphakic (large PCR with inadequate posterior capsule support)
     - Avoid silicone lenses in PCR – higher rate of endophthalmitis
     - Consider IOL capture in CCC for stability
   - Checklist at the end of operation
     - Obvious vitreous at pupil borders?
     - Inject miotic agent → round pupil observed?
     - Traction at wound edge with weck sponge → peaking of pupil? (Marionette sign)
     - Inject air bubble → regular round bubble observed?
     - Sweep iris → movement in AC
   - Postoperative – risk of
     - Endophthalmitis
     - Glaucoma
     - Inflammation
     - Bullous keratopathy
     - Suprachoroidal hemorrhage
     - CME
     - RD

"Suprachoroidal hemorrhage is a rare but blinding complication of cataract extraction."

Suprachoroidal Hemorrhage

1. **Risk factors**
   - Ocular factors
     - Glaucoma
     - Severe myopia
     - PCR during surgery
   - Patient factors
     - HPT
     - Chronic lung disease
     - Obese patient with short thick neck

2. **Clinical signs**
   - Progressive shallowing of AC
   - Increased IOP
   - Prolapse of iris
   - Vitreous extrusion
   - Loss of red reflex

   - Dark mass behind pupil seen
   - Extrusion of all intraocular contents

3. **General principles of management**
   - Intraoperative
     - Stop surgery
     - Immediate closure with 4/0 silk suture (use superior rectus stitch)
     - IV mannitol
     - Posterior sclerostomy
       - Controversial and may exacerbate bleeding
   - Postoperative
     - Risk of glaucoma (need timolol) and inflammation (need predforte)
     - May need to drain blood later on (vitrectomy)

> **Exam tips:**
> - **The risk factors are nearly identical to that for PCR!**

Q | **How do You Manage a Dropped Nucleus During Phacoemulsification?**

"The management of a dropped nucleus depends on the **stage** of the operation, the **amount** of the lens fragment dropping into the vitreous and whether **vitreoretinal** surgical help is available."

Dropped Nucleus

1. **Why in phacoemulsification, but not in ECCE?**
   - PCR more difficult to see in phacoemulsification
   - High pressure AC system (infusion solutions)

2. **Types of dropped nucleus**
   - Prior to nucleus removal
     - Whole nucleus drop
     - Runaway capsulorrhexis or during hydrodissection
   - During nucleus removal
     - Nuclear fragment drop
     - Phacoemulsification of posterior capsule, puncture or aspirate capsule
   - After nucleus removal
     - PCR is associated with vitreous loss but no nuclear drop
     - Management similar to PCR in ECCE

3. **General principle of prevention**
   - Good sized and shaped capsulorrhexis
   - Careful hydrodissection
   - Clear endpoints in nuclear management
   - Recognition of occult PCR

4. **Management**
   - Stabilize AC with viscoelastics and remove phacoprobe. Enlarge wound
   - Inject viscoelastics under nucleus if possible
   - Retrieve fragments with vectis/forceps/posterior assisted techniques
     - Controversial: May increase vitreous traction and risk of retinal breaks
   - Either close wound and remove fragments at later date, or proceed with immediate vitrectomy and nucleus removal

> **Notes**
> - "What are the signs of an impending nuclear drop?"
>   - Runaway capsulorrhexis
>   - "Pupil snap" sign (pupil suddenly constricts)
>   - Difficulty in rotation of nucleus
>   - Nuclear tilt
>   - Receding nucleus

"Postoperative endophthalmitis is a rare but blinding complication after cataract surgery."
"The management depends on **isolation** of organism, intensive **medical** treatment and **surgical** intervention if necessary."

Classification and Microbial Spectrum

Classification	Types	Incidence	Microbial spectrum	Onset
Endogenous	• Generalized septicemia • Localized infections (endocarditis, pyelonephritis, osteomyelitis)		• *Klebsiella* and gram negatives • Depending on source	
Exogenous	• Postoperative (cataract)	• 0.1%	• *S. epidermidis* (70%) • *S. aureus*, *Streptococcus* • Gram negatives • *Propionibacterium* species (chronic)	• 1–14 days
	• Postoperative (glaucoma)	• 1%	• *Streptococcus* • *Hemophilus influenze*	• Early to late
	• Post traumatic	• 5–10%	• *S. epidermidis* • *S. aureus* • *Bacillus* • Gram negatives	• 1–5 days

Postoperative Endophthalmitis

1. **Clinical features**
   - Pain
   - Decreased VA
   - Lid edema and chemosis
   - Corneal haze
   - AC activity, hypopyon, fibrin
   - Absent red reflex
   - Vitritis

2. **General principles of management**
   - Prevention
     - Preoperatively: Only irrigation of conjunctival sac with 5% povidone iodine has been shown to reduce endophthalmitis risk
       - Other measures like antibiotics not proven but commonly employed
     - Intraoperatively:
       - ESCRS multi-center study on intra-cameral antibiotic prophylaxis showed that use of intra-cameral cefuroxime (1 mg/0.1 ml) was associated with **5x** reduced risk of endophthalmitis

   - Vitreous tap to isolate organism (see below)
   - Medical treatment
     - Intravitreal antibiotics
     - Intensive fortified topical antibiotics
     - Systemic antibiotics (controversial)
     - Steroids (controversial – usually better given systemically)
   - Surgical treatment
     - Vitrectomy
       - Endophthalmitis vitrectomy study (*Arch Ophthalmol* 1995; **113**:1479)
         - 420 patients with post cataract surgery endophthalmitis
         - Randomly assigned to either early vitrectomy vs vitreous tap and IV antibiotics vs topical and intravitreal antibiotics.
         - Results: Immediate vitrectomy only beneficial in patients with perception of light vision or worse. No benefit of IV antibiotics

Exam tips:
- Be careful, "postoperative endophthalmitis" is not the same as "endophthalmitis" (the latter includes endogenous and post-traumatic endophthalmitis).
- The incidence after cataract surgery is 1 in 1,000 (0.1%) but is 10 times higher in glaucoma surgery (1%) and 100 times higher after trauma (5–10%).

Q How do You Perform a Vitreous Tap?

"I would perform a vitreous tap in the operating room under sterile conditions."
"First I would prepare the antibiotics and culture…."

Vitreous Tap

1. **Perform in OR under sterile conditions**
2. **Prepare antibiotics and culture media before procedure**
   - 0.2 ml of antibiotic
     - Cephazolin 2.5 mg in 0.1 ml
     - Vancomycin 1 mg in 0.1 ml
     - (Alternatives: Amikacin 0.4 mg in 0.1 ml, ceftazidime 2.25 mg in 0.1 ml)
   - Topical LA, clean eye with iodine
3. **Procedure**
   - Use 23G needle mounted on Mantoux syringe with artery forceps clamped 10 mm from tip of needle

- Enter pars plana from temporal side of the globe, 4 mm behind limbus, directed towards center of vitreous
  - If no fluid aspirated, reposition or consider use of hand-held automated vitrector
- Withdraw 0.2 ml of vitreous, remove syringe and inject pus/contents onto culture media
- Inject 0.2 ml of antibiotics

Q Tell me about Posterior Capsule Opacification (PCO) after Cataract Surgery.

"Posterior capsule opacification is a common complication after cataract surgery."
"There are 3 types of PCO…."

Management of PCO

1. **Types of PCO**
   - Proliferation of epithelium (Elschnig's pearls and Soemmering's ring)
   - Primary opacification of capsule
   - Primary fibrosis of capsule
2. **Problems with PCO**
   - Visual dysfunction (VA, contrast, color)
   - Decrease view of fundus – management of
     - Diabetic retinopathy
     - RD
   - IOL decentration with capsular phimosis
3. **Risk factors for PCO**
   - Young patient
   - DM, uveitis
   - Retained lens matter during surgery
   - IOL design (controversial) – square edged designs reduce PCO risk

4. **General principles of management**
   - Intraoperative stage – prevention of PCO
     - Surgical factors
       - Complete removal of soft lens matter
       - Polish posterior capsule
       - Consider primary posterior capsulotomy (pediatric cataract)
     - IOL design factors
       - Acrylic IOL (lower risk because more IOL/posterior capsule apposition)
       - Posterior bowing of optic (more IOL/posterior capsule apposition)
       - Laser barrier ridges (prevent epithelium from migrating behind IOL)
       - Heparin-coated IOL (not proven)
5. **Postoperative treatment**
   - Nd:YAG capsulotomy [timing]

Q **What are the Causes of Raised IOP/Low IOP/Shallow AC after Cataract Surgery?**

"Management depends on the severity and cause of the shallow AC...."
"The severity is graded as follows (see page 82)."
"The possible causes of shallow anterior chamber are...."

IOP	Shallow AC	Deep AC
High	• Malignant glaucoma • Suprachoroidal hemorrhage • Pupil block glaucoma	• Retained viscoelastics • Retained soft lens matter • Inflammation, hyphema
Low	• Wound leak • Choroidal effusion	• Ciliary body shutdown • Retinal detachment

Exam tips:
• **Very similar causes to shallow AC after trabeculectomy (see page 82).**

Q **How do You Control Postoperative Corneal Astigmatism?**

Corneal Astigmatism after Cataract Surgery

1. **Preoperative stage**
   • Assess amount of astigmatism
     • Use keratometry readings (not manifest refraction because astigmatism may be due to lenticular astigmatism)
   • Consider astigmatism of the other eye (with- or against-the-rule astigmatism)
   • Plan surgery (ECCE vs phacoemulsification)

2. **Intraoperative — prevention**
   • ECCE
     • Decrease size of incision
     • Less diathermy
     • Place IOL centrally
     • Wound closure/suture techniques
       · Regularly placed sutures, short, deep bits
       · If there is overlapping of wound edges, sutures are too tight (with-the-rule astigmatism)
   • Phacoemulsification
     • Site of incision
       · Temporary or superior incision (based on preoperative astigmatism)
       · Cornea, limbal or scleral tunnel (less astigmatism with scleral tunnel)

   • Avoid wound burns
   • Limbal relaxing incisions
   • Corneal relaxing incisions (less predictable)
     · Newer technique: Femtosecond assisted keratotomy for greater predictability
   • Toric IOLs: Currently correct up to 3D astigmatism
     · Prerequisites:
       · Astigmatically neutral/predictable incision
       · Stable in the bag IOL fixation

3. **Postoperative management**
   • Manipulate frequency of steroid drops
     • With-the-rule astigmatism → more steroids (delay healing, wound will slide)
     • Against-the-rule → less steroids (increase healing and fibrosis)
   • Selective suture removal according to astigmatism
   • Toric contact lens
   • Photorefractive keratectomy/excimer laser procedures
   • Accurate keratotomy

SUBLUXED LENS AND MARFAN'S SYNDROME

Overall yield: ✪✪✪ **Clinical exam:** ✪✪✪✪✪ **Viva:** ✪✪ **Essay:** ✪✪ **MCQ:** ✪✪✪

Q **Opening Question:** What are the Causes of Subluxed or Dislocated Lens?

"Subluxed lens can be classified into 2 groups: Primary or secondary."

Classification of Subluxed Lens

1. **Primary**
   - Idiopathic
   - Familial ectopic lentis (usually AD)

2. **Secondary**
   - Systemic disorders
     - Marfan's syndrome
     - Other connective tissue disorders (Weil Marchesani, Stickler's, Ehler Danlo's syndromes)
     - Metabolic disorders (homocystinuria, hyperlysinema)

- Ocular developmental disorders
  - Big eyes and cornea (megalocornea, high myopia, bulphthalmos)
  - Iris anomalies (aniridia, uveal coloboma, corectopia)
- Ocular diseases/acquired
  - Trauma
  - Uveitis
  - Hypermature cataracts, pseudoexfoliation syndrome
  - Anterior uveal tumors (ciliary body melanoma)

> **Exam tips:**
> - **The classification is identical for congenital glaucoma (page 57) and congential cataract (page 9)!**

Q What are the Symptoms and Signs of Subluxed or Dislocated Lens?

Clinical Features

1. **Symptoms**
   - Fluctuating vision
   - Difficulty in accommodation
   - Monocular diplopia
   - High monocular astigmatism

2. **Signs**
   - Phacodonesis

- Iridodonesis (better seen with undilated pupil)
- Deep or uneven AC
- Uneven shadowing of iris on lens
- Superior or inferior border of lens and zonules seen
- Acute ACG

Q How would You Manage a Patient with Subluxed Lens?

"I would need to assess the **cause** of the subluxation and manage both the **ocular** and **systemic** problems."
"If the lens is dislocated into the AC...."

Management of Subluxed Lens

1. **Dislocation**
   - Into AC
     - **Ocular emergency**, immediate surgical removal
   - Into vitreous
     - Lens capsule intact and no inflammation, consider leaving it alone
     - Lens capsule ruptured with inflammation, surgical removal indicated (pars plana lensectomy)

2. **Subluxed lens**
   - If asymptomatic, conservative treatment (spectacles or contact lens)
   - Surgical removal indicated if there is
     - Lens-induced glaucoma
     - Persistent uveitis
     - Corneal decompensation
     - Cataract
     - Severe optical distortion (despite conservative treatment)
   - Surgical techniques
     - Standard ECCE/phaco (minimal subluxation, intact zonules)
     - ICCE (moderate subluxation, weaken zonules)
     - ICCE with anterior vitrectomy (associated with vitreous loss)

- Phaco with devices for capsular stabilization
  - Surgical pearls:
    - Intact CCC is critical to successful implantation of capsular stabilization devices
    - CCC initiation may be difficult — use sharp needle
    - Start CCC small, use shear method to control size
    - Aim is to implant CTR as late as possible during surgery, ideally after nucleus removed (CTR is bulky and difficult to implant smoothly when lens still present)
      - Temporary capsular stabilization during surgery can be achieved with capsular tension segments and iris/capsular hooks
    - Lower phaco parameters
    - Use chop techniques to minimize zonular stress
  - <1 quadrant zonulysis: Capsular tension ring (CTR)
  - 1–2 quadrants zonulysis: Cionni 1L modified CTR
  - >2 quadrants zonulysis: Cionno 2L modified CTR

Q What are the Clinical Features of Marfan's Syndrome?

"Marfan's syndrome is a systemic connective tissue disorder."
"There are characteristic systemic and ocular features."

Marfan's Syndrome

1. **Systemic features**
   - AD inheritance
   - Skeletal
     - Tall and long arms (inappropriately long armspan to height)
     - Fingers (arachnodactyly, joint laxity)
     - High arched palate
     - Scoliosis and pectus abnormalities
     - Hernias
   - Cardiac
     - Mitral valve prolapse
     - Aortic aneurysm, aortic incompetence and aortic dissection

2. **Ocular features**
   - Anterior segment
     - Subluxed lens (bilateral, upward, symmetrical)
     - Glaucoma (angle anomaly)
     - Keratoconus
     - Hypoplasia of dilator pupillae (difficult to dilate pupils)
   - Posterior segment
     - Axial myopia
     - RD

Clinical approach to Marfan's syndrome

"On SLE, there is bilateral upward dislocation of lens."
"However, the lens is not cataractous and the zonules can be seen inferiorly."

Look for
- Corneal evidence of keratoconus
- Dilated pupil
- Systemic features
  - High arched palates
  - Arachnodactyl, joint flexibility
  - Tall, wide armspan, scoliosis, chest deformity

I'd like to
- Check the IOP
- Perform a gonioscopy
- Refract the patient (high myopia)
- Examine the fundus (myopic changes and RD)
- Examine the cardiovascular system (aortic incompetence, mitral valve prolapse)
- Evaluate family members (for Marfan's syndrome)

Exam tips:
- Listen to the question, "What are the CLINICAL FEATURES?" which is different from "What are the OCULAR features?"

Q **What are the Differences between Marfan's Syndrome, Homocystinuria and Weil Marchesani Syndrome?**

	Marfan's	Homocystinuria	Weil Marchesani
Inheritance	AD	AR	AD
Intellect	Normal	Mental retardation	Mental retardation
Fingers	Arachnodactyly	—	Short stubby fingers
Osteoporosis	—	Severe	—
Vascular complications	—	Severe	—
Cardiac	Severe	—	—
Lens subluxation	Upwards	Downwards	Downwards
	Zonules present	Zonules absent	Microspherophakia
Accommodation	Intact	Lost	—

Section 2

GLAUCOMA AND GLAUCOMA SURGERY

LIMBUS, CILIARY BODY AND TRABECULAR MESHWORK

Overall yield: ✪ ✪ ✪ ✪   **Clinical exam:**   **Viva:** ✪ ✪ ✪ ✪   **Essay:** ✪ ✪ ✪   **MCQ:** ✪ ✪ ✪ ✪

Q Opening Question: Where is the Limbus?

"The limbus is the structure between the cornea and the sclera."
"It can be defined in 3 ways…."

Limbus

1. **Anatomical limbus:**
   - Anterior limit of limbus formed by a line joining end of Bowman's and end of Descemet's (Schwalbe's line)
   - Posterior limit is a curved line marking transition between regularly arranged corneal collagen fibres to haphazardly arranged scleral collagen fibres

2. **Pathological limbus:**
   - Anterior limit same as in one

   - Posterior limit formed by line perpendicular to surface of conjunctival epithelium about 1.5 mm behind end of Bowman's membrane

3. **Surgical limbus:**
   - Annular band 2 mm wide with posterior limit overlying scleral spur
   - Divided into:
     - Anterior blue zone (between Bowman's and Schwalbe's line)
     - Posterior white zone (between Schwalbe's line and scleral spur)

> **Exam tips:**
> - **Some of the most commonly asked anatomy or physiology questions in the examinations.**

Q What is the Anatomy of the Ciliary Body?

"The ciliary body is a triangular structure located at the junction between the anterior and posterior segment."
"Anatomically it is part of the uveal tract."

Ciliary Body

1. **Function of the ciliary epithelium**
   - Secretion of aqueous humor by ciliary nonpigmented epithelium (NPE)
   - Accommodation
   - Control of aqueous outflow
   - Part of BLOOD-AQUEOUS Barrier:
     - Formed by tight junctions between NPE (as well as nonfenestrated iris capillaries)
     - Maintain clarity of aqueous humor required for optical function
   - Secretion of hyaluronic acid into vitreous

2. **Gross anatomy**
   - Ciliary body, iris and choroid comprise vascular uveal coat
   - Ciliary body:
     - 6 mm wide ring in inner lining of globe
     - Extending from ora serrata posteriorly to scleral spur anteriorly
     - **Triangular** in cross section:
       - Anterior surface (uveal portion of trabecular meshwork)
       - Outer surface (next to sclera, potential suprachoroidal space between ciliary body and sclera)
       - Inner surface (next to vitreous cavity)
         - Smooth pars plana (posterior 2/3)
         - Ridged pars plicata (anterior 1/3)
           - Pars plicata 70 ciliary processes

3. **Blood supply**
   - Arterial supply:
     - **Seven anterior ciliary arteries** and **two long posterior ciliary arteries**
     - Anastomosis of the two forms the major arterial circle of iris
       - Located at base of the iris within ciliary process stroma
   - Venous drainage
     - Ciliary processes venules drain into pars plana veins, which drain into vortex system

4. **Nerve supply**
   - Main innervation from branches of **long posterior ciliary** and **short ciliary nerves**
   - Parasympathetic fibers from Edinger-Westphal nucleus to sphincter pupillae as follows:
     - Edinger-Westphal nucleus

   - III CN
   - Branch to IO muscle
   - Ciliary ganglion
   - Short ciliary nerves
   - Sphincter pupillae
   - Sympathetic fibers from superior cervical ganglion to ciliary body as follows:
     - Superior cervical ganglion
     - Ciliary ganglion
     - Short ciliary nerves
     - Muscle and blood vessels of ciliary body
   - Sensory fibers from ciliary body to CNS as follows:
     - Ciliary body
     - Long posterior ciliary nerves
     - Nasociliary nerve
     - Ophthalmic division of V CN
     - Brainstem

5. **Microscopic anatomy**
   - Histologically divided into three parts:
     - Ciliary epithelium (double layer)
     - Ciliary stroma
     - Ciliary muscle
       - Longitudinal, radial and circumferential
   - **Inner nonpigmented epithelium (NPE)**
     - Direct contact with aqueous humor
     - Columnar cells with numerous organelles
     - Extension of sensory retina with basal membrane, an extension of inner limiting membrane
   - **Outer pigmented epithelium (PE)**
     - Between NPE and stroma
     - Cuboidal cells, with numerous melanosomes, fewer organelles compared to NPE
     - Extension of RPE with basal membrane, an extension of Bruch's membrane
   - NPE and PE lie apex to apex
   - Different types of intercellular junction join NPE and PE:
     - Tight junctions between NPE (with nonfenestrated iris vessels) form **BLOOD-AQUEOUS Barrier**
     - Desmosomes found between internal surfaces of NPE cells
     - Gap junctions found between NPE and PE

Exam tips:
- Compare and contrast the two epithelial layers (nonpigmented vs pigmented epithelium). Note that while the pigmented epithelium is an extension of the RPE (as expected), it is NOT part of the BLOOD-AQUEOUS Barrier (unexpected, as the RPE forms the blood retinal barrier).

Q What is the Anatomy of the Trabecular Meshwork?

"The trabecular meshwork is located at the angle of the anterior chamber, beneath the limbus."
"Its main function is drainage of aqueous."

Trabecular Meshwork

1. **Gross anatomy**
   - Triangular in shape:
     - Base located at scleral spur
     - Anterior tip located at Schwalbe's line (= termination of Descemet's)

2. **Microscopic anatomy**
   - Three zones (from innermost to outermost):
     - **Uveal** meshwork:
       - From root of iris to Schwalbe's line
       - 70 μm in diameter (least resistance to flow)
   - **Corneoscleral** meshwork:
     - From scleral spur to Schwalbe's line
     - 35 μm in diameter (moderate resistance)
   - **Juxtacanalicular:**
     - Lines the endothelium of Schlemm's canal
     - 7 μm in diameter (highest resistance to flow)

Exam tips:
- The pore diameter in the juxtacanalicular meshwork is 10 times smaller than the uveal meshwork, while the corneoscleral meshwork is 2 times smaller.

Q What are the Blood Ocular Barriers? When are They Breached?

"There are two blood ocular barriers…."
"They are breached in certain circumstances…."

Blood Ocular Barriers

1. **Classification**
   - Blood-aqueous barrier (BAB):
     - Nonfenestrated iris capillaries
     - Tight junctions between ciliary nonpigmented epithelium (NPE)
   - Blood retinal barrier (BRB):
     - Nonfenestrated retinal capillaries
     - Tight junctions between RPE
   - Ciliary processes and choroidal capillaries are fenestrated and do not contribute to barrier

2. **Breach of the barriers**
   - Physiological:
     - Defect in BRB exists at level of optic disc:
       - Water-soluble substances may enter ON head by diffusion from extravascular space in choroid
   - Endocrine modifications:
     - Rapid, reversible increments in permeability via secretion of hormones (histamine, serotonin, bradykinin, etc.)
   - Pathological:
   - Defect in BRB in vascular diseases:
     - Diabetic retinopathy and hypertensive retinopathy
     - BRVO, CRVO
   - Defect in BAB and BRB after cataract or other intraocular surgery
   - Defect in BAB and BRB in ocular tumors
   - Defect in BAB and BRB in ocular inflammatory or infectious diseases

AQUEOUS HUMOR AND INTRAOCULAR PRESSURE

Overall yield: ✪ ✪ ✪ ✪ ✪ **Clinical exam: Viva:** ✪ ✪ ✪ ✪ ✪ **Essay:** ✪ ✪ ✪ **MCQ:** ✪ ✪ ✪ ✪

Q Opening Question: What is the Aqueous Humor?

"The aqueous humor is the fluid in the anterior (AC) and posterior chamber (PC)."
"It has the following properties…."
"And its functions include, first, the maintenance of…."
"The aqueous humor is formed in the PC by…."

Aqueous Humor

1. **Properties**
   - Clear fluid
   - Composition:
     - No cells and less than 1% of proteins compared to plasma
     - Same sodium and chloride, slightly lower potassium and **30%** lower bicarbonate than plasma
     - **Thirty times** higher ascorbate than plasma
   - Refractive index (RI) = **1.33**
     - Therefore, diverges light (!) because RI of cornea: 1.37
   - Volume in AC and PC = **0.30 ml**
     - 0.25 ml in AC
     - 0.05 ml in PC
   - Rate of secretion = **3 ul/min** (therefore takes 100 min to completely reform AC and PC!)

2. **Three functions**
   - Maintains volume and IOP
   - Nutrition for avascular ocular tissue:
     - Posterior cornea, trabecular meshwork, lens and anterior vitreous

   - Optical role

3. **Formation and outflow**
   - **Three formation** mechanisms from ciliary body process (nonpigmented epithelium):
     - Active transport (most important)
     - Ultrafiltration
     - Diffusion
   - **Three outflow** mechanisms:
     - Trabecular meshwork/pressure dependent flow
       - 90% of outflow
       - Related to IOP via Goldman equation (see below)
     - Uveoscleral/pressure independent flow:
       - 10% of flow
       - Aqueous enters ciliary body into the suprachoroidal space and vortex veins
       - Rate of aqueous flow quite constant and independent of IOP
     - Other routes
       - Iris veins
       - Retinal veins
       - Via the cornea

> **Exam tips:**
> - **Notice the importance of number "3" in aqueous humor physiology!**
> - **Another possible question is, "What are the differences between aqueous and plasma?"**

Q What is the Goldman Equation?

"The Goldman equation states that the IOP is determined by three interrelated factors."

The Goldman Equation:

1. **Goldman equation states that the following factors determine IOP**
   - IOP = F/C + Pr
   - Rate of aqueous secretion (F, in μl/in)
   - Level of episcleral venous pressure (Pr, in mmHg)

- Resistance encountered in outflow channel (R in ul/min/mmHg):
  - Resistance to flow related to facility of outflow
  - R = 1/C, where R is resistance and C is facility of outflow

Q How does IOP Vary?

"The IOP can have long term variation and short term fluctuations, and are affected by drugs."

IOP Variation

1. **Long term variations**
   - Age:
     - Increase with age
   - Blood pressure:
     - Increase with BP but not linearly
   - Body weight:
     - Increase with increase in body mass
   - Climate:
     - Increase in winter

2. **Short term fluctuations**
   - CVP changes
     - Change in body position and valsalva maneuver
   - Diurnal variation:
     - Increase in morning
     - Normal variation = 4 mmHg (>10 mmHg in glaucoma)
     - Correlates with increase in endogenous cortisol and catecholamines
     - Accentuated in POAG
   - Eye movement
     - Clinically important in restrictive ophthalmopathy (e.g. thyroid eye disease, pseudotumor)
   - Exercise:
     - Decrease in IOP
     - Correlated to metabolic acidosis and changes in extracellular fluid volume and osmolality

3. **Pharmacological effects**
   - Miotics
     - Generally decreases IOP
     - Effects:
       - Contraction of iris sphincter
       - Contraction of ciliary muscle pulls scleral spur, leading to change in trabecular meshwork and increase in outflow
     - Direct parasympathomimetics (pilocarpine, carbachol) and indirect (phospholine iodide)
   - Mydriatics:
     - Generally increases IOP
     - Effects
       - Allows peripheral portion of anterior iris stroma to move forward towards inner aspect of uveoscleral meshwork, leading to decrease in trabecular outflow facility
   - Others:
     - Beta adrenergic blockers (e.g. timolol) reduces production of aqueous and IOP
     - Carbonic anhydrase inhibitors (e.g. diamox) affects membrane transport of bicarbonate and water across ciliary epithelium, thereby reducing production of aqueous and IOP
     - Hyperosmotic agents (e.g. mannitol, glycerol) elevates blood osmolality with resulting fluid shift out of the vitreous
     - Steroids (page 36)

> **Exam tips:**
> - **The variations can be easily remembered as A, B, C, D, E and F (pharmacological)!**

"Tonometry is the measurement of the IOP."
"There are three types of tonometry…."

Tonometry

1. **Applanation tonometry**
   - Determines force necessary to flatten a **fixed area** of cornea
   - Based on the Imbert-Fick principle:
     - Force required to flatten an area of a perfect sphere is proportional to pressure inside sphere
   - Goldman tonometer:
     - Double prism in tonometer tip to facilitate visualization
     - Tonometer tip has diameter of 3.06 mm
       - Surface tension of tear meniscus = corneoscleral rigidity (cancels each other)
     - End point occurs when inner border of two semicircular halves of tear meniscus touch one another
     - IOP measured in mmHg
   - Air puff tonometer:
     - Non-contact
     - Pressurized air current directed against a fixed area of cornea
     - Not reliable in extremes

2. **Indentation tonometry**
   - Determines extent of indentation of cornea by **fixed weight**
   - Schiotz tonometer
     - Plunger with known weight indents cornea
       - Weights of 5.5, 7.5 or 10 g

   - Method:
     - Patient in supine position
     - Topical anesthetic
     - Tip of plunger allowed to rest on surface of eye forcing an indentation
     - Depth of indentation registered on scale in mm
     - IOP in mmHg read off from conversion chart

3. **Combined applanation–indentation tonometry**
   - Mackay-Marg tonometer:
     - Contains a spring-mounted plunger and surface footplate
       - Plunger has 1.5 mm area that protrudes 10 µm through center of footplate
     - Initially plunger indents cornea (indentation)
     - End point occurs when plunger indents enough to be flushed with footplate (applanation)
   - Other examples (e.g. tonopen)

4. **Tonometry that reduces the influence of the corneal biomechanical properties**
   - Dynamic control tonometry (DCT)
   - Ocular response analyzer tonometry (ORA)

OPTIC DISC CHANGES IN GLAUCOMA

Overall yield: ✪ ✪   **Clinical exam:** ✪ ✪ ✪   **Viva:** ✪ ✪   **Essay:** ✪   **MCQ:** ✪

Q **Opening Question:** What are the Optic Disc Changes in Glaucoma?

"Optic disc changes in glaucoma can be divided into specific and less specific signs."
"Specific signs include an increase in cup disc ratio (CDR)...."

Optic Disc Changes In Glaucoma

1. **Specific signs**
   - Optic disc cupping:
     - Large optic cup (vertical CDR 0.7 or more)
     - Asymmetry of optic cup (difference of CDR 0.2 or more)
     - Progressive enlargement of optic cup
     - Does not obey the "ISNT" rule
   - Focal signs:
     - Notching of rim
     - Regional pallor
   - Splinter (Drance) hemorrhage
   - Nerve fiber layer thinning
2. **Less specific signs:**
   - "Lamellar dot" sign
   - Nasalization of vessels
   - Peripapillary crescent (Beta zone)
   - Barring of circumlinear vessels

Exam tips:
- **There are four cup signs, four focal signs and four less specific signs.**

Q What are the Clues that a Large Optic Cup is Physiological?

Physiological Cupping

1. **Optic disc:**
   - No progression in cupping
   - Symmetrical cupping
   - Follows "ISNT" rule
   - Optic disc may be large
   - No focal changes or vessel abnormalities
2. **Associated with consistently normal IOP and VF**

"The imaging techniques can be classified into anterior segment and posterior segment techniques...."

Imaging Techniques in Glaucoma

1. **Anterior segment**
   - Ultrasound biomicroscopy:
     - Evaluate angle of AC and ciliary body
     - Requires contact of ultrasound probe with ocular surface
     - Indications:
       - Angle closure glaucoma
       - Malignant glaucoma
       - Plateau iris syndrome
   - Anterior segment optical coherence tomography (AS-OCT):
     - Evaluates angle of AC, but penetration insufficient for imaging the ciliary body
     - Advantages:
       - Non-contact modality – no distortion of AC angle
       - More objective than gonioscopy
       - Faster and easier to obtain images compared to ultrasound biomicroscopy
     - Disadvantages:
       - Scleral spur not easily identified in at least 20% of AS-OCT images
       - Unable to image ciliary body
       - Quality of vertical images inferior to horizontal images

2. **Posterior segment**
   - Stereoscopic optic disc photography (stereodisc photography):
     - Document optic disc changes
     - Advantages:
       - Cheap and simple
       - More objective than clinical evaluation
   - Glaucomascope:
     - Computer raster stereography where a series of equidistant parallel lines are projected onto optic disc at an oblique angle. Deflection of lines gives an indication of depth of optic cup
     - Advantage:
       - More quantitative than stereodisc photos
     - Needs minimal pupil size of 4 mm and clear media
   - Confocal scanning laser ophthalmoscopy: Heidelberg Retinal Tomograph (HRT):
     - Sequential images of coronal sections of optic disc are obtained via laser

- HRT software automatically defines a reference plane:
  - Cup: Structures below reference plane
  - Rim: Structures above reference plane
- Optic nerve head analysis (HRT-III)
  - Stereometric parameters:
    - Linear cup/disc ratio
    - Cup shape measure
    - Rim area
    - Rim volume
    - Height variation contour
    - Mean RNFL thickness
    - Disc size
  - Moorfields Regression Analysis (MRA)
  - Glaucoma Probability Score (GPS)
  - Progression analysis
- Advantages:
  - Higher resolution
  - Miotic pupils and media clarity not important
  - Automated definition of disc margin (HRT-III)
  - Superior to OCT in detecting progression
- Disadvantages:
  - Physiologic variability of optic nerve head configuration high
  - Poor accuracy in:
    - Tilted discs
    - Very large or small discs
    - Peripapillary atrophy
- Optical coherence tomography:
  - Image formation based on optical backscatter, similar to "ultrasound B scan of optic disc"
  - Advantages:
    - Highest resolution
    - Noncontact, noninvasive
    - Miotic pupils and media clarity not important
  - Disadvantages:
    - Time domain OCT inferior to HRT in detecting glaucoma progression
    - Glaucoma software for spectral domain OCT still in initial phases and expensive
    - RNFL reduced in other conditions e.g. myopia

THE VISUAL FIELDS

Overall yield: ✪ ✪ ✪ ✪ **Clinical exam:** **Viva:** ✪ ✪ ✪ ✪ **Essay:** ✪ ✪ ✪ **MCQ:** ✪ ✪ ✪ ✪

Q **Opening Question:** What is the Visual Field? What is an Isopter? And What is a Scotoma?

"The visual field (VF) is one of the functional components of vision."
"It is defined as the area that is perceived **simultaneously** by a **fixating** eye."

Visual Field Basics

1. **Definition:**
   - Area that is perceived simultaneously by a fixating eye
   - Not 2- but 3-dimensional
   - "Island of vision in a sea of darkness" (Traquair's definition)

2. **Limits:**
   - 60° nasally, 50° superiorly, 90–110° temporally, 70° inferiorly
   - Blind spot 15° temporal to fixation

3. **Isopter**
   - **Line in VF** connecting points with same **visual threshold**
   - Encloses an area within which a target of a given size and intensity is visible

4. **Scotoma and VF defect**
   - Scotoma
     - Absolute or relative decrease in retinal sensitivity **within** VF, bounded by areas of normal retinal sensitivity
   - VF defect
     - Absolute or relative decrease in retinal sensitivity **extending** from edge of VF

5. **Luminance and visual threshold**
   - Luminance:
     - Intensity of light
     - Apostilb (asb) is an **absolute** unit of luminance
       - Normal human range: 2 to 9,000 asb
       - Humphrey VF can measure from 0.08 to 10,000 asb
     - Decibel (dB) is a **relative** unit of luminance
       - Inverse log scale
       - 10,000 asb = 0 dB; 1 asb = 40 dB
   - Visual threshold:
     - Luminance of stimulus which is perceived 50% of time
     - The brighter the stimulus needed to be perceived, the lower the visual threshold
   - **Therefore, bright stimulus = high asb = low dB = low visual threshold**

Exam tips:
- See also the visual field examination in neuroophthalmology (page 255).

Q What is Perimetry? What are the Types and Advantages of Each?

"Perimetry is the **quantification** of the VF."
"It can be divided into...."

Perimetry Basics

1. **Classification**
   - Campimetry (flat surface):
     - **Tangent screen:**
       - Manual and kinetic
       - Test central 30°
       - Subject seated 1 or 2 meters from black screen
       - Target is presented by examiner
   - Perimetry (curved surface):
     - **Lister:**
       - Manual and kinetic
       - Extend beyond 30° (peripheral fields)
     - **Goldman** bowl perimeter:
       - Manual and kinetic or static
       - Hemispherical bowl with radius of 33 cm (subject at 33 cm)
       - Stimuli has different intensities (1–4) and sizes (I–V)
       - Extend beyond 30° (peripheral fields)
   - **Humphrey visual field analyzer (HVF):**
     - Automated and static
     - Test central 30°

2. **Advantages of automated (over manual):**
   - More quantitative
   - No examiner bias
   - Constant monitoring of fixation
   - Automated re-testing of abnormal points
   - Computer software for analysis

3. **Advantages of static (over kinetic):**
   - More objective and quantitative
   - More sensitive to shallow scotomas
   - Random presentation of stimuli (less anticipation of subject)
   - Faster

> **Exam tips:**
> - Comparison between Goldman and HVF is a common question.

Q What are the Uses of Visual Field in Ophthalmology?

"VF is used for diagnosis and follow-up of ophthalmic conditions."

Uses of Visual Field

1. **Diagnosis of**
   - Glaucoma
   - Optic nerve diseases (optic neuritis, anterior ischemic optic neuropathy, toxic neuropathy)
   - Unexplained visual loss
   - Malingering patients

2. **Follow-up of**
   - Glaucoma
   - Tumors (pituitary adenoma)

Q Tell me about the Humphrey Visual Field Analyzer.

"Humphrey visual field analyzer is an **automated static** perimetry."
"Maps the VF by quantifying the **visual threshold** of the retinal at predetermined locations."

Humphrey Visual Field Analyzer

1. **Basic**
   - Automated static perimetry
   - Stimuli (size = Goldman size III with duration of 0.2 s)
   - Background illumination = 31.5 asb

2. **Test strategies**
   - Full threshold strategy:
     - Uses the "4–2 bracketing" algorithm at each retinal point
   - Stimuli intensity increases in 4 dB steps until threshold is crossed (patients see stimuli)
   - Threshold is recrossed with stimuli intensity decreasing in 2 dB steps
   - Test pattern:
     - 24–2 test pattern:
       - Test central 24° of fixation and on either side of meridian (24–2) as opposed to tests on meridians as well (24–1)
     - 30–1 or 30–2 (Test central 30° of fixation)

- Related threshold strategies:
  - Full threshold with prior data:
    - Faster, uses prior VF data, presents each point at 2 dB higher than patient's previous threshold values and tests each point in 2 dB decrement
  - Fast threshold:
    - Even faster, presents entire field at 2 dB higher than patient's previous threshold

values and then tests only abnormal points
- Suprathreshold test strategy:
  - Fast screening test
  - Presents stimuli at 6 dB higher than expected threshold
  - Each point is recorded as normal vs abnormal

Q How do You Read the Humphrey Visual Field?

"This is a HVF for the left and right eyes respectively."
"Done on January 2nd, 1999, using the 24–2 threshold test pattern…."
"First, the reliability indices are…."

Evaluating the HVF

1. **Reliability indices**
   - Fixation loss:
     - Positive response to blind spot stimulation
     - "Moving eyes around"
     - Normal: Less than 20%
   - False positive:
     - Positive response but no stimuli
     - "Happy clicker"
     - Normal: Less than 33%
   - False negative:
     - Negative response with brighter than threshold stimuli
     - "Falling asleep"
     - Normal: Less than 33%
   - Other clues:
     - Short-term fluctuation significantly raised
     - "Clover leaf pattern" on grayscale (inattentiveness with time)
     - Increased eye (upstroke) or lid (downstroke) movement on eye tracker line

2. **Global indices**
   - Mean deviation (MD):
     - Average deviation of each point from age-corrected normal (e.g. −5 dB MD means that on average, each point has a 5 dB lower threshold than normal)
     - Minus is bad
   - Pattern standard deviation (PSD):
     - Standard deviation of each point from age-corrected normal
     - Measures the variability/irregularity of field (e.g. a high PSD indicates irregular field)
     - Plus is bad

- Short-term fluctuation (SF):
  - Retests 10 pre-selected points and calculates differences between original test and retest thresholds
  - Measures consistency
  - One of earliest signs of glaucoma (patient sometimes sees it and sometimes does not)
  - May also be indicator of reliability
- Corrected pattern standard deviation (CPSD):
  - PSD corrected for SF
  - Measures localized variability/irregularity (a high CPSD indicates localized irregularity)
- Glaucoma hemifield test (GHT):
  - 5 clusters of points in upper and lower half of VF are compared
  - Early indicator of glaucoma

3. **Figures**
   - Raw numeric values and grayscale:
     - Threshold at each point (e.g. 25 dB at that point means visual threshold is 25 dB)
   - Total deviation:
     - Age-corrected normal minus raw threshold value (e.g. −2 dB at that point means visual threshold is 2 dB less than what is normal at that point)
     - Similar to MD
   - Pattern deviation:
     - Total deviation adjusted upwards or downwards to pick up localized defects
     - Measures localized defects
     - Similar to CSPD

Interpretation

MD	CSPD	Total deviation plot	Pattern deviation plot	Diagnosis
Normal	Normal	Clean	Clean	Normal
Abnormal	Normal	Many abnormal points	Clean	Generalized loss of sensitivity (e.g. cataract)
Normal	Abnormal	Many abnormal points	Similar abnormal points	Localized defect (e.g. glaucoma)
Abnormal	Abnormal	Many abnormal points	Less abnormal points but not clean	Both generalized and localized defects

Exam tips:
- You may be given a HVF printout to read. You need to be systematic and not jump at the obvious VF defect seen.
- Remember Mean deviation = Minus is bad. Pattern standard deviation = Plus is bad.

Q What are the Visual Field Defects in Glaucoma?

"The VF defects can be divided into early and late."

Glaucoma Visual Field Defects

1. **Early:**
   - Paracentral nasal defect
   - Nasal step/temporal wedge
   - Scotoma in Bjerrum's area (10–20° of fixation)
   - Siedal's scotoma (defect extending from blind spot)

2. **Late:**
   - Arcuate defect/double arcuate
   - Temporal island with central vision
   - Central vision only (tunnel vision)

Q What are the Newer VF Techniques?

Newer Perimetry Techniques

1. **SITA (Swedish Interactive Thresholding Algorithm)**
   - Aims to increase speed without losing accuracy
   - SITA Standard:
     - Full version comparable to standard threshold algorithm in sensitivity and accuracy **twice** but as fast
   - SITA Fast:
     - Similar to suprathreshold algorithm in sensitivity and accuracy but twice as fast
   - How SITA works:
     - Smart questions and smart pacing
     - All factors considered as test occurs, producing estimate of threshold at each point
     - Uses normal age-corrected threshold values as starting point
     - Real time calculation and re-calculation of threshold values as test proceeds
   - Knows when to quit when standardized amount of information is obtained
   - Uses all information from every point

2. **SWAP (Short Wavelength Automated Perimetry)**
   - Blue on yellow perimetry
   - **Blue-yellow ganglion** cells first lost in glaucoma
   - SWAP detects abnormal VF 2–5 years before white on white VF abnormal
   - The presence of cataracts may affect the accuracy of SWAP

3. **Frequency doubling perimetry**
   - Low spatial frequency sinusoidal grating undergoing high temporal frequency flicker
   - Tests **magnocellular** pathway, which appears to be first lost in glaucoma
   - Possible screening tool for future

TOPIC 5

GONIOSCOPY

Overall yield: ✪✪✪   **Clinical exam:**   **Viva:** ✪✪✪   **Essay:** ✪   **MCQ:** ✪✪✪

Q Opening Question: What is Gonioscopy?

"Gonioscopy is an evaluation of the AC angle."
"It overcomes total internal reflection…."
"There are two types of lens used to evaluate the angle."

Gonioscopy

1. **Principle**
   - Light from AC angle exceeds critical angle at cornea-air interface, undergoes total internal reflection and cannot be seen
   - Goniolens has similar refractive index as cornea and alters cornea-air interface to allow light to pass from AC through cornea into lens
   - Critical angle of new interface between lens and air is not exceeded and therefore images from angle can be visualized
   - Indirect goniolens provide mirror image of angle, while direct lens provide actual view of angle

2. **Indirect goniolens**
   - Goldman goniolens:
     - Diameter of 12 mm
     - Stabilizes globe and therefore good for argon laser trabeculoplasty
     - Needs coupling fluid
     - 2-mirror lens angled at 62°
     - 3-mirror lens:
       - Largest mirror at 73° (visualize posterior pole to equator)

   - Second largest at 67° (visualize equator to retinal periphery)
   - Smallest (semicircular) at 59° (visualize angles)
   - Zeiss goniolens:
     - Diameter of 9 mm and flatter than cornea
       - Can be used for **indentational** gonioscopy
     - Lack stability and therefore not good for argon laser trabeculoplasty
     - 4-mirror angled at 64°
       - Can see entire extent of angle
     - No coupling fluid needed
       - Better visualization
   - Posner 4-mirror and Sussman 4-mirror lens (modified Zeiss with handle)

3. **Direct goniolens**
   - Diagnostic:
     - Koeppe (prototype diagnostic goniolens):
       - Stable
       - Entire extent of angle can be viewed
   - Surgical:
     - Barkan (prototype surgical goniolens), Medical Workshop, Thorpe and others

Exam tips:
- **Candidates seldom answer the principle of gonioscopy well.**
- **The comparison between Goldman and Zeiss is another favorite question.**

"Gonioscopy is an evaluation of the AC angle."
"A systematic evaluation of the structures of the angle is done as follows...."

Gonioscopic Examination

1. **Grade the angle (see below)**
   - Standard gonioscopy
   - Indentational gonioscopy
     - Differentiate appositional closure from synechial closure

2. **Assess the structures**
   - Anterior displacement of Schwalbe's line
     - Posterior embryotoxon
   - Trabeculum pigmentation:
     - **P** seudoexfoliation and pigment dispersion syndrome
     - **I** ritis
     - **G** laucoma (post angle closure glaucoma)
   - **M** elanomosis of angles (oculodermal melanosis)
   - **E** ndocrine (diabetes and Addison's syndrome)
   - **N** evus (Cogan Reese syndrome)
   - **T** rauma
- Peripheral anterior synechiae
- Blood in Sclemms' canal (raised episcleral venous pressure):
  - Carotid cavernous fistula
  - Sturge-Weber syndrome
  - Superior vena cava obstruction
  - Ocular hypotony
  - Post gonioscopy

Exam tips:
- **The differential diagnoses for trabecular pigmentation can be remembered by the mnemonic "PIGMENT"!**

Notes
- Compared to iris processes, peripheral anterior synechiae are denser, more irregular and extend beyond scleral spur

"The angle is graded according to classification systems such as...."

Grading of Angle

Shaffer system (1–V. 4)	Scheie's system (I–IV)
Grade 4 (40°) Ciliary body seen	Grade I
Grade 3 (30°) Scleral spur seen	Grade II
Grade 2 (20°) Trabeculum seen	Grade III
Grade 1 (10°) Schwalbe's line seen	Grade IV
Grade 0 (closed angle) Iridocorneal contact	

Spaeth system
Angular approach (degrees)
Curvature of peripheral iris
Regular (normal)
Steep (risk of closure)
Queer (aphakia, pigmentary glaucoma, subluxed lens)
Iris insertion
A = Above Schwalbe's line
B = Below Schwalbe's line
C = At scleral spur
D = Anterior part of ciliary body
E = Ciliary body

Q How do You Clinically Assess the AC Depth?

"We can clinically assess separately the central or peripheral AC at the slit lamp."

Clinical AC Depth Assessment

1. **Peripheral (Van Herick's method):**
   - Narrow slit beam from 60°
   - Beam aligned vertically and directed just inside limbus
   - Distance between corneal endothelium and iris compared with corneal thickness
     - AC considered shallow when this distance is <1/4 corneal thickness

2. **Central (Redman-Smith method):**
   - Narrow slit beam from 60°
   - Beam is aligned horizontally and focused between the corneal endothelium and lens
   - Adjust width of slit:
     - Align the nasal end of "corneal slit" with temporal end of "lens slit"
     - This length is measured in mm
   - AC depth = length of slit (mm) + 1.1 + 0.5

CONGENITAL GLAUCOMAS

Overall yield: ✪ ✪ ✪   **Clinical exam:**   **Viva:** ✪ ✪ ✪   **Essay:** ✪ ✪   **MCQ:** ✪ ✪ ✪

Q **Opening Question:** What are the Causes of Congenital Glaucomas?

"Congenital glaucoma can be classified into two groups: Primary or secondary."
"Secondary causes include…."

Classification of Congenital Glaucoma

1. **Primary:**
   - Congenital (birth), infantile (1–2), juvenile (2–16)

2. **Secondary:**
   - Systemic disorders:
     - Chromosomal disorders
     - Metabolic disorders (Lowe's syndrome, Zellweger's syndrome)
   - Phakomatoses (Sturge-Weber syndrome)
   - Ocular developmental disorders:
     - Anterior segment dysgenesis, aniridia
     - Congenital ectropian uvea, nanophthalmos
   - Ocular diseases:
     - Retinoblastoma, ROP, persistent hyperplastic primary vitreous, trauma, uveitis

Exam tips:
- **The classification is exactly the same as for congenital cataracts (page 9)!**

Q What are the Causes of Cloudy Cornea at Birth?

"Cloudy corneas can be caused by many different disorders."
"They can be classified based on the size of the eye."

Cloudy Cornea at Birth

1. **Large eye:**
   - Congenital glaucoma
   - Mesenchymal dysgenesis

2. **Small eye:**
   - Microphthalmos
   - Severe prenatal infection
   - Mesenchymal dysgenesis

3. **Normal size eye:**
   - Diffuse opacity:
     - Congenital hereditary endothelial dystrophy
     - Congenital hereditary stromal dystrophy
     - Sclerocornea
     - Mucopolysaccharidosis
     - Mucolipidosis
     - Interstitial keratitis
     - Congenital glaucoma

- Regional opacity
  - Linear:
    - Forceps injury
    - Congenital glaucoma (Haab's striae)
- Round:
  - Infective keratitis
  - Peter's anomaly
  - Localized mesenchymal dysgenesis

Exam tips:
- **Differential diagnosis of cloudy cornea at birth:**

S – **Sclerocornea**
T – **Trauma**
U – **Ulcer**
M – **Metabolic disease**
P – **Peter's anomaly**
E – **Endothelial dystrophy**
D – **Descemet's membrane breaks**

Q **How do You Manage Congenital Glaucomas?**

"The management of congenital glaucoma is difficult."
"And involves a **multidisciplinary team** approach."
"The important **issues** include…."
"A complete history and physical examination, usually under anesthesia, is needed."

Management of Congenital Glaucoma

1. **Issues in management**
   - Assessing **etiology** and **inheritance** of congenital glaucoma
   - Managing **systemic** problems of secondary congenital glaucoma
   - Deciding on **type** of surgery (corneal diameter as a guide):
     - <13 mm: Goniotomy/trabeculotomy
     - >14 mm: Trabeculotomy/trabeculectomy/ valve implant
     - >16 mm: Cyclodestructive procedures (usually very poor prognosis)
   - Managing associated ocular problems and **amblyopia**:
     - Refractive errors
     - Corneal opacity
     - Cataract
     - Squint

2. **Physical examination**
   - Symptoms:
     - Tearing
     - Photophobia
     - Blepharospasm
     - Red eye
     - Poor vision
   - Signs:
     - **A** xial myopia
     - **B** uphthalmos
     - **C** loudy cornea
     - **D** escemet's breaks (Haab's striae)
     - **D** iameter of cornea enlarged
     - **D** isc cupping
     - **E** xamination under anesthesia
   - Examination under anesthesia:
     - Ketamine anesthetic (other agents like isoflurane, halothane give falsely low IOP)
     - IOP (tonopen or Perkins)
     - Opthalmoscopy (disc)
     - Gonioscopy (Koeppe)
     - Refraction (retinoscopy)
     - Corneal diameter (horizontal and vertical)

Exam tips:
- **Like management of congenital cataracts (page 9), this is a fairly difficult question to handle.**
- **Provide precise opening statements to capture spectrum of related problems.**

Q What is Goniotomy and Trabeculotomy?

"Goniotomy and trabeculotomy are surgical operations for congenital glaucoma."

Treatment Options for Congenital Glaucoma

1. **Goniotomy**
   - Establish communication between AC and Schlemm's canal
   - Indications:
     - Usually in children **< 3 years**
     - Common conditions: Primary congenital glaucoma, Sturge-Weber's syndrome, Lowe's syndrome
   - Requires **clear cornea**
   - Procedure:
     - Incision made at superficial layer of meshwork, **midpoint** of trabecular band (midpoint of Schwalbe's line and scleral spur)
     - Each sweep for 120°
     - Iris should drop posteriorly
     - Repeat from opposite side
   - Results:
     - Good initial results (85% success)
     - However, 40% need re-operation
     - Repeated up to three times

2. **Trabeculotomy**
   - Establish communication between AC and Schlemm's canal by removal of a portion of trabecular meshwork (goniotomy ab externo)
   - Indications:
     - Usually in children **> 3 years**
     - Common conditions: Juvenile glaucoma, Axenfeld's anomaly, Peter's anomaly
     - Poor corneal **visibility**
   - Procedure:
     - Scleral flap fashioned, usually inferotemporal region (preserve superotemporal conjunctiva for trabeculectomy later)
     - Radial incision made over Schlemm's canal until it is inserted
     - Check location of Schlemm's canal by threading 5/0 nylon into canal
     - Trabeculotome inserted into canal and rotated into AC, tearing meshwork

   - Withdraw trabeculotome and introduce it in the opposite direction
   - Result:
     - Similar results as goniotomy but conjunctiva violated

3. **Trabeculodialysis**
   - Similar to goniotomy
   - Usually for children with secondary glaucoma from inflammation (**Juvenile chronic arthritis**)
   - Differs from goniotomy in that knife cuts are made at **Schwalbe's line**
   - Meshwork is pushed inferiorly using flat side of blade and is disinserted from scleral spur

4. **Trabeculectomy**
   - Needs mitomycin C/5 fluorouracil application
   - Problems with trabeculectomy in children
     - Thick Tenon's
     - Thin sclera
     - Difficulty in identifying limbus
     - Higher rates of scarring and trabeculectomy failure
     - Risk of endophthalmitis
   - Chronic post-op hypotony frequent

5. **Glaucoma drainage implants**
   - Mitomycin C or 5-fluorouracil application usually indicated in congenital glaucoma
   - Some advocate the use of glaucoma drainage implants as a primary surgical intervention in congenital glaucoma, due to the problems with trabeculectomy in children
   - Often more than one implant needed
   - Indication: Refractory primary congenital glaucoma
   - Complications (similar to those in adults):
     - Hypotony
     - Tube exposure
     - Endophthalmitis
     - Corneal decompensation
     - Persistent Iritis

6. **Cyclodestruction**
   - Indications:
     - Painful blind eye
     - Glaucoma refractory to other forms of treatment
     - Patient not fit for surgery
   - Complications:
     - Chronic hypotony/phthisis
     - Vision loss
     - Cataracts

7. **Medical therapy**
   - Problems
     - Not very effective

   - Compliance:
     - **Toxicity, especially systemic toxicity**
     - Alpha2 agonists: Bradycardia, hypotension, apnea (cross blood-brain barrier in children)
     - Prostaglandin analogues and miotics: Often ineffective in congenital glaucoma
     - Beta blockers: Asthma, bradycardia
     - Side effects are usually very different from those of adults (e.g. failure to thrive, bed wetting, abnormal school behavior)

Q **What are Mesodermal Dysgeneses?**

"Mesodermal dysgeneses are a group of congenital disorders."
"Which involves the cornea, iris and AC angle."
"And frequently associated with congenital glaucoma."

Mesodermal Dysgeneses and Aniridia

	Axenfeld's anomaly	Rieger's anomaly and syndrome	Peter's anomaly	Aniridia
Inheritance	• AD	• AD	• AD	• AD • AR (Mental retardation) • Sporadic (Wilm's tumor)
Iris	• Posterior embryo-toxon • Iris strands	• Posterior embryo-toxon • Iris hypoplasia, corectopia, polycoria, ectropion uvea	• Posterior embryo-toxon • Iris hypoplasia, corectopia, polycoria, ectropion uvea	• Aniridia
Cornea			• Corneal opacity • Keratolenticular adhesions • Corneal plana, sclerocornea	• Corneal opacity • Keratolenticular adhesions • Corneal plana, sclerocornea
Others			• Cataract	• Cataract • Foveal hypoplasia • Nystagmus • Choroidal coloboma
Glaucoma	• Glaucoma rare	• Glaucoma in 50%	• Glaucoma in 50%	• Glaucoma in 50%
Systemic	• None	• Dental and facial malformations in **Reiger's syndrome**	• None	• Wilm's tumor in AR trait

Clinical approach to mesodermal dysgenesis

"The most obvious abnormality is the presence of posterior embryotoxon."
"There are also diffuse areas of iris atrophy, corectopia, ectropian uvea."

Look for
- *Corneal opacity (Peters plus syndrome)*
- *Lenticular opacities – anterior polar cataracts (Peters syndrome)*
- *Keratolenticular adhesions (Peters plus syndrome)*
- *Abnormality in fellow eye (bilateral condition)*
- *Maxillary hypoplasia, teeth (hypodontia, microdontia)*

"This young patient has mesodermal dysgenesis."

I'll like to
- *Check IOP*
- *Perform gonioscopy*
- *Assess optic disc*
- *Look at visual fields*
- *Assess family members for similar condition*

 Clinical approach to aniridia

"The most obvious abnormality is the absence of iris…."

Look for
- *Corneal opacity, microcornea, sclerocornea*
- *Limbal dermoid*
- *Lenticular opacities*
- *Keratolenticular adhesions*
- *Check fellow eye (bilateral condition)*
- *Nystagmus*

"This young patient has aniridia."

I'll like to
- *Check IOP*
- *Perform gonioscopy*
- *Check fundus (foveal and disc hypoplasia, choroidal coloboma)*
- *Assess the family members for similar condition*
- *If sporadic, refer to renal physician to exclude Wilm's tumor*

Exam tips:
- Another name is iridocorneal dysgenesis. Do not confuse this with the iridocorneal endothelial syndromes (ICE).
- Aniridia is NOT part of the spectrum, but included in the table for comparison.
- Remember that Wilm's tumor is associated with AR type of aniridia.

TOPIC 7

OPEN ANGLE GLAUCOMAS

Overall yield: ✪✪✪✪   **Clinical exam:** ✪   **Viva:** ✪✪✪   **Essay:** ✪✪✪   **MCQ:** ✪✪✪✪

Q Opening Question: What is Glaucoma?

"Glaucoma is a specific type of optic neuropathy."
"With characteristic optic disc changes and VF abnormalities."
"The major risk factor is an increase in IOP."
"Glaucoma can be classified into open and closed angle and also as primary and secondary…."

Glaucoma

1. **Definition**
    *   Optic neuropathy with characteristic optic disc changes and VF abnormalities
    *   IOP is one of the risk factors

2. **Classification**
    *   Open angle glaucoma (OAG):
        *   Primary (POAG)
        *   Secondary:
            *   Paratrabecular (membrane)
    *   Trabecular (pigment dispersion, pseudoexfoliation syndrome, neovascular glaucoma)
    *   Post-trabecular (raised episcleral venous pressure)
    *   Angle closure glaucoma (ACG):
        *   Primary (PACG)
        *   Secondary:
            *   Posterior pushing forces (posterior synechiae, phacomorphic glaucoma)
            *   Anterior pulling forces (peripheral anterior synechiae, neovascular glaucoma)

Q What is the Pathogenesis of Primary Open Angle Glaucoma?

1. **Genetics**
    *   MYOC: Myocilin (GLC1A), associated with juvenile open angle glaucoma and ~4% of adults with POAG
    *   OPTN: Optineurin (GLC1E)
    *   Other loci: GLC1B, GLC1C etc.

2. **Pressure-dependent (mechanical) factors**
    *   Increased IOP → compression and backward bowing of lamina cribrosa → obstruction of axoplasmic transport → ganglion cell death

3. **Ischemic factors (especially significant for NTG)**
    *   Vascular perfusion compromise (DM, HPT, migraine, Raynaud's phenomenon)

*   Abnormal blood coagulability
*   Nocturnal hypotension, significant blood loss

4. **Neurodegenerative factors**
    *   Primary ON damage leads to release of glutamate, which interacts with cell receptors that leads to an increase in intracellular calcium levels
    *   This triggers cell death via apoptosis and leads to further release of glutamate and a vicious cycle occurs

"Steroid response is the change in IOP with steroid administration."

Steroid Response

1. **Definition**
   - Based on 6-week course of topical betamethasone, there are three groups of persons:
     - High responders (>30 mmHg):
       · 5% of population
       · 90% of POAG
       · 25% of POAG relatives
     - Moderate responder (22–30 mmHg):
       · 35% of population
     - Low responder (21 mmHg or less):
       · 60% of population

2. **Risk in IOP dependent on:**
   - Strength of steroids
     - Strong steroids (dexamethasone, betamethasone and prednisolone, etc.) more likely to produce IOP rise than weak steroids (fluorometholone etc.)
   - Route of administration:
     - Systemic steroids less likely to produce IOP rise
   - Duration, frequency and dose

3. **Mechanism**
   - Decrease phagocytosis
   - Interfere with transport in trabeculum
   - Decrease in prostaglandin activity

Q What are the Factors Which Influence the Management of Open Angle Glaucoma?

"The factors which will influence the management of a patient with open angle glaucoma include...."

Factors that Determine the Management of Open Angle Glaucoma

1. **Severity and progression of disease:**
   - IOP level (most important factor)
   - Optic nerve head changes
   - Visual field changes
   - Ocular risk factors (CRVO, Fuch's endothelial dystrophy, retinitis pigmentosa)

2. **Patient factors:**
   - Age
   - Race (blacks higher rate of progression)
   - Family history of blindness from glaucoma
   - Only eye or fellow eye blind from glaucoma
   - Concomitant risk factors (DM, HPT, myopia, other vascular diseases)
   - Compliance to follow-up and medication use
   - Socioeconomic status (costs of drugs vs surgery)

Resources Available to the Patient
   - Surgery for POAG in places which has no resources for long term follow-up

Exam tips:
- Similar to factors affecting management of cataract and glaucoma (page 25).
- A very useful approach to many different glaucoma questions. For example, the examiner may ask, "How do you manage a 70-year-old man with uncontrolled POAG in one eye and is blind in the other eye from advanced POAG?"

Q **What is the Relationship between IOP and Glaucoma? What are Ocular Hypertension and Normal Tension Glaucoma (NTG)?**

"Ocular hypertension is defined as IOP >95th percentile of the normal distribution in that population (see below)." "NTG is defined as…. (see below)."

Spectrum of POAG, Ocular Hypertension and NTG

IOP	Optic disc	VF	Diagnosis	Clinical approach
Increased	*Abnormal*	*Abnormal*	Glaucoma (POAG)	
Normal	*Abnormal*	*Abnormal*	NTG	Exclude POAG with diurnal IOP variation Exclude optic neuropathy Decide on treatment approach
Increased	Normal	Normal	Ocular hypertension	Determine risk of POAG Decide on treatment approach
Normal	Normal	*Abnormal*	Glaucoma suspect	Exclude either POAG or NTG
Normal	*Abnormal*	Normal	Glaucoma suspect	Exclude either POAG or NTG
Normal	Normal	Normal	Normal	

Q **What is Ocular Hypertension (OHT)? How do You Manage OHT?**

"Ocular hypertension is defined as an IOP >95th percentile of the normal distribution in that population."
"The ON and VF are normal."
"But the IOP is consistently >21 mmHg."
"The management has to be individualized."
"I would discuss the management options with the patient: He can either be observed or glaucoma treatment can be commenced."
"I would be more inclined to start treatment if these risk factors for developing POAG are present: …."

Ocular Hypertension

1. **Natural history**
   - VF loss about 2% per year
   - Treatment decreases VF loss to 1% per year
   - However, mean years from initial VF loss to death (12 years in whites, 16 years in blacks)
   - Therefore elderly patient with OHT rarely becomes blind even without treatment!

2. **Risk factors for developing POAG (Ocular Hypertension Treatment Study)**
   - Age of patient (older)
   - Larger vertical CDR
   - Higher IOP
   - Thinner CCT (<555 µm) greater PSD on HVF
   - Family history of glaucoma (though not significant in OHTS)
   - Myopia, migraine, hypertension were not found to be risk factors
   - DM was protective against development of POAG

3. **Management**
   - Establish baseline and follow-up **optic disc** appearance (stereodisc photos, HRT)
   - Establish baseline and follow-up **VF** (to detect progression and to improve patient reliability)
   - Determine central corneal thickness (CCT)
   - Patient's preference is an important factor in the management

> **Notes**
> - Refer to the Collaborative Normal Tension Glaucoma Study (*Am J Ophthalmol* 1998;126:487–497)
> - Multi-center randomized controlled trial to determine whether a substantial drop in IOP would halt/slow the progression of NTG

"Normal tension glaucoma is a common form of POAG."
"In which the ON and VF changes are characteristic of POAG."
"But the IOP is consistently <21 mmHg."
"The management of NTG is difficult and controversial."
"It includes establishing the diagnosis and follow-up for progression of disease."
"The findings of the Collaborative Normal Tension Glaucoma Study (CNTGS) suggest that NTG is often non-progressive. When VFD or optic nerve damage is progressive, medical and surgical treatment is indicated."
"Some patients progress despite treatment, suggesting that factors other than IOP may play a more important role in optic nerve damage."

Normal Tension Glaucoma

1. **Clinical examination and diagnostic approach**
   - **Aim**
     - Exclude other types of glaucoma:
       - POAG with *diurnal variation*? (daily changes) Intermittent ACG?
       - Old secondary glaucoma?
     - Exclude optic neuropathy:
       - Compressive optic neuropathy (consider neurological consultation and CT scan)
       - Congenital disc anomalies
       - Anterior ischemic optic neuropathy
       - Radiation and toxic optic neuropathy
   - **History**
     - Risk factors for NTG:
       - Severe vascular compromise (shock, major accidents, major surgery)
       - Vascular diseases (DM, HPT, migraine, smoking, Raynaud's disease)
     - Family history of POAG
     - Intermittent ocular pain (intermittent ACG)
     - Radiotherapy, TB treatment (optic neuropathy)
   - Establish baseline and follow-up **optic disc** appearance (stereodisc photos, HRT)
   - Establish baseline and follow-up **VF** (to detect progression and to improve patient reliability)
   - Determine CCT to exclude artificially low IOP readings

   - If there are reliable and progressive optic disc and VF changes, consider **phasing**:
     - If raised IOP found, treat as POAG
     - If normal IOP with wide diurnal fluctuation found, treat as for NTG
     - If normal IOP with no fluctuation, exclude optic nerve disease, and consider **neurological consultation and CT scan**
   - If neurological consultation and CT scan are normal, treat as for NTG

2. **Treatment**
   - No proven treatment
   - Maintain IOP as low as possible (latanoprost and other new drugs):
     - CNTGS found that decreasing IOP by 30% reduced rate of VF progression from 35% to 12%
   - Treat associated vascular risk factors (DM, HPT)
   - Systemic vasodilator and Calcium channel blockers (nifedipine, namodipine, lisinopril)
   - Neuroprotective agents (betoptic, brominidine, akatinol/memantine)
   - Trabeculectomy
     - Has been shown in some studies to preserve VF in NTG

Notes
- "What optic discs changes are more common in NTG compared with POAG?"
- Greater rim thinning
- Peripapillary crescent more common
- Splinter hemorrhage more common
- Optic disc pallor more than cupping
- Optic disc pits more common

Notes
- "What VF changes are more common in NTG compared to POAG?"
- VF loss closer to fixation
- Steeper slopes

	Early Manifest Glaucoma Trial	Advanced Glaucoma Intervention Study	Collaborative Initial Glaucoma Treatment Study
Aim	To compare the effects of immediate treatment (Betaxolol and ALT) vs no/late treatment on the progression of newly detected POAG To determine the extent of IOP reduction attained by treatment and explore factors that can influence glaucoma progression	To assess the long-term outcome of intervention sequences (TAT vs ATT) in eyes that have failed initial medical treatment for glaucoma	To compare long-term effect of treating newly diagnosed POAG with standard medical treatment (meds → ALT → trab) vs filtration surgery (trab → ALT → meds)
Design	Multicenter, randomized controlled trial	Multicenter, randomized controlled trial	Multicenter, randomized controlled trial
Inclusion	Newly diagnosed and untreated POAG	POAG uncontrolled by medication	Newly diagnosed and untreated POAG
Endpoint	Glaucoma progression (visual field and optic disc)	Visual acuity, visual field	Visual acuity, visual field, IOP, quality of life
Results	25% reduction in IOP reduced progression from 49% to 30% at 4 years	Black patients tended to preserve vision with ATT while whites did better with TAT Eyes with IOP <18 mmHg did not progress on the visual fields over 6 years	Both groups had substantial and sustained reduction in IOP (surgical group had IOP about 2–3 mmHg lower) No substantial difference in VF or quality of life between the 2 groups

"The Ocular Hypertension Treatment Study (OHTS) showed CCT to be a powerful predictor of the development of glaucoma."

"Eyes with CCT <555 μm had a threefold greater risk of developing glaucoma than those who had CCT >588 μm."

1. **Importance of CCT:**
   - Thicker corneas cause falsely higher IOP readings, and thinner corneas cause falsely lower IOP readings
   - Thin CCT may be an independent risk factor for the development of glaucoma (evidence lacking)

2. **Measurement of CCT:**
   - Ultrasound pachymetry: Contact required, accuracy dependent on technician's expertise
   - Scanning slit topography (Orbscan): Non-contact, higher readings compared to pachymetry
   - Specular microscopy: Provides pachymetric measurements and specular microscopy simultaneously

3. **Tonometry that reduces the influence of the corneal biomechanical properties:**
   - Dynamic control tonometry (DCT)
   - Ocular response analyzer tonometry (ORA)

ANGLE CLOSURE GLAUCOMA

Overall yield: ✪✪✪✪ **Clinical exam:** ✪ **Viva:** ✪✪✪ **Essay:** ✪✪✪ **MCQ:** ✪✪✪✪

Q Opening Question: What is Primary Angle Closure Glaucoma? How do You Get Angle Closure?

"Primary Angle Closure Glaucoma (PACG) is a specific type of glaucoma."
"Aqueous outflow is blocked as a result of closure of the angles."
"The risk factors can be divided into patient and ocular factors."

Primary Angle Closure

1. **Pathogenesis risk factors**
   - Patient factors:
     - Age (increases with age)
     - Sex (females)
     - Race (more common in orientals, Eskimos)
   - Ocular factors:
     - Anatomical:
       - Shallow AC
       - Narrow angle
       - Relative anterior location of iris-lens diaphragm
       - Risks increases with increasing lens thickness, small corneal diameters and short axial lengths (hypermetropia)
   - Physiological
     - Relative pupil block:
       - Mid-dilated pupil (semi-dark lighting)
       - Autonomic neuropathy (loss of pupil hippus)

2. **Stages**

Stages	Clinical presentation	Treatment options
Primary Angle Closure Suspect	• Iridotrabecular contact of 180 degrees or more Normal IOP, no peripheral anterior synechiae (PAS)	• Consider no treatment vs benefit of Laser PI
Primary Angle Closure	• Iridotrabecular contact of 180 degrees or more • Raised IOP or PAS present	• Laser PI for both eyes • Medical treatment or surgery if IOP still raised
Primary Angle Closure Glaucoma	• Iridotrabecular contact of 180 degrees or more • Glaucomatous optic neuropathy and visual field loss	• Laser PI for both eyes • Medical treatment or surgery if IOP still raised
Acute PAC	• Acute presentation	• Acute management • Laser PI • Surgery might be required

Exam tips:
- **The pathogenesis of PACG is usually not well answered. There must be a clear and systematic plan.**

Q **What are the Mechanisms of Angle Closure?**

"Pupil block is the most common mechanism of angle closure."
"However, mechanisms other than pupil block are now increasingly recognized...."

Mechanisms of Angle Closure

1. **Pupil block (most common)**
2. **Abnormalities anterior to iris**
   - PAS
   - ICE syndrome: Abnormal endothelial cells
   - Rubeotic glaucoma: Neovascular membranes
3. **Abnormalities of iris and ciliary body**
   - Plateau iris

   - Iris and ciliary body cysts
   - Thick peripheral iris, peripheral iris roll
4. **Abnormalities of lens**
   - Thick intumescent lens: Phacomorphic glaucoma
   - Subluxed lens
5. **Abnormalities posterior to lens**
   - Malignant glaucoma

Notes
- Causes of raised IOP post PI for angle closure:
- Plateau iris
- PAS
- Steroid response
- Non-patent PI
- Malignant glaucoma
- Subluxed lens

Q **What is the Plateau Iris Syndrome?**

"Plateau Iris syndrome is a form of angle closure glaucoma."
"There is no pupil block but the ciliary body is anteriorly positioned and the iris is inserted anteriorly."
"With characteristic clinical features."

Plateau Iris Syndrome

1. **Clinical features:**
   - Younger patient
   - Less hypermetropic (may be **myopic**)
   - AC normal depth, flat iris plane
   - Gonioscopy
     - Iris inserted anteriorly (A or B under Spaeth classification, page 56)

   - **Angle crowding** (keyword)
   - Indentation gonioscopy does not open angles ("double hump sign")
2. **Treatment:**
   - Laser PI should still be performed (plateau iris syndrome is diagnosed only after PI)
   - Laser iridoplasty

Clinical approach to angle closure glaucoma

"On examination, the AC is shallow…."

Look for
- *Pigmented deposits on the endothelium of cornea, which is otherwise clear*
- *Shallow AC, especially peripheral AC*
- *Iris:*
  - *Widespread iris atrophy (spiral atrophy)*
  - *Patent laser PI at superonasal quadrant*
  - *Old laser iridoplasty scars*
  - *Posterior synechiae on pupil margin*
  - *Pupil may be dilated and fixed (sphincter ischemia)*
- *Glaukomflecken (grayish opacities)*
- *Trabeculectomy blebs*

"This patient has a previous attack of angle closure glaucoma."

I'll like to
- *Check IOP*
- *Perform a gonioscopy*
- *Assess optic disc*
- *Look at VF*

SECONDARY GLAUCOMAS

Overall yield: ✪✪✪✪✪ **Clinical exam:** ✪✪✪✪ **Viva:** ✪✪✪ **Essay:** ✪✪✪ **MCQ:** ✪✪✪✪

Q Opening Question: What are the Causes of Neovascular Glaucoma?

"Neovascular glaucoma is a secondary glaucoma."
"Can be either open angle or closed angle."
"The most common etiologies are diabetic retinopathy, CRVO and ocular ischemia."
"Management is extremely difficult and prognosis is usually very poor."
"Treat underlying condition and the glaucoma."

Etiology of Neovascular Glaucoma:

- **R** etinopathy and **R**etinal vein occlusion (proliferative diabetic retinopathy, CRVO)
- **R** etinal detachment
- **U** veitis
- **B** RVO
- **E** ales disease
- **O** cular ischemic syndrome
- **T** rauma
- **I** ntraocular tumors (choroidal melanoma)
- **C** arotid cavernous fistula

 Clinical approach to neovascular glaucoma

"On examination of the anterior segment, the most obvious abnormality is at the iris."
"New vessels are seen at the pupil border at 3 o'clock…."

Look for
- *Ciliary injection*
- *Cornea clarity*
- *AC activity (microscopic hyphema) and AC depth*
- *Trabeculectomy/filtering shunt*
- *Iris:*
  - *Peripheral anterior synechiae at limbus*
  - *Posterior synechiae on pupil margin*
  - *Pupillary distortion and ectropion uveae*
  - *Pupil may be fixed and dilated*
- *Lens clarity (cataract)*

"This patient has Rubeosis iridis."

I'll like to
- *Check IOP*
- *Perform gonioscopy (new vessels and peripheral anterior synechiae at the angle)*

(Continued)

Exam tips:
- **A very good anterior segment examination case.**
- **Remember the etiology by the mnemonic, "RUBEOTIC."**

Q How would You Manage this Patient?

"Management of this condition is **difficult** and **prognosis** is usually very poor."
"I'll need to manage both the **underlying disease** and the neovascular **glaucoma** in both eyes."
"This will depend on the patient's **visual potential** and whether there is significant **pain**...."
"In the case of good visual potential, I'll...."

Management of Neovascular Glaucoma

1. **Scenario 1: Good visual potential**
   - Treat underlying condition (PRP for DM retinopathy and CRVO)
   - Control IOP with medications
   - Consider early surgical filtering operation if IOP not controlled
     - Shunts
     - Modified trabeculectomy with MMC
   - Cyclodestructive procedure as a last resort

2. **Scenario 2: Poor visual potential**
   - Not in pain
     - Treat underlying condition
     - Symptomatic relief (steroids, timolol, atropine)
   - In pain with high IOP
     - Control IOP with medication
     - Cyclodestructive procedure early

Q Tell me about Pigment Dispersion Syndrome and Pseudoexfoliation.

"Pigment dispersion syndrome is a type of secondary open angle glaucoma."
"Pseudoexfoliation syndrome is a type of secondary open angle glaucoma."

Pigment Dispersion Syndrome and Pseudoexfoliation Syndrome

	Pigment dispersion syndrome	Pseudoexfoliation syndrome
Demographics	- 30–50 years (a **decade** younger) - Men - Related to **myopia** - White race	- 60 years - Men and women - Related to **aortic aneurysms** (abnormal basement membrane) - Scandinavian countries
Pathogenic mechanisms	- **Posterior bowing** of iris - Constant rubbing of posterior pigment iris and zonules - **Release of pigments** - Trabecular block	- Systemic disease of abnormal **basement membrane** (skin, viscera, eyes) - Secretion of amyloid-like material (oxytalon) in AC - Deposit in zonules and trabeculum - Trabecular block

(Continued)

	Pigment dispersion syndrome	Pseudoexfoliation syndrome
Clinical features	• **Krukenberg's** spindle • Deep AC, with iris bowing posteriorly (**reverse pupil block**) • Iris atrophy in **periphery** of iris • Pigment deposit on lens (Zentmayer's line)	• **Pseudoexfoliative material,** dandruff-like appearance throughout AC • Pupil difficult to dilate • Iris atrophy at **edge** of pupil margin • Deposit on lens is characteristic (target-like appearance, called hoarfrost ring) • Lens subluxation (weak zonules)
Gonioscopy	• Heavily pigmented over **entire** angle • **Queer** iris configuration	• **Sampaolesi's line** (pigmented line anterior to Schwalbe's line) • Pseudoexfoliative material
Treatment	• Glaucoma risk: 10% at 5 years, 15% at 15 years • Bilateral disease: 90% • Good prognosis • Medical treatment same as POAG • Argon laser trabeculoplasty **more effective** • Pilocarpine and laser PI may work sometimes (reverse pupil block) • Trabeculectomy same as POAG	• Glaucoma risk: 1% per year (5% in 5 years, 15% in 15 years) • Bilateral disease: 30% • Fair prognosis • Medical treatment not very effective • Argon laser trabeculoplasty **more effective** in the short term • Trabeculectomy same as POAG • Cataract surgery is particularly difficult: • Weakened zonules • Small pupil • Raised IOP (risk of suprachoroidal hemorrhage)

Q Tell me about Uveitic Glaucoma.

"Uveitic glaucoma is a type of secondary glaucoma."
"Management can be difficult and involves controlling both the inflammation and the raised IOP."

Uveitic Glaucoma

1. **Mechanisms of raised IOP**
   - Angle closure with pupil block (seclusion pupillae)
   - Angle closure without pupil block (PAS)
   - Open angle glaucoma
   - Steroid responders
   - Specific hypertensive uveitis syndromes:
     - Fuch's heterochromic uveitis
     - Posner-Schlossman syndrome

2. **Management**
   - Controlling inflammation:
     - Steroids: Topical, periocular, intravitreal or systemic
   - NSAIDS: Topical, systemic
   - Immunomodulators
   - Lowering IOP
     - Medication:
       - β-blockers, α_2 agonists and carbonic anhydrase inhibitors are first-line agents
       - Relatively contraindicated: Miotics, prostaglandin analogues (though can be used cautiously in stable, well-controlled uveitis)
       - Hyperosmotic agents (e.g. mannitol): Rapid reduction of IOP in acute settings
     - Surgery:
       - When IOP is not well-controlled with medication

- Ensure inflammation is well-controlled before surgery: Consider preoperative steroids
- Higher risk of complications: Hypotony, inflammation, malignant glaucoma, choroidal effusion
- Trabeculectomy: With antimetabolites (5FU, MMC)

- Glaucoma drainage devices: Increasingly used for uveitic glaucoma
- Laser:
  - Longer duration of steroids post-laser
  - PI: When pupil block present
  - TCP: Use with caution because high rates of hypotony post-TCP
  - No role for ALT

Q **Tell me about Lens-Induced Glaucomas.**

"Lens-induced glaucomas are a group of common secondary glaucomas."
"They are classified into…."

Lens-Induced Glaucomas

1. **Classification**
   - Phacomorphic:
     - Secondary ACG
     - Intumescent lens causing pupil block
   - Phacolytic:
     - Secondary OAG
     - Hypermature cataracts, leakage of lens proteins through an **intact** capsule
   - Phaco-antigenic:
     - Secondary OAG
     - Autoimmune granulomatous reaction to exposed lens proteins from a **ruptured** capsule

   - Lens particle glaucoma:
     - Secondary OAG
     - Following cataract extraction, capsulotomy or trauma. Lens particles obstruct trabecular meshwork
   - Lens subluxation and dislocation

2. **Management**
   - Phacomorphic:
     - Manage acute attack like for acute PACG
     - Avoid miotics
     - If IOP is not controlled, carry out urgent cataract surgery

---

Notes

Possible questions:
- *"How would you manage this patient if he had a symptomatic cataract?"*
- *"How would you remove this patient's cataract?"*

 Clinical approach to trabeculectomy patients

"This patient has had a trabeculectomy operation."
"The bleb is at 10 o'clock and is avascular, not inflamed…."

Look for signs of
- *Post acute angle closure glaucoma:*
  - *Pigments on endothelium*
  - *Shallow AC*
  - *Spiral iris atrophy*
  - *Glauckomflecken*
  - *Laser PI*
- *Pigment dispersion syndrome:*
  - *Krukenberg's spindle*
  - *Deep AC*

- • *Peripheral iris atrophy*
- • *Posterior bowing of the iris*
- • *Pigmentary deposits on lens*
- • *Pseudoexfoliation syndrome:*
  - • *Pigments on endothelium*
  - • *Deep AC*
  - • *Gray white dandruff-like deposits at the pupil border*
  - • *Iris atrophy at pupil border*
  - • *Hoarfrost ring*
  - • *Subluxed lens*

I'll like to
- • *Check IOP*
- • *Perform gonioscopy (pigmentation, Sampaolesi's line and pseudoexfoliation material)*
- • *Assess optic disc*
- • *Perform VF*
- • *Phacolytic and phaco-antigenic glaucoma*
  - • *Medical control of IOP*
  - • *Semi-elective cataract surgery*

Q What are the Effects of Intraocular Hemorrhage?

Intraocular Hemorrhage

1. **Hyphema**
   - • Acute glaucoma (trabecular blockage)
   - • Chronic glaucoma (trabecular damage)
   - • Corneal blood staining (hemosiderin)

2. **Hemosiderosis bulbi**

3. **Ghost cell glaucoma**

4. **Vitreous hemorrhage**
   - • Synchysis scintillans
   - • Tractional retinal detachment

5. **Expulsive suprachoroidal hemorrhage**

> Exam tips:
> - • Remember that size affects rebleeding rate, both of which affect IOP levels, and all three increase risk of corneal blood staining!
> - • Therefore, surgical intervention is targeted specially at these complications.

Q How do You Manage a Patient with Hyphema?

"Hyphema is commonly caused by blunt ocular injury, but may also occur under other circumstances."
"The main management issues are…."

Hyphema

1. **Etiology**
   - • Trauma (blunt, penetrating)
   - • Spontaneous:
     - • Vascular abnormalities (rubeosis and its causes, page 68)
   - • Tumors
   - • Clotting disorders (sickle cell, anticoagulant treatment, blood dyscrasias)

2. **Clinical classification**
   - • Microscopic
   - • Grade I (<1/3 AC volume)

- Grade II (1/3–4/5 AC volume)
- Grade III (>1/2 AC volume)
- Grade IV (total)

3. **Problems and complications**
   - Rebleeding:
     - Dependent on **size** of hyphema
     - Grade I hyphema (25% will rebleed)
     - Grade III hyphema (75% will rebleed)
   - Increased IOP
     - Dependent on **size** and **rebleeding**
   - Corneal blood staining
     - Dependent on **size**, **IOP** and **rebleeding**

4. **Indications for surgical treatment**
   - Ocular factors (Ann Ophthalmol 1975;7: 659–662):
     - Corneal blood staining
     - Total hyphemas with IOP >50 mmHg for 5 days (to prevent optic nerve damage)
     - Hyphemas that are initially total and do not resolve below 50% at 6 days with IOP ≥ 25 mmHg (to prevent corneal blood staining)

- Hyphemas that remain unresolved for 9 days (to prevent PAS)
- Patient factors:
  - Risk of glaucoma damage (elderly, glaucoma patient, vascular diseases)
  - Sickle cell anemia
  - Risk of corneal blood staining and amblyopia (children)

5. **Management**
   - Conservative:
     - Bed rest, head elevation
     - Topical steroids and cycloplegic agents
   - Others:
     - Topical glaucoma medication
     - Aminocaproic acid
     - Tranexamic acid
     - Avoid aspirin
   - Types of surgical treatment:
     - AC paracentesis and washout
     - Clot expression and limbal delivery
     - Automated hyphectomy

Q Tell me about Angle Recession Glaucoma.

"Angle recession glaucoma is a complication of blunt ocular trauma."
"The main management issues are...."

Angle Recession Glaucoma

1. **Definition:**
   - Angle recession: Rupture of **anterior surface** of ciliary body, extending between longitudinal and oblique/circular fibers
   - Cyclodialysis: Disinsertion of **longitudinal fibers** of ciliary body from scleral spur
   - Iridodialysis: Rupture of **iris diaphragm** at iris base from ciliary body

2. **Risk of glaucoma:**
   - More than 50% of patients with gross traumatic hyphema have angle recession but only 10% develop glaucoma
   - Risk of glaucoma depends on extent of recession (risk significant if >180°)
   - Mechanism: Trabecular damage (not the recession itself)

Exam tips:
- **Know the difference between angle recession, iridodialysis and cyclodialysis.**

Q Tell me about Aphakic Glaucoma.

"Aphakic glaucoma is a difficult glaucoma to manage."

Aphakic Glaucoma

1. **Mechanisms**
   - Irido-vitreal/pupillo-vitreal block (secondary ACG)

- Vitreal-trabeculectomy contact (secondary OCG)
- Vitreal-peripheral iridectomy block

2. Prevention

- Two or more peripheral iridectomies during surgery
- Extensive anterior vitrectomy during surgery

3. Treatment

- Miose pupils with pilocarpine
- Decrease production (diamox, mannitol)
- High risk trabeculectomy

 Clinical approach to iridocorneal endothelial (ICE) syndromes

"On examination of the anterior segment of this middle aged lady."
"There are diffuse areas of iris atrophy seen."

Look for

- *Corectopia, ectropion uvea, peripheral anterior synechiae*
- *Iris nevus (Cogan-Reese's syndrome)*
- *Corneal edema (Chandler's syndrome)*
- *Lenticular opacities*
- *Trabeculectomy blebs*
- *Symptoms in fellow eye (should be normal)*

"This patient has iridocorneal endothelial syndrome."

I'll like to

- *Check IOP*
- *Perform gonioscopy*
- *Assess optic disc*
- *Look at VF*

Exam tips:
- **Remember ICE as consisting of Iris nevus, Chandler's syndrome (with Corneal involvement) and Essential iris atrophy!**

MEDICAL TREATMENT OF GLAUCOMA

Overall yield: ✪✪✪ **Clinical exam:** **Viva:** ✪✪✪ **Essay:** ✪✪ **MCQ:** ✪✪✪✪✪

Q Opening Question: What is the Ideal Drug for Glaucoma?

"The ideal drug carries certain characteristics…."

Ideal Drug

1. Effective (in lowering IOP)
2. Active on multiple fronts (decrease production, increase outflow, neuroprotective)
3. Minimal side effects
4. Convenient dosage regiments
5. Relatively inexpensive

Exam tips:
- This is a good approach to most "What is the ideal steroid for uveitis?" or "What is the ideal antibiotic for endophthalmitis?"

Q What are the Current Drugs Available for Treatment of Glaucoma?

"Current drugs available can be divided into their effectiveness in lowering IOP…."

Effectiveness in lowering IOP	Examples
Class I (30% reduction in IOP)	Beta blockers Latanoprost Alpha 2 agonist (brimonidine) Unoprostone
Class II (20%)	Pilocarpine Dorzolamide Alpha agonist (apraclonidine) Beta 1 blockers (betoptic)
Class III (10%)	Propine Other older alpha agonists

Exam tips:
- One of the most important pharmacological questions in the examinations.
- Classify according to IOP effect, mode of action (difficult) or traditional vs new drugs.

Q What are the Traditional Drugs for Treatment of Glaucoma?

Traditional Drugs

Drug	Pharmacodynamics	Effectiveness/Advantages	Side effects
Beta blockers (timolol, betaxolol, carteolol, metipranolol)	• **Decrease aqueous production** • Twice daily dosage (T1/2 = 12 hours • Concentration: 0.25 and/or to 0.5%)	• **Class I** prototype • **30% drop** in IOP in 80–90% of patients (e.g. 24 to 16 mmHg) • Good compliance • Additive effects with pilocarpine but not with sympathetic agents • Cheap	• Mild local side effects (decrease corneal sensation, allergic reaction, cicatricial conjunctivitis) • Severe systemic side effects (pulmonary bronchospasm, bradycardia, hypoglycemia) • Common systemic side effects (lethargy, decreased libido, depression)
Miotics (pilocarpine)	• **Increase aqueous drainage** (miosis with opening of angle and contraction of longitudinal fibers of ciliary body) • Works only if sphincter pupillae is not ischemic • Four times daily dosage • Concentration: 1–16%	• **Class II** prototype • **20% drop** in IOP • Additive effects with beta blockers and sympathetic agents • Cheap	• Miosis (impairment of night vision) • Myopia and headache (spasm of accommodation from circular muscle contraction) • Retinal detachment (longitudinal muscle contraction) • Uveitis (increased permeability for blood-aqueous barrier) • Angle closure glaucoma
Sympathetic agents (adrenaline and propine)	• **Decrease aqueous production** (alpha 2 effect) • **Increase aqueous drainage** (beta 2 effect) • Twice daily dosage • Concentration: 0.5%, 1%, 2% (adrenaline) • Concentration: 0.1% (propine)	• **Class III** prototype • **10% drop** in IOP • Additive with pilocarpine but not with beta blockers • Cheap	• Allergic conjunctivitis (20% in one year, 50% in 5 years) • Angle closure glaucoma • Adrenachrome deposition • Aphakic cystoid macular edema • Risk factor for trabeculectomy failure

(Continued)

Drug	Pharmacodynamics	Effectiveness/Advantages	Side effects

Carbonic anhydrase inhibitors (acetazola-mide)	• **Decrease aqueous production** (inhibit carbonic anhydrase)
	• Oral/IV
	• Concentration: 250 mg/500 mg
		• Effect independent of IOP levels
		• Useful for short term treatment
			• Tingling of fingers and toes
			• Renal (metabolic acidosis, hypokalemia and renal stones)
			• Gastrointestinal symptoms
			• Stevens-Johnson syndrome
			• Malaise, fatigue, weight loss
			• Bone marrow suppression (aplastic anemia)
			• Contraindications:
			  • Sulphur allergy
			  • Kidney or liver disease
			  • Sickle cell anemia
			  • Renal stones
			  • G6PD
			  • Pregnancy or lactation

Hyperosmotic agents (glycerol, mannitol, isosorbide)	• Dehydrates vitreous
	• Oral/IV
	• Concentration:
	  • Glycerol and isosorbide 1g/kg
	  • Mannitol 20% 1g/kg
		• Rapid onset: Peak action within 30 minutes for mannitol	• Cardiovascular overload (use with caution when cardiovascular or renal disease present)
			• Urinary retention
			• Nausea
			• Headache
			• Backache
			• Alteration of mental state, confusion

Exam tips:
• The side effects of adrenaline can be remembered by "A."

Q What are the New Drugs for Treatment of Glaucoma?

New Drugs

Drug	Pharmacodynamics	Effectiveness/Advantages	Side effects
Latanoprost (Xalatan) Travoprost (Travatan) Bimatoprost (Lumigan)	• PGF2 alpha agonist • **Increase uveoscleral outflow** • Once nightly dosage (T1/2 = 12 hours) • Concentration: 0.005%	• Better or as effective as timolol (depending on which study) • **Class I** drug. 30% drop in IOP in 80–90% of patients (e.g. 24 to 16 mmHg) • IOP effect at night • Good compliance • Additive effects with other medications • Effective for 2 years with no drift	• Little systemic SE (T1/2 in plasma = 7 s): occasional headache/URTI symptoms • Conjunctival injection (10% will complain of redness, 30% objective injection) • Inflammation (contraindicated in uveitis) • Hypertrichosis (increase in length, number and thickness) • Iris pigmentation (melanin deposition, no melano-cytic hyperplasia, therefore no risk of melanoma) • Cystoid macular edema (pseudophakics/aphakics) • Expensive
Brimonidine (Alphagan) Apraclonidine (Iopidine)	• Alpha 2 agonist – three effects: 1. Decreases aqueous production 2. Increase uveoscleral outflow 3. Neuroprotective • Twice daily dosage • Concentration: 0.2% • Rapid onset (30 min)	• **Class I** drug • Alpha 2 selectivity – aqueous production suppression (without vasoactivity effects of alpha 1) • Less side effects compared with older non-specific alpha agonists (apraclonidine) 1. Tachyphylaxis (30%) 2. Chemosis and stinging (30%) • Additive effects with other medications	• Allergic blepharoconjunctivitis (10%) • Corneal irritation (10%) • Dry mouth (10%)

(Continued)

92   The Ophthalmology Examinations Review

(Continued)

Drug	Pharmacodynamics	Effectiveness/Advantages	Side effects
Dorzolamide (Trusopt) Brinzolamide (Azopt)	• Topical carbonic anhydrase inhibitor • Only 1/3 as effective as oral • Three times daily dosage • Concentration: 0.2%	• **Class II** drug • Less side effects compared with oral	• Injection and stinging (30%) • Less effective than timolol • **Corneal opacification** in compromised corneas (inhibits endothelial pump function) • Less systemic SE compared to acetazolamide
Unoprostone (Rescula)	• PGF2 alpha metabolite agonist: 1. Increase conventional outflow 2. Increase uveoscleral outflow • Twice daily dosage • Concentration: 0.12%	• **Class I** drug • As effective as timolol • May also increase optic nerve head perfusion	• Similar to latanoprost

Combination Eyedrops:

1. Cosopt: Timolol + dorzolamide
2. Xalacom: Timolol + latanoprost
3. TimPilo: Timolol + pilocarpine
4. Combigan: Timolol + alphagan
5. Duotrav: Timolol + travoprost

LASER THERAPY FOR GLAUCOMA

Overall yield: ✪ ✪ ✪ ✪ **Clinical exam:** **Viva:** ✪ ✪ ✪ **Essay:** ✪ **MCQ:** ✪ ✪ ✪ ✪

Q Opening Question: What are the Uses of Lasers in Glaucoma?

"Lasers can be used for **diagnostic** and **therapeutic** purposes."
"Therapeutic use can be divided anatomically into…."

Diagnostic

1. **Confocal scanning laser ophthalmoscope (optic nerve head evaluation)**

2. **Laser retinal doppler flowmetry (optic nerve head perfusion)**

Therapeutic

Anatomical site	Procedure name	Type of laser	Indications	Notes
Iris	Peripheral iridotomy (PI)	Nd:YAG or sequential Argon-YAG	• PACG • Narrow, occludable angles • Secondary ACG (phacomorphic, uveitic)	Settings: Argon (1.1 W, 0.05 s, 50 μm) followed by Nd:YAG (2–3 mL) Lens: Abraham's syndrome or Wise's syndrome
	Laser iridoplasty	Argon	• Medically unresponsive PACG • Angle crowding • Plateau iris • Laser PI block • Prior to ALT in POAG with narrow angles	Laser 1 ring around iris (stretches angles and dilates pupil to relieve pupil block)
	Laser pupilloplasty	Argon	As in laser iridoplasty	Laser 3 rings around pupils (dilates pupil to relieve pupil block)

(Continued)

Anatomical site	Procedure name	Type of laser	Indications	Notes
Angles	Laser trabeculoplasty (ALT)	Argon	Temporizing procedure that tends to fail in the long term. Less effective than medications and surgery in VF preservation • Medically unresponsive POAG • Pigment dispersion and pseudoexfoliation • Elderly patient not fit for surgery	Settings: Argon (0.2 W, 0.1 s, 50 µm) Extent: 180 or 360° Number of shots: 40 1/3 of patients do not respond at all Average decrease in IOP ~ 30% (replaces one eyedrop)
	Selective laser trabeculoplasty (SLT)		Does not cause structural/coagulative damage to TM unlike ALT	Settings: 400 µm, 0.6–1.2 mJ, 3 ns Extent and number of shots: 45–55 spots over 180°

Anatomical site	Procedure name	Type of laser	Indications	Notes
	Laser trabeculo-coagulation	Argon	Neovascular glaucoma	Laser new vessels at iris
Ciliary body	Ciliary body ablation 1. Transscleral cyclophotocoagulation (TCP) 2. Transpupillary cyclophotocoagulation 3. Endoscopic cyclophotocoagulation	Diode (1.8–2 W) Continuous wave YAG (8–9 W)	Refractory glaucomas • Neovascular • Uveitic • Traumatic • Failed trabeculectomy • Congenital	Why not cryotherapy? Advantages of laser, lower risk of: • Phthisis bulbi • Sympathetic ophthalmia • Chemosis and pain
Sclera	Laser sclerostomy	Holium YAG	POAG	Makes 300 µm hole in sclera Little collateral damage because using picoseconds pulses High incidence of failure
	Laser suture lysis	Argon	Post trabeculectomy (Useful 1–3 weeks after trabeculectomy to improve filtration)	Settings: Argon (0.2 W, 0.1 s, 50 µm) Lens: Hoskins
Vitreous	YAG capsulotomy for malignant glaucoma	YAG	Malignant glaucoma	Settings: YAG (2–2.5 mJ, 1 pulse per burst) Lens: Capsulotomy lens

Q How do You Perform Cyclodestruction Using Laser?

"I would use a **diode laser** to perform a transscleral cyclophotocoagulation (TCP)."

Diode TCP

1. **Procedure:**
   - Retrobulbar anesthesia
   - Contact fiber-optic probe
   - Settings:
     - 1.8 to 2 W
     - 1–2 s
     - 30–40 shots
   - Extent: 360° 1–3 mm from limbus, sparing 3 and 9 o'clock areas
   - Hear "pop" sound (microablation of ciliary body epithelium)

2. **Post-procedure:**
   - Analgesics
   - Steroids
   - Check IOP 3 weeks later

3. **Complications:**
   - Pain
   - Hypotony, phthisis bulbi
   - Inflammation, iritis
   - Scleral thinning
   - Decrease in VA
   - Hyphema
   - Malignant glaucoma

Q When do You Perform a Laser Peripheral Iridotomy (PI)?

"The laser peripheral iridotomy is indicated for therapeutic and prophylactic purposes."

Indications for a Laser Peripheral Iridotomy

1. **Therapeutic:**
   - PACG (acute ACG, intermittent ACG, chronic ACG)
   - POAG with narrow angles
   - Secondary ACG (irido-IOL block, irido vitreal block, subluxed lens with pupil block)

2. **Prophylactic:**
   - Fellow eye of patient with PACG
   - Narrow occludable angles

Q How do You Perform a Laser PI?

"I would perform a Nd:YAG laser PI as follows…."
or "I would perform a sequential Argon YAG laser PI as follows…."

Procedure for Laser Peripheral Iridotomy

1. **Prepare the patient:**
   - Miosed pupil with 2% pilocarpine
   - Instil 1% apraclonidine 1 hour before procedure
   - Topical anesthetic and position patient at laser machine

2. **Argon blue green laser settings: 1.1 W, 0.05 s, 50 μm**

3. **Abraham's iridotomy lens**

4. **Location of PI:**
   - Upper nasal iris (to avoid diplopia and macular burn)
   - 1/3 distance from limbus to pupil
   - Iris crypt if possible
   - Apply 20–30 burns until iris is penetrated

5. **Signs of penetration:**
   - Plomb of iris pigments
   - Deepening of AC

- Retroilluminate to see patent PI
- Gonioscopy to see opened angles

6. **Nd:YAG laser setting: 2.5 mJ, 3–5 shots:**
    - PI size should ideally be 300–500 μm

7. **Post-procedure:**
    - Instil 1% apraclonidine
    - Check IOP 1 hour later
    - Topical steroids for 1 day

Notes
- "What are the unique features of Abraham's iridotomy lens?"
- Contact lens with +66D lenticule
- Stabilizes globe during procedure
- High magnification
- Increases cone angle and energy at site by 4x:
    - Therefore, the spot area is effectively reduced 4× and radius reduced 2× (square root of 4) (i.e. 50 μm spot size is reduced to 25 μm)
    - In addition, the energy around the cornea and iris reduced by 4×

Q **What are the Complications of a Laser PI?**

Complications

1. **Contiguous damage:**
    - Cornea
    - Cataract

2. **Iris:**
    - Iris bleeding
    - Iritis
    - Increased IOP

3. **Malignant glaucoma**
4. **Monocular diplopia**

Exam tips:
- **Remember "MIC."**

SURGICAL TREATMENT FOR GLAUCOMA

Overall yield: ✪✪✪✪✪ **Clinical exam:** **Viva:**✪✪✪✪ **Essay:**✪✪ **MCQ:** ✪✪✪✪

Q **Opening Question:** What are the Indications for Trabeculectomy in Glaucoma?

"There are no absolute indications for trabeculectomy...."
"In general...."
"Common scenarios include...."

Indications

1. **Treatment should be individualized with no fixed rule**

2. **General principle: When IOP is raised to a level where there is evidence of progressive VF or ON changes which will threaten quality of visual function, despite adequate medical treatment**

3. **Common scenarios include:**
   - Uncontrolled POAG with maximal medical treatment:
     - **Failure** of medical treatment (IOP not controlled with progressive VF or ON damage)
     - **Side effects** of medical treatment

- **Noncompliance** with medical treatment
- Additional considerations:
  - Young patient with good quality of vision
  - One-eyed patient (other eye blind from glaucoma)
  - Family history of blindness from glaucoma
  - Glaucoma risk factors (HPT, DM)
- Uncontrolled PACG after laser PI and medical treatment
- Secondary OAG or ACG

Q How does Medical Therapy Compare with Surgical Therapy in Glaucoma?

"It is difficult to compare medical with surgical treatment, with new research showing both having advantages and disadvantages. We can compare the two in four major areas...."

	Medical treatment	Surgical treatment
Effectiveness	• 40% respond readily and consistently to low dose medicine • 50% eventually require complex medical regimen, adjuvant ALT and filtration surgery	• 5–10% poor response to medical treatment in first instance and require surgery • Improved surgical technique has led to 80–90% success rates • Better control of IOP (delay VF/ON progression) • Increase morbidity associated with delaying surgery until evidence of VF/ON damage
Cost	• Cheaper initially, but accumulates over years • In the United States, cost of bilateral surgery = cost of 8 years of topical medication	• Actual cost may be less in the long term

Safety/Problems	• Poor compliance with multiple medications
	• Less control of IOP with continuing ON damage
	• Minor side effects is troublesome
	• Major side effects can occur:
	  • Aplastic anemia (with diamox)
	  • Respiratory and cardiac side effects (beta blockers)
	  • Increase risk of bleb failure (with chronic topical eyedrop use)
		• Even after surgery, may require adjuvant medical treatment
		• No long term proof that good IOP control alone will stop ON damage (IOP only one risk factor)
		• Usually no minor side effects
		• Major side effects (common):
		  • Anesthetic and surgical morbidity
		  • Risk of endophthalmitis and malignant glaucoma
		  • Shallow AC, hypotony, progression of cataracts

Quality of life	• Poorer quality of life (with use of multiple eyedrops)	• Better quality of life

Exam tips:
• As expected, this topic will be a constant debate with new research findings every month. Stick to a conservative approach but keep an open mind about new ideas.

"I would perform a trabeculectomy as follows."

Trabeculectomy

1. **Preparation:**
   - Retrobulbar anesthesia
   - Inferior corneal traction suture with 7/0 silk

2. **Conjunctival flap:**
   - Superonasally or superotemporally
   - Fornix or limbal based flap (stick to one approach, see below)
   - Dissect Tenons with Wescott scissors
   - Remove all episcleral tissue

3. **Scleral flap:**
   - Outline flap with diathermy
   - Size 4 x 3 mm
   - Cut with beaver blade 1/2 to 2/3 scleral thickness
   - Dissection with crescent blade until surgical limbus is seen (page 41)
     - "Where is the surgical limbus?"

4. **Paracentesis performed at distant location**

5. **Sclerostomy:**
   - Enter AC through scleral flap with a beaver blade
   - Excise 2 × 1 mm block of sclera with Kelly's punch or Vanna scissor

6. **Peripheral iridectomy:**
   - Prevent blockage of sclerectomy site by iris

7. **Closure:**
   - Scleral flap sutured with 8/0 vicryl or 10/0 nylon
   - Reform AC and check aqueous egress
   - Conjunctiva sutured with 8/0 vicryl

> **Exam tips:**
> - As in cataract surgery, be concise but accurate with the steps, as if you had done the procedure a hundred times. Say, "I will perform a superotemporal limbal-based conjunctival flap" instead of "conjunctival flap."

> **Notes**
> - Why perform a paracentesis?
>   - Decompress AC prior to sclerectomy
>   - Reform AC later
>   - Check aqueous egress later

Fornix-based vs Limbal-based Conjunctival Flap

	Fornix-based	**Limbal-based**
Advantages	• Faster to create and close • Good exposure • Easier to identify limbal landmarks • Less dissection (less bleeding and risk of button hole) • Avoids posterior conjunctival scarring (limits posterior filtration of aqueous)	• Easier to excise Tenon's • Less risk of wound leak and flat AC • No limbal irregularity (dellen) • Allows adjunctive use of anti-metabolites with less corneal toxicity
Disadvantages	• Increase risk of flat AC • Harder to excise Tenon's • IOP control not as good as with limbal-based flap	• Slower and more surgical experience needed • Poorer exposure • Risk of button hole higher

Q What are the Complications of a Trabeculectomy?

"The complications can be divided into intraoperative, early postoperative and late postoperative."

Complications

1. **Intraoperative (not common, usually due to poor surgical techniques):**
   - Suprachoroidal hemorrhage (most important complication, as in cataract surgery)
   - Button hole in conjunctival flap
   - Subconjunctival hemorrhage from bridle suture
   - Hyphema

2. **Early postoperative:**
   - **Flat AC and malignant glaucoma (see below)**
   - Endophthalmitis
   - Hyphema
   - Suprachoroidal hemorrhage
   - "Wipe-out" syndrome
   - Cystoid macular edema

3. **Late postoperative:**
   - **Filtration failure (see below)**
   - Endophthalmitis, blebitis
   - Cataract progression
   - VF loss progression
   - Refractive errors
   - Hypotony

Q How do You Manage a Shallow AC after a Trabeculectomy?

"Management involves an assessment of the **severity of shallowing** and the **etiology**."
"This depends on the **IOP** and presence/absence of a **bleb**."

Shallow AC

1. **Grades of shallow AC:**
   - Grade I: Irido-corneal touch (can afford to be conservative)
   - Grade II: Pupillo-corneal touch
   - Grade III: Lenticulo-corneal touch (need to intervene surgically)

2. **Etiology**

IOP	Bleb	Differential diagnoses	Management
High	• No bleb • Siedal's sign +ve	• Malignant glaucoma • Suprachoroidal Hb • Pupil block glaucoma	• See below • Fundus examination (dark brown mass) • Dilate pupil (AC may deepen) • Enlarge surgical PI with laser
Low	• No bleb +ve • Siedal's sign +ve	• Wound leak	Conservative: • Usually will resolve within 24 hours • Decrease steroids and increase antibiotics (gentamicin) to induce scarring • Dilate pupil with mydriatic (atropine) • Decrease aqueous production (timolol and diamox) • Pressure pad/bolster • Simmon's shell/oversized (flex) contact lens Surgical: • Resuture
	• Good bleb • Siedal's sign –ve	• Excessive filtration	Conservative: • Decrease steroids, increase antibiotics, dilate pupil and decrease aqueous production • Pressure pad/bolster • Inject gas (air or SF6) or viscoelastic into AC • Injection of autologous blood into bleb • Compression mattress suture Surgical: • Resuture

How do You Manage a Malignant Glaucoma?

"Malignant glaucoma is a serious complication of glaucoma surgery."
"Management involves an assessment of the **severity** (grades of AC shallowing)."
"And can be **conservative** or **surgical**."

Malignant Glaucoma

1. **Conservative:**
   - Topical mydriatics (atropine)
   - Lower IOP (diamox and osmotic agents)
   - Enlarge PI
   - Nd:YAG laser to disrupt anterior vitreous face (see laser therapy, page 78)

2. **Surgical:**
   - **Chandler's** procedure (see vitreous tap, page 33):
     - 19G needle inserted into vitreal cavity, about 12 mm from tip to drain 1–1.5 ml of aqueous and separate solid vitreous from trapped aqueous
   - Vitrectomy

Q **How do You Manage a Filtration Failure?**

"Management involves an evaluation of the **causes** of failure."
"And can be conservative or surgical."

Filtration Failure

1. **Etiology**
   - Early:
     - Blockage by ocular components (lens, iris, Descemet's membrane, vitreous, scleral remnants)
     - Blockage by surgical intervention (blood, viscoelastic)
   - Late:
     - Subconjunctival fibrosis
2. **Conservative**
   - Increase topical steroids
   - Medical control of IOP
   - Scleral depression at posterior lip of scleral flap

   - Digital massage
   - Laser suture lysis:
     - Done usually at 1–3 weeks after surgery (see laser therapy, page 78)
   - Needling of bleb:
     - Done usually at 6 weeks after surgery
     - Topical anesthetics under sterile conditions
     - Approach from unoperated conjunctiva with 27G needle
     - May be combined with 5 FU injection
3. **Surgical**
   - Revision of trabeculectomy/new trabeculectomy with antimetabolites

> **Notes**
> - Risk factors for subconjunctival fibrosis = indications for antimetabolite used

---

Q **What are the Indications for Using Antimetabolites in Trabeculectomy?**

"Antimetabolites are used in trabeculectomy when a **high risk of failure** with the conventional operation is anticipated."
"This is related to either **patient** or **ocular** factors."

Indications for Antimetabolites

1. **Patient factors:**
   - Young (<40 years)
   - Black race
   - Previous chronic medical therapy (especially with Adrenaline)

   - Previous failed trabeculectomy
   - Previous conjunctival surgery (e.g. pterygium surgery)
2. **Ocular factors:**
   - Secondary glaucomas (neovascular and uveitic glaucoma)

- Traumatic glaucomas
- Aphakic/pseudophakic glaucomas
- Iridocorneal endothelial syndromes (ICE)

- Congenital/pediatric glaucomas
- Conjunctival scarring

> **Notes**
> - What additional measures must be taken in trabeculectomies with antimetabolites?
> - Prevent antimetabolites from entering eye:
>   - Limbal-based flaps
>   - Watertight wound (interrupted non-absorbable conjunctival sutures)
>   - Careful dissection to prevent button hole formation

Q Tell me about Antimetabolites Used in Glaucoma Surgery.

	5 Fluorouracil (5 FU)	Mitomycin C (MMC)
Pharmacology	• Fluorinated **pyrimidine** analogue • Binds intracellular thymidylate synthetase (inhibits thymidine and DNA synthesis) • Affects only cells in **mitotic phase** of cell cycle • In the eye, inhibits fibroblast proliferation and delays fibrosis	• Natural antibiotic compound/**alkylating agent** • Cross-links with DNA strands by formation of covalent bonds • Affects cells in **all phases** • Kills fibroblast permanently and stop fibrosis
Dosage	• Intraoperative dose: 25–50 mg/ml • Postoperative drops: 5 mg/ml for 1 week	• Intraoperative dose: 0.2–0.4 mg/ml
Results	• Improves success rate of filtration operation	• No randomized trial results • Better than 5 FU?
Complications	• Corneal epithelial toxicity • Hyphema • Wound leak • Infection	• Prolonged hypotony • Avascular bleb • Endothelial, ciliary body and retinal damage • Hyphema • Wound leak • Infection

> **Exam tips:**
> - Refer to three-year follow-up of the Fluorouracil Filtering Surgery Study (*Am J Ophthalmol* 1993;115:82–92).

Q What is the Fluorouracil Filtering Surgery Study?

"The Fluorouracil Filtering Surgery Study is a multicenter prospective randomized clinical trial which evaluates the effectiveness of adjuvant subconjunctival 5 FU following trabeculectomy."

1. **Inclusion criteria**
   - 213 patients considered to be at a higher risk of surgical failure on the basis of having previous cataract extraction or previous failed filtering surgery in a phakic eye

2. **Treatment**
   - Trabeculectomy with adjuvant postop subconjunctival 5 FU injections vs trabeculectomy alone

3. **Outcome**
   - Treatment failure defined as:
     - Reoperation to decrease IOP, or
     - An IOP > 21 mmHg with or without adjuvant IOP-lowering medications

4. **Results**
   - Treatment failure at 3 years: 51% with 5 FU vs 74% without 5 FU
   - Complications associated with 5 FU:
     - Corneal epithelial erosions
     - Early wound leaks

5. **Conclusion**
   - 5 FU indicated after trabeculectomy only in patients at high risk of failure

---

Q Tell me about Filtering Shunts.

"Filtering shunts are communications between AC and sub Tenon's space."
"They are indicated when a **high risk of failure** with the conventional operation is anticipated."
"This is related to either **patient** or **ocular** factors."
"The shunts can be divided into…."
"The complications include…."

Filtering Shunts

1. **Indications**
   - Patient factors:
     - Previous failed trabeculectomy
     - Previous major anterior segment surgery
   - Ocular factors:
     - Secondary glaucomas (neovascular and uveitic glaucoma)
     - Traumatic glaucomas
     - Aphakic/pseudophakic glaucomas
     - Iridocorneal endothelial syndromes (ICE)
     - Pediatric glaucomas

2. **Type of shunts**
   - Vary with shape and size
   - Valves (Krupin-Denver, Ahmed) vs no valves (Molteno, Baerveldt)
   - Material: PMMA, silicon, polypropylene

3. **Complications**
   - Intraoperative:
     - Hyphema
     - Lens damage and cataract
     - Globe perforation
     - Muscle disinsertion and laceration
   - Postoperative:
     - Functional (excessive drainage, blockage of tube by blood and uveal tissue)
     - Mechanical (corneal endothelial decompensation, cataract)
     - Diplopia due to extraocular muscle limitation
     - Bleb encapsulation over footplate → poor drainage
     - Late endophthalmitis

4. **Efficacy compared to trabeculectomy**
   - Tube vs Trabeculectomy Study (*Am J Ophthalmol* 2009;148:670–684)
   - Tube shunt surgery had a higher success rate compared to trabeculectomy with MMC during first 3 years of follow-up
   - Both procedures associated with similar IOP reduction and use of supplemental medical therapy at 3 years
   - Postoperative complications higher following trabeculectomy with MMC relative to tube shunt surgery, but most complications were transient and self-limited

Exam tips:
- **The indications are nearly IDENTICAL to that of antimetabolite use.**

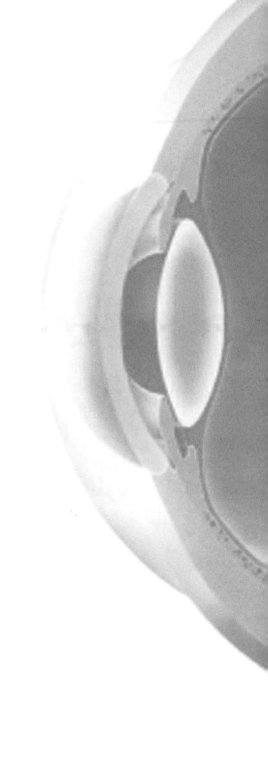

Section 3

CORNEAL AND EXTERNAL EYE DISEASES

THE CORNEA

Overall yield: ✪ ✪ ✪ ✪   **Clinical exam:**   **Viva:** ✪ ✪ ✪ ✪   **Essay:** ✪ ✪   **MCQ:** ✪ ✪ ✪ ✪

Q **Opening Question:** What is the Anatomy of the Cornea?

"The cornea is a transparent structure in the anterior segment of eye…."

Anatomy of the Cornea

1. **Gross anatomy**
   - General dimensions:
     - 11.5 mm horizontal diameter
     - 10.5 mm vertical diameter
     - 1 mm thick periphery
     - 0.5 mm thick centrally
     - Anterior surface radius 7.7 mm
     - Posterior surface radius 6.8 mm

2. **Microscopic anatomy**
   - Five layers:
   - Epithelium:
     - **Stratified squamous, nonkeratinized, nonsecretory epithelium** (keyword)
     - 5–6 layers deep
     - Superficial cells have microvilli (needs tears to keep cornea smooth)
     - Basement membrane — strongly attached to Bowman's layer
   - Bowman's layer:
     - 8-12 μm
     - Acellular
     - Consists of interwoven type IV collagen fibrils which are anterior condensation of substantia propia
     - **Incapable of regeneration**, replaced by fibrous tissue if damaged (i.e. scars)

   - Ends abruptly at limbus
   - Deep layers appear to merge into stroma
   - Stroma (substantial propia):
     - 90% of cornea thickness, 400 μm centrally
     - 80% water
     - Glycosaminoglycans in extracellular matrix
       - Three major fractions:
         - Keratan sulphate (50%)
         - Chondroitin phosphate (25%)
         - Chondroitin sulphate (25%)
   - Descemet's membrane:
     - **Basement membrane of the endothelium** (keyword)
     - 10 μm thick
     - Secreted and regenerated by endothelial cells
     - Type IV collagen fibrils
     - Hassall-Henle bodies
     - Terminates abruptly at limbus (Schwalbes line)
   - Endothelium:
     - Single layer, polygonal, cuboidal cells
     - Tight junctions (control of corneal hydration)
     - Microvilli
     - **Incapable of regeneration: Repair occurs by cellular hypertrophy and sliding**
     - Line passages of trabecular meshwork

Exam tips:
- **One of the most common basic science questions in life viva and MCQ examinations.**

Q **What is the Function of the Cornea?**

Physiology of Cornea

1. **Three main functions:**
   - Light transmission (400–700 nm light)
   - Light refraction:
     - Total refractive power of cornea 43 D (70% of eye's refractive power)
     - Refractive index of cornea 1.376
   - Protection
2. **Corneal metabolism:**
   - Energy needed for maintenance of transparency and dehydration

- Glucose:
  - Cornea obtains glucose mainly from **aqueous**
  - Tears and limbal capillaries appear to provide minimal contribution
  - Glucose can be stored in epithelium as glycogen
  - ATP obtained through glycolysis and Kreb's cycle
- Oxygen:
  - Endothelium acquires oxygen from **aqueous**
  - Epithelium acquires oxygen from either **capillaries** at the limbus or precorneal film

Q **Why is the Cornea Transparent?**

"Corneal transparency is due to a combination of factors including…."

Cornea Transparency

- **Relative dehydration** of cornea due to:
  - Anatomic integrity of endothelium and epithelium
  - Endothelial pump removes fluids from stroma
  - Evaporation of water from tear increases osmolarity of tear, which draws water from cornea

- Normal intraocular pressure (if too high, relative hydration occurs)
- Relative **acellularity**, lack of blood vessels and pigments
- **Regular matrix structure** of corneal fibrils:
  - Destructive interference of light occurs
- Consistent **refractive index** of all layers

> **Exam tips:**
> - **Variations to questions include "What are the factors which keep the cornea dehydrated?"**

Q **What is the Nerve Supply of the Cornea?**

"The cornea is innervated by the V CN."

Nerve Supply

- V CN
- Ophthalmic division
- Long posterior ciliary nerves gives off:
  - Annular plexus at limbus

- Subepithelial plexus just below Bowman's membrane
- Intraepithelial plexus

CONGENITAL CORNEAL ABNORMALITIES

Overall yield: ✸   **Clinical exam:**   **Viva:**   **Essay:** ✸   **MCQ:** ✸

Q **Opening Question:** What are the Congenital Abnormalities of the Cornea?

Megalocornea

1. **Corneal diameter > 13 mm (or 12 mm at birth):**
   - Buphthalmos must first be excluded (no axial myopia, no cornea opacity, normal IOP)
   - Distinction between simple megalocornea (large cornea without structural abnormalities and associated ocular malformations) and anterior megalophthalmos (large cornea with structural abnormalities/ocular malformations)

2. **Inheritance: AD (simple megalocornea) or SLR (anterior megalophthalmos)**

3. **Clinical features (anterior megalophthalmos):**
   - Congenital
   - Males (90%)
   - Bilateral (80%), symmetrical, nonprogressive
   - Normal cornea
   - Normal thickness and endothelial cell density
   - No Descemet's rupture (i.e. no Haab's straie)
   - Normal posterior segment
   - Normal visual development

4. **Ocular associations (anterior megalophthalmos):**
   - Astigmatism
   - Atrophy of iris stroma
   - Ectopic lentis and cataract
   - Glaucoma (but not congenital glaucoma!)

5. **Systemic associations (anterior megalophthalmos):**
   - Down's
   - Connective tissue diseases (Marfan's syndrome, Ehlers-Danlos syndrome)
   - Craniosynostosis (Apert's syndrome)
   - Alport's syndrome

   - Facial hemiatrophy
   - Dwarfism

Microcornea

1. **Corneal diameter < 10 mm**

2. **May occur as:**
   - Isolated cornea abnormality
   - Nanophthalmos (small but normal eye)
   - Microphthalmos (small and abnormal eye)

3. **Inheritance: AD, AR, sporadic**

4. **Ocular associations:**
   - Shallow AC
   - Glaucoma
   - Hyperopia
   - Persistent hyperplastic primary vitreous
   - Congenital cataract
   - Anterior segment dysgenesis
   - Optic nerve hypoplasia

5. **Systemic associations:**
   - Dwarfism
   - Achondroplasia
   - Myotonic dystrophy
   - Fetal alcohol syndrome

Cornea Plana

1. **Flat cornea:**
   - Radius of curvature **< 43D** (may be 20–30D)
   - Pathognomonic when corneal curvature is the same as adjacent sclera!

2. **Inheritance: AD, AR, sporadic**

3. **Bilateral, peripheral opacification of cornea**
4. **Ocular associations:**
   - **Sclerocornea**
   - Microcornea
   - Congenital cataract
   - Glaucoma

Sclerocornea

1. **Diffuse scarring and vascularization of cornea**
2. **Epithelium thickened, Bowman's membrane absent**

3. **May be AD/sporadic**
4. **Classification:**
   - Isolated sclerocornea: No other abnormalities
   - Sclerocornea plana: With flat cornea (mean K < 38D)
   - Peripheral sclerocornea with anterior chamber cleavage abnormalities: Peter's, Rieger's anomalies
   - Total sclerocornea

Q   **Tell me about Goldenhar's Syndrome.**

Clinical Features

1. **Ocular features:**
   - Megalocornea
   - **Coloboma** of iris and lids
   - Squint, **Duane's** syndrome
   - Fundus — optic nerve hypoplasia, coloboma
   - Refractive errors

2. **Systemic features:**
   - Wide mouth
   - Maxillary and mandibular hypoplasia
   - **Preauricular tags** and hearing loss
   - Vertebral defects

CHEMICAL INJURY

Overall yield: ✹ ✹ ✹   **Clinical exam:**   **Viva:** ✹ ✹ ✹ ✹   **Essay:** ✹ ✹   **MCQ:** ✹ ✹

Q **Opening Question:** What are the Complications of Chemical Injuries?

"Chemical injuries are ocular emergency."
"They can be mild or potentially blinding."

Complications of Chemical Injury

1. **Acute problems:**
   - Corneal abrasion and perforation
   - Infection
   - Glaucoma

2. **Long-term problems:**
   - Ocular surface:
     - Trichiasis, distichiasis, entropion
     - Cicatricial conjunctivitis, dry eyes, symblepharon, ankyloblepharon

- Cornea:
  - Persistent epithelial defect
  - Limbal stem cell failure and persistent ocular surface disease
  - Stromal scar
- Intraocular complications:
  - Glaucoma
  - Diffuse trabecular damage iritis
  - Cataract

Classification of Chemical Injury (Hugh's Classification)

Grade	Signs	Prognosis
1	Corneal epithelial damage No limbal ischemia	Excellent
2	Corneal hazy but iris details seen Ischemia <1/3 of limbus	Good
3	Corneal hazy but iris details hazy Ischemia <1/2 of limbus	Fair
4	Opaque cornea Ischemia >1/2 of limbus	Poor

Updated classification (ref Dua H *et al, Br J Ophthalmol* 85(11):1379

- Updated grading scheme with *prognostic* value
- 6 grades
- Main criteria for classification:
  - Extent of limbal **staining** (vs ischemia): Staining of greater value in predicting epithelial recovery

- Area of bulbar and forniceal conjunctival staining: Conjunctiva important in ocular surface stabilization when limbus severely compromised

Exam tips:
- **One of the few true ocular emergencies.**
- **Need to know difference between "acidic" and "alkaline" injuries.**

Notes:
- "What are the possible mechanisms of glaucoma?"
  - Acute shrinkage of collagen
  - Uveitis, trabeculitis
  - Lens-induced inflammation
  - Peripheral anterior synechiae
  - Steroid response

Q **How do You Manage a Patient with Severe Chemical Injury?**

"Chemical injury is an ocular emergency…."

Management of Chemical Injury

1. **Acute management**
   - Irrigate eyes immediately copious amounts of sterile fluid (normal saline preferred):
     - Remove particulate matter
     - Debride devitalize tissues
   - Start antimicrobial treatment
   - Start steroids immediately (to decrease mediators of inflammation and stabilize lysosome in white blood cells)
     - Minimize steroids after 10 days (because steroids decrease fibroblast and collagen synthesis)
     - Alternatively, medroxyprogesterone can be used (no anti-anabolic effects)

2. **Manage epithelial defect**
   - Conservative:
     - Tear substitutes and lubricants
     - Vitamin C (antioxidant, cofactor in collagen synthesis)
     - Ascorbate or citrate (antioxidant, cofactor in collagen synthesis)
     - N acetylcysteine (collagenase inhibitor, contributes to cross-linkages and maturation of collagen)
     - Sodium EDTA (collagenase inhibitor — calcium chelator, calcium required for collagenase activity)
     - Bandage contact lens
   - Surgical:
     - Punctal occlusion in severe dry eyes
     - Lid closure (taping, pressure pad, tarsorraphy)
     - Tissue glue
     - Conjunctival flap
     - Lysis of conjunctival adhesions (glass rods)

3. **Long-term management**
   - Ocular surface reconstruction:
     - Lid surgery (cicatricial entropion, trichiasis and distichiasis)
     - Conjunctival replacement (AMT or cultivated conjunctiva)
     - Ocular surface surgery
       - Principles:
         - Removal of dysplastic epithelium
         - Wide excision of fibroblastic undergrowth
         - Judicious diathermy
         - Epithelial replacement (autografts/allografts/cultivated transplants)
   - Cornea:
     - Keratoplasty (limbal, lamellar, penetrating)
   - Intraocular:
     - Antiglaucoma treatment
     - Cataract surgery
   - Controversial:
     - Retinoic acid (promote surface keratinization)
     - Fibronectin (growth factor)
     - Epidemal growth factor
     - Subconjunctival heparin (to facilitate limbal reperfusion)

"Cicatricial conjunctivitis can be divided into…."

Cicatricial Conjunctivitis

1. **Infectious:**
   - Adenovirus
   - Herpes simplex
   - Trachoma
   - *Corynebacterium diphtheriae*
   - Beta hemolytic streptococcus

2. **Noninfectious:**
   - Autoimmune:
     - Ocular cicatricial pemphigoid
     - Steven-Johnson syndrome
   - Vernal/atopic keratoconjunctivitis
   - Dermatological:
     - Ocular rosacea
     - Scleroderma
   - Neoplasia:
     - Squamous cell carcinoma, Bowen's disease
   - Trauma:
     - Mechanical, chemical injury
   - Others:
     - Long-term timolol use

CORNEAL OPACITY, SCARRING AND EDEMA

Overall yield: ✪✪✪   **Clinical exam:** ✪✪✪   **Viva:** ✪   **Essay:** ✪   **MCQ:** ✪✪✪

Q **Opening Question:** What are the Causes of Corneal Scarring?

"Corneal scarring can be divided into the location of the scarring...."

Corneal Scarring

1. **Superior cornea:**
   - Superior limbic keratoconjunctivitis
   - Trachoma
   - Vernal keratoconjunctivitis

2. **Central cornea:**
   - Disciform keratitis
   - Keratoconus (hydrops)
   - Fuch's endothelial cell dystrophy
   - Bullous keratopathy
   - Lipid keratopathy
   - Band keratopathy

3. **Inferior cornea:**
   - Neurotrophic keratopathy
   - Exposure keratopathy
   - Marginal keratitis

4. **Diffuse scarring:**
   - Interstitial keratitis
   - Trauma
   - Ocular surface diseases (Stevens-Johnson syndrome, ocular cicatricial pemphigoid)
   - Trachoma

 Clinical approach to a superior corneal scar

"This patient has stromal scarring seen at the superior half of the cornea...."

Look for
- *Trachoma:*
  - *Trichiasis, entropion of upper lid*
  - *Herbert's pits*
  - *Evert upper lid (Arlt's line)*
- *Vernal keratoconjunctivitis:*
  - *Punctate epitheliopathy, macroerosions, shield ulcers, plaque, subepithelial scar*
  - *Trantas dots*
  - *Pseudogerontoxon (cupid's bow)*
  - *Evert upper lid (giant papillae)*
- *Superior limbic keratoconjunctivitis:*
  - *Superior conjunctival injection*
  - *Punctate epitheliopathy, corneal filaments*

Clinical approach to central corneal scar or edema

"This patient has a central corneal stromal scar/edema."
"The visual axis is involved."

Look for
- *Disciform keratitis:*
  - *Lid scarring (usually very subtle)*
  - *Epithelial edema*
  - **Descemet's folds**
  - *Wessley ring*
  - *Keratic* **precipitates**
  - *AC activity*
- *Keratoconus:*
  - *Parastromal thinning*
  - *Vogt's straie*
  - **Fleischer's ring**
  - *Prominent corneal nerves*
- *Fuch's endothelial cell dystrophy:*
  - *Epithelial edema*
  - *Subepithelial scarring*
  - *Stromal thickening*
  - **Corneal guttata**
- *Pseudophakic bullous keratopathy:*
  - *Epithelial bullae*
  - **IOL**

I'll like to
- *Check corneal sensation (disciform keratitis)*
- *Check IOP (Fuch's endothelial dystrophy, disciform keratitis)*

Q **How do You Manage a Patient with Bullous Keratopathy?**

"Management of bullous keratopathy depends on the **etiology**, **severity** and **visual potential** and whether patient has symptoms of **pain**."
"In mild cases, conservative treatment is usually adequate... ."
"In severe cases, if the visual potential is good... ."
"On the other hand, if the visual potential is poor and the eye is painful... ."

Bullous Keratopathy

1. **Etiology:**
   - Pseudophakic bullous keratopathy
   - Fuch's endothelial cell dystrophy
   - End-stage glaucoma
   - Long-standing inflammation
   - Chemical burns

2. **Conservative treatment:**
   - Lubricants
   - Hypertonic saline
   - Lower intraocular pressure
   - Avoid steroids
   - Therapeutic contact lens
   - Hair-dryer

3. **Surgical treatment:**
   - If good visual potential, consider optical keratoplasty
   - If poor visual potential and eye is painful, consider palliative procedures for pain relief:
     - Tarsorrhaphy, botox to lids
     - Conjunctival flap (see page 139)
     - Retrobulbar alcohol
     - Enucleation (very last resort)

Exam tips:
- Very similar approach to management of neovascular glaucoma! (see page 69).
- See also management of Fuch's endothelial dystrophy (page 113) and glaucoma and cataract (page 25).

CORNEAL ULCERS

Overall yield: ✪✪✪ **Clinical exam:** **Viva:** ✪✪✪✪ **Essay:** ✪✪ **MCQ:** ✪✪✪✪

Q Opening Question No. 1: How do You Manage a Patient with a Corneal Ulcer?

"Corneal ulcer is a potentially blinding condition which needs immediate ophthalmic management."

Management of Corneal Ulcer

1. **Admit patient if necessary**
2. **Identify predisposing factors:**
   - Contact lens wear
   - Ocular trauma
   - Ocular surface disease
   - Systemic immunosuppression
3. **Perform a corneal scrape for microbiological analyses**

4. **Intensive topical antibiotic treatment:**
   - Gutt. gentamicin 15 mg/ml hourly (or gutt tobramycin)
   - Gutt. cephazolin 50 mg/ml hourly (or gutt cefuroxime)
5. **Systemic antibiotic treatment if:**
   - Ulcer near limbus (scleral extension)
   - Perforated ulcer (endophthalmitis)

Exam tips:
- **"Prepare specific antibiotic regimes with exact dosage and frequency of treatment"** gentamicin frequently does not sound as impressive as "I would prescribe topical gentamicin 15 mg/ml hourly for the next 24 hours."

Q When will You Consider Using Monotherapy with Antibiotics?

- Cautious in using monotherapy
- Broad spectrum antibiotic (e.g. gutt. ciprofloxacin)
- Indications:
  - Small, peripheral ulcer

- Culture positive
- Organism is NOT *Pseudomonas or Streptococcus*
- Organism sensitive to antibiotics
- Patient follow-up and compliance good

Q When will You Consider Using Steroids?

- Use of steroids is controversial, extreme caution needed
- Use only after adequate antimicrobial treatment
- Indications:
  - Culture positive

- Sensitive to antibiotics
- Responding clinically
- Ulcer has been sterilized
- Patient follow-up and compliance good

- Stop antibiotics for 24 hours
- Rescrape and/or corneal biopsy
  - Steps in corneal biopsy:
    - LA or GA
    - Corneal tissue on standby (for tectonic replacement)
    - Dermatological trephine with biopsy area encompassing base and active edge of ulcer
- Specimen divided and sent for microbiological analyses and histological staining
- Re-start intensive antibiotics
- Consider other diagnosis (e.g. sterile ulcers?)
- Consider penetrating keratoplasty

Q What are the Causes of Sterile Ulcers?

Sterile Ulcers

1. **Post infection (treated, resolved)**
   - Herpes (metaherpetic ulcer)
   - Bacterial
   - Fungal
2. **Nearby (contiguous) ocular surface inflammation**
   - Lids and lashes (entropian, ectropian, trichiasis, lid defects)
   - Skin (Stevens-Johnson syndrome, ocular pemphigoid, ocular rosacea)
   - Lacrimal gland (keratoconjunctivitis sicca)
3. **Neurotrophic keratitis**
   - DM
   - V CN palsy
   - Herpes zoster
4. **Exposure keratitis**
   - VII CN palsy

- Lagophthalmos
- Proptosis
5. **Nutritional keratitis (Vitamin A deficiency)**
6. **Neoplasia (acute leukemia)**
7. **Immune-mediated**
   - Connective tissue diseases:
     - Rheumatoid arthritis
     - Wegener's granulomatosis
     - Systemic lupus erythematosis
     - Polyarteritis nodosa
   - Mooren's, Terrien's
   - Marginal keratitis
   - Allergic conjunctivitis
8. **Iatrogenic/trauma**
   - Postsurgical, topical eyedrops
   - Chemical, thermal, radiation injury

Exam tips:
- **Remember "N"on "I"nfected ulcers.**

Q **Opening Question No. 2:** Tell me about Fungal Keratitis

"Fungal keratitis is a potentially blinding condition which needs immediate ophthalmic management."

Fungal Keratitis

1. **Types of fungi:**
   - **Filamentous** fungi (multicellular, hyphae present):
     - **Septate** (most common cause of fungal keratitis)
       - Monilial (*Fusarium, Aspergillus, Penicillium*)
       - Dermatiaceous (*Curvularia*)
     - **Nonseptate** (cause orbital infections)
       - *Mucor, Rhizopus*

- **Yeasts** (unicellular, no hyphae)
  - *Candida, Cryptococcus*
- **Dimorphic** (filamentous at 25° and yeasts at 37°):
  - *Blastomyces, Coccidioides* (orbital infections, rarely affect cornea)
2. **Predisposing factors:**
   - Ocular trauma (filamentous), particularly with organic matter (e.g. vegetation, soil)
   - Ocular surface disease and systemic immunosuppression (yeasts)

3. **Clinical features:**
   - Grayish white ulcer
   - Elevated
   - Indistinct borders, feathery edges
   - Satellite lesions
   - Ring infiltrate
   - Endothelial plaque (may be pigmented)

4. **Stains:**
   - Indian ink
   - Gram stain
   - Giemsa
   - Periodic acid shift
   - Methanamine silver

Exam tips:
- Another common variation is, "Tell me about fungal keratitis."

Q How do You Treat Fungal Keratitis?

"Fungal keratitis is a potentially blinding condition which needs immediate ophthalmic treatment."
"It is difficult to treat, requires multiple drugs, long duration of treatment and may involve surgery."

Treatment

1. **All medication work by interfering with ergosterol metabolism (keyword)**

2. **Polyenes**
   - Amphotericin B:
     - Forms complex with ergosterol that destabilizes the fungal wall
     - Good for **yeasts**
     - Epithelial debridement may improve penetration (highly lipophilic)
     - Unstable, rapid degradation to light
     - Systemic toxicity: Renal, anemia, fever
   - Natamycin:
     - Mechanism of action similar to amphotericin B
     - Good for **filamentous** fungi

3. **Imidazoles**
   - Act by interfering with CYP450 mediated pathways in ergosterol synthesis
   - Miconazole, fluconazole, ketoconazole
   - Voriconazole:
     - Relatively new agent with good oral bioavailability (96%) and ocular penetration
     - Effective in cases that have failed therapy with other agents
     - Toxicity: Transient visual disturbances, liver, renal

4. **Flucytosine**
   - Converted to 5 Fluorouracil
   - Adjunct treatment

Q **Opening Question No. 3:** What are the Characteristics of Acanthamoeba Keratitis?

"Acanthamoeba keratitis is a potentially blinding condition which needs immediate treatment."

Acanthamoeba Keratitis

1. **Microbiology**
   - Protozoan:
     - Active trophozoite form
     - Dormant cystic form
       - Highly resistant to hostile environment (e.g. chlorinated water)

2. **Predisposing factors:**
   - Contact lens wear
   - Ocular trauma

3. **Clinical features:**
   - In early cases, **mimics herpetic epithelial keratitis**

   - **Pain** (severe and disproportionate to lesion) (keyword)
   - Multifocal infiltrates and microabscess
   - **Ring infiltrate** (keyword)
   - **Keratoneuritis** (keyword)
   - Complication: Scleritis, secondary bacterial keratitis

4. **Stains:**
   - Giemsa
   - Calcofluor white
   - Acridine orange

5. **Culture (nonnutrient agar with *E. coli* lawns)**

"Acanthamoeba keratitis is a potentially blinding condition which needs immediate treatment."
"It is difficult to treat, needs multiple drugs, long duration of treatment and may involve surgery."

Treatment:

1. **Aminoglycosides:**
   - Neomycin (but not gentamicin)

2. **Biguanides (disrupts DNA):**
   - Polyhexamethylene biguanide (PHMB)
   - Chlorhexidine

3. **Diamidines (disrupts cell membrane):**
   - Propamidine isethionate (brolene)
   - Hexamidine

4. **Imidazoles:**
   - Econazole

Exam tips:
- Notice the answer to this question is identical to the answer to the question on fungal keratitis treatment.
- The drugs are difficult to remember. A simple mnemonic is "ABCDE."

HERPETIC EYE DISEASES

Overall yield: ✹✹✹ **Clinical exam:** ✹✹✹✹ **Viva:** ✹✹ **Essay:** ✹✹ **MCQ:** ✹✹✹

Q **Opening Question:** What is the Difference between the Ocular Manifestations of Herpes Simplex vs Herpes Zoster?

"Herpes simplex is caused by the virus herpes simplex virus type 1."
"Herpes zoster is caused by the virus zoster varicella virus."
"The different manifestations can be divided into…."

	Herpes simplex	Herpes zoster
Age pattern	• Primary — < 5 years • Recurrent — Middle ages	• Elderly • Immunosuppressed
Skin manifestations:		
1. Dermatome	• Incomplete	• Complete
2. Bilaterality	• Rarely	• Never
3. Pain	• Less	• More
4. Postherpetic neuralgia	• Rare	• Common
5. Skin scarring	• Rare	• Common
Ocular manifestations		
1. Dendritic keratitis	• Central • Large • Well-defined dendrite • Central ulceration (stains with Fluorescein) • Terminal bulbs	• Peripheral • Small • Broad, stellate-shaped • Raised, plaque-like (stains with Rose Bengal) • No terminal bulbs

2. Spectrum	1. Blepharoconjunctivitis:
	  • Follicular
	  • Cicatricial
	2. Epithelial disease:
	  • Dendritic ulcer
	  • Geographic ulcer
	  • Marginal ulcer
	  • Neurotrophic/metaherpetic ulcer
		Each stage has skin, ocular and neural complications
		A) Acute herpes zoster
		  1. Episcleritis/scleritis
		  2. Conjunctivitis
		  3. Keratitis:
		    • Punctate epithelial keratitis
		    • Microdendrite
		    • Nummular keratitis

(Continued)

Herpes simplex	Herpes zoster
3. Stromal keratitis: 　• Necrotizing keratitis 　　• Interstitial (immune) keratitis 4. Endothelitis: 　• Disciform 　• Diffuse 　• Linear 5. Corneal complications: 　• Pannus, stromal vascularization and scarring 　• Trophic keratitis 　• Lipid keratopathy 6. Acute uveitis 7. Episcleritis/Scleritis 8. Acute retinal necrosis	• Disciform keratitis 4. Anterior uveitis 5. Acute retinal necrosis B) Chronic herpes zoster 　1. Mucous secreting conjunctivits 　2. Keratitis: 　　• Nummular keratitis 　　• Disciform neurotrophic 　　• Neutrophic and exposure keratitis 　　• Mucous plaque

---

Q **What are the Results of the Herpetic Eye Disease Study?**

1. **Three components: To assess effectiveness of:**
   • Topical steroids in stromal keratitis in patients on topical antivirals — **safe and effective** in stromal keratitis (*Ophthalmol* 1994; 101: 1871)
   • Oral Acyclovir (400 mg 5x/day) in stromal keratitis in patients on topical steroids and topical antivirals — **no benefit** in stromal keratitis (*Ophthalmol* 1994; 101; 1871)
   • Oral Acyclovir (400 mg 5x/day) in uveitis in patients on topical steroids and topical

   antivirals — **effective** in uveitis (*Ophthalmol* 1996; 114: 1065)
2. **Additional trial:**
   • Oral **Acyclovir** (400 mg bd for 1 year after resolution of ocular HSV) in preventing recurrence of HSV — **decreased** rate of recurrence of ocular HSV (all disease types), especially important after resolution of stromal keratitis (*New Engl J Med* 1998; 339: 306)

Q **What are the Causes of Iris Atrophy?**

"The causes of iris atrophy include…."

Causes of Iris Atrophy

1. **Iatrogenic (postoperative)**
2. **Injury to iris**
3. **Inflammation:**
   • Herpes simplex (sectoral atrophy), herpes zoster
   • Fuch's uveitis, Posner Schlosmann syndrome
4. **Increased IOP (glaucoma):**
   • Post angle closure glaucoma (spiral atrophy)

   • Iridocorneal endothelial syndromes (scattered atrophy with corectopia, pseudopolycoria)
   • Pigment disperson syndrome (atrophy at periphery of iris)
   • Pseudoexfoliation syndrome (atrophy at pupil border)
5. **Ischemia:**
   • Anterior segment ischemia

Exam tips:
- Be careful, this clinical sign can be easily missed.
- The causes can be remembered by "I"ris atrophy.

Q **What are the Causes of Corneal Hypoesthesia?**

"Corneal hypoesthesia can be physiological or pathological."

Corneal Hypoesthesia

1. **Physiological:**
   - Increasing age
   - Peripheral cornea
   - In the morning
   - Brown eyes

2. **Pathological**
   - Congenital:
     - Riley Day syndrome
     - Congenital corneal hypoesthesia
     - Corneal dystrophies (Reis Buckler dystrophy, lattice dystrophy)

- Acquired:
  - Diabetes mellitus
  - Leprosy
  - Herpes simplex
- Iatrogenic:
  - Topical eyedrops (timolol, atropine, sulphur drugs)
  - Surgery (limbal section ECCE, penetrating keratoplasty, epikeratophakia)
  - Contact lens wear

PERIPHERAL ULCERATIVE KERATITIS

Overall yield: ✪✪✪   **Clinical exam:** ✪✪✪   **Viva:** ✪✪   **Essay:** ✪   **MCQ:** ✪✪✪

Q Opening Question: What are the Causes of Peripheral Ulcerative Keratitis?

Causes of Peripheral Ulcerative Keratitis

1. **Systemic**
   - Connective tissue diseases:
     - Rheumatoid arthritis (RA)
     - Systemic lupus erythematosus
     - Wegener's granulomatosis
     - Polyarteritis nodosa (PAN)
     - Relapsing polychondritis
   - Sarcoidosis
   - Leukemia

2. **Ocular**
   - Infective:
     - Bacterial, viral, acanthamoeba, fungi
   - Noninfective:
     - Mooren's ulcer
     - Terrien's marginal degeneration
     - Marginal keratitis
     - Pellucid marginal degeneration
     - Acne rosacea
     - Exposure keratopathy
     - Neurotrophic keratopathy
     - Trauma

Exam tips:
- Peripheral ulcerative keratitis (or PUK) differential diagnoses can be classified either as systemic and ocular or infective and noninfective.
- PUK is a limbal-based disease with inflammatory changes in the limbus; therefore, it is more "immune"-related than "infective."
- See also "Connective tissue diseases and the eye" (page 34).

Clinical approach to peripheral ulcerative keratitis

"The most obvious lesion in this patient is peripheral corneal thinning seen at the interpalpebral region."

Look for
- *Mooren's ulcer:*
  - ***Overhanging*** *central edge of ulcer*
  - *Stromal white infiltrate central edge of ulcer*
  - ***Epithelial defect***
  - *Cataract*

- Terrien's marginal degeneration:
  - **Gradual** outer slope and central steep slope (but **not** overhanging)
  - Intact epithelium
  - Gray white demarcation line central edge of thinning
- Other eye:
  - Unilateral (Mooren's ulcer)
  - Bilateral (Terrien's, connective tissue diseases)
- **Scleral** involvement (important sign):
  - Scleritis (connective tissue diseases)
  - No scleral involvement (Mooren's ulcer, Terrien's marginal degeneration)
- Exclude:
  - **Blepharitis** (marginal keratitis)
  - Skin hyperemia, telangiectasia, papule, nodules, rhinophyma (rosacea)
  - Systemic features:
    - Hands (RA)
    - Malar rash (systemic lupus erythematosus)

I'll like to
- Examine fundus for evidence of vasculitis, optic neuropathy (connective tissue diseases)
- Examine patient for systemic signs (connective tissue diseases)

Q How would You Manage a Patient with PUK?

"I would like to investigate the specific etiology of the PUK and manage accordingly."

Management of PUK

1. **Investigation**
   - Ocular:
     - Scrapings for culture and sensitivity
   - Systemic:
     - CBC, ESR
     - VDRL, FTA
     - ANA, dsDNA
   - C-ANCA
   - RF
   - CXR
   - Mantoux test

2. **Treatment**
   - Systemic steroids
   - Immunosuppressives

Q How do you Differentiate Terrien's Marginal Degeneration from Mooren's Ulcer?

Terrien's Marginal Degeneration vs Mooren's Ulcer

Terrien's marginal degeneration	Mooren's ulcer
1. Early onset:	1. Two forms:
• Males (75%)	• Early onset: Progressive, bilateral
• Bilateral	• Later onset: Limited, unilateral
2. Symptoms:	2. Symptoms:
• Little pain and redness	• Severe pain and redness
3. Clinical features:	3. Clinical features:
• Starts at **superior** and **inferior** quadrant	• Starts at **interpalpebral cornea**
• Epithelium intact	• **Epithelial** defect

(Continued)

Terrien's marginal degeneration	Mooren's ulcer
• Sloping inner edge of "ulcer" with **lipid line** and **bridging vessels**	• **Overhanging** inner edge of ulcer
• No clear interval	• **Clear interval** between lumbus and ulcer
• Low risk of perforation	• Risk of **perforation**
• Eye not inflamed	• Eye is inflamed
• Otherwise eye is normal	• **Cataract, glaucoma** may be present

Q How do You Manage a Patient with Mooren's Ulcer?

"The management of Mooren's ulcer depends on the severity of disease."
"And involves both medical and surgical treatment."

Stepwise Treatment Approach for Mooren's Ulcer

- Step 1: Topical steroids
- Step 2: Oral steroids and immunosuppressives
- Step 3: Conjunctival excision/recession
- Step 4: Tectonic Lamellar keratoplasty/ penetrating keratoplasty

Q Tell me about Acne Rosacea.

"Acne rosacea is a skin disease of idiopathic origin."
"It commonly occurs in middle-age women."
"It has both skin and ocular manifestations."

Acne Rosacea

1. **Skin involvement:**
   - Persistent erythema
   - Telangiectasia
   - Papules, pustules
   - Hypertrophy of sebeceous glands
   - Rhinophyma

2. **Ocular involvement:**
   - Blepharitis almost always develops at some time
   - Severe lesions occur in region of 3%
     - 20% eyes involved first
     - 50% skin involved first
     - 25% simultaneous skin and eye involvement
   - Eyelids:
     - Recurrent blepharitis
     - Meibomitis
     - Styes, Chalazoins

- Conjunctiva:
  - Papillary conjunctivitis
- Cornea:
  - Punctate epithelial keratitis
  - Stromal keratitis, peripheral thinning, vascularization
  - Subepithelial opacification
  - Ulceration, scarring and melting

Treatment

- Oral tetracycline:
  - Effective for both skin and ocular lesions
  - Basis of therapeutic response unknown, **not** related to antibacterial effect on *Staph aurevs*
  - Ampicillin and Erythromycin also found to be effective
  - Possible to taper and stop therapy but recurrence is high (50%)
  - Also given topically

INTERSTITIAL KERATITIS

Overall yield: ✪ ✪   **Clinical exam:** ✪ ✪ ✪   **Viva:** ✪   **Essay:**   **MCQ:** ✪

Q Opening Question: What is Interstitial Keratitis?

"Interstitial keratitis is a **nonsuppurative**, chronic inflammation of the stroma."
"**Without** primary involvement of the epithelium or endothelium."
"The common causes include…."

Causes of Interstitial Keratitis

1. **Infective**
   - Congenital (or acquired) syphilis
   - TB
   - Leprosy
   - Herpes
   - Onchocerciasis
   - Lyme disease
2. **Noninfective**
   - Cogan's disease (associated with polyarteritis nodosa)
   - Sarcoidosis

 Clinical approach to interstitial keratitis

"On examination of the anterior segment…."
"There is midstromal corneal opacity."
"Involving the visual axis."
"There are ghost vessels seen within the lesion."

Look for
- *Mutton fat keratic precipitates (TB, syphilis, leprosy, sarcoid)*
- *AC activity*
- *Lens opacity*
- *Fellow eye — bilateral (congenital syphilis)*

I'll like to
- *Check corneal sensation (herpes, leprosy)*
- *Check fundus for: Optic atrophy, salt and pepper retinopathy (syphilis)*
- *Ask for history of deafness, tinnitis, vertigo (Cogan's dystrophy)*
- *Systemic examination for rheumatic conditions*
- *Investigate for cause:*
  - *CBC, ESR*
  - *CXR*
  - *Mantoux test*
  - *VDRL, FTA*
  - *Connective tissue screen (polyarteritis nodosa)*

CORNEAL DYSTROPHY

Overall yield: ✪✪✪✪✪ **Clinical exam:** ✪✪✪✪✪ **Viva:** ✪✪✪ **Essay:** ✪✪ **MCQ:** ✪✪✪✪

Q | Opening Question: What are Corneal Dystrophies? How are They Different from Corneal Degenerations

"Corneal dystrophies are a group of **inherited**, **noninflammatory** corneal conditions characterized by...."
"Corneal degenerations are a group of **sporadic**, **age-related** corneal conditions characterized by...."

Dystrophy	Degeneration
Inherited, noninflammatory condition of cornea	Sporadic, age-related condition of cornea
1. Inherited, AD (1)	1. Sporadic
2. Early onset	2. Late onset
3. Nonprogressive/slowly progressive	3. Progressive
4. Clinical features:	4. Clinical features:
• Bilateral	• Unilateral or bilateral
• Symmetrical	• Asymmetrical if bilateral
• Axial, do not extend to periphery (2)	• Peripheral
• One layer of cornea	• Different corneal layers
• Otherwise eye is normal	• Other age-related changes present

- Except for Macular (AR)
- Except for Macular and Meesmann's Dystrophy
  (Extends to periphery)

Q | What are the Pathological Features of Epithelial Corneal Dystrophies?

"Epithelial dystrophies affect the epithelium, basement membrane (BM) and Bowman's membrane of the cornea."

	Microcystic (map-dot-fingerprint)	Reis-Buckler	Meesmann's
Inheritance	• AD (Incomplete penetrance)	• AD	• AD
Pathology	• Abnormal epithelial cells with microcysts	• Granular deposis in BM that stain with Masson's trichrome	• Periodic acid shift positive substance deposited in BM
	• Thickened BM		
	• Duplication of BM		
	• Fibrillar material deposited between BM and Bowman's membrane		

(Continued)

	Microcystic (map-dot-fingerprint)	Reis-Buckler	Meesmann's
Clinical features	• Recurrent corneal erosion (RCE) in 10%; most asymptomatic • Lesions look like dots, cysts, lines, fingerprint, maps	• RCE • Honeycomb appearance • Corneal hypoesthesia	• Photophobia • Tiny epithelial cysts extend to periphery
Treatment	• Conservative • Treat RCE	• One of earliest to require PKP • Highest risk of recurrence after PKP	• Conservative

Q **What are the Pathological Features of Stromal Corneal Dystrophies?**

"Stromal corneal dystrophies affect the stroma of the cornea."
"There are three classical types...."

	Lattice	Granular	Macular

Inheritance Pathology	• AD
	• **Amyloid** material
	• Stains:
	  • **Congo red**
	  • PAS positive
	  • Birefringent
	  • Dichroism
	  • Crystal violet metachromasia
		• AD
		• **Hyaline** material
		• Stains **Masson trichrome**
			• AR
			• **Mucopolysaccharides**
			• Stains **Alcian blue**

Clinical features	• RCE • Linear, branch-like pattern • Intervening stroma clear • Peripheral stroma clear	• RCE • Bread-like crumbs • Intervening stroma clear • Peripheral stroma clear	• Decreased VA • Gray opaque spots • Stroma diffusely cloudy • Peripheral stroma involved

Notes	• Type 2:
	  • Patients older
	  • VA better
	  • Systemic amyloidosis associated
	  • Less numerous lines
	  • Lines more peripheral
	  • PKP rarely needed
		• Type 2
		  • Patients older
		  • VA better
		  • Larger ring-shaped lesions
			• Occurs in much younger patients compared with the other two stromal dystrophies

Treatment	• Treat RCE • PKP by 40 years	• PKP needed **early**	• PKP needed **very early** • Highest recurrence rate of stromal dystrophies

Exam tips:
• **Common clinical and viva examination**
• **Remember the mneumonic, "Marilyn Monroe Always Gets Her Man in L A City" = "Macular Mucopolysaccharides Alcian Granular Hyaline Masson Lattice Amyloid Congo"**

"Amyloid is an eosinophilic hyaline substance with some characteristic staining characteristics."
"The manifestations can be classified as...."

Amyloidosis

1. **Staining characteristics**
   - Congo red positive
   - Birefringent and dichroism
   - Crystal violet metachromasia
   - Fluorescence in ultraviolet light with thioflavin T stain
   - Typical filamentous structure on electron microscopy
2. **Classification**
   - Primary localized amyloidosis:
     - Most common form of ocular amyloidosis
     - Conjunctival involvement
     - **Lattice dystrophy**
   - Primary systemic amyloidosis
   - Secondary localized amyloidosis:
     - Long standing ocular **inflammation** e.g. trachoma, interstitial keratitis
   - Secondary systemic amyloidosis:
     - Long standing chronic systemic diseases e.g. RA, leprosy

"Crystalline dystrophy of Schnyder is a stromal dystrophy associated with abnormal cholesterol metabolism."
"The clinical features include...."

Crystalline Dystrophy of Schnyder

- AD
- Localized abnormality in cholesterol metabolism
- Minute crystals in stroma
- Stromal haze
- Associated with corneal arcus and Vogt's limbal girdle
- Associated with hypercholesterolemia in 50%
- Stain: Oil Red O

"Endothelial dystrophies affect the Descemet's membrane and endothelium of the cornea."
"There are three classical types...."

	Fuch's endothelial dystrophy	Posterior Polymorphous dystrophy (PPMD)	Congenital Hereditary Endothelial dystrophy (CHED)
Inheritance	• AD	• AD or AR	• AR
Pathology	• Abnormal deposition of collagen material in Descemet's membrane	• Focal thickening of Descemet's membrane • Multilayering of endothelium (pseudoepithelium)	

Clinical features	• Middle aged women
	• **4 signs:**
	  • Corneal guttata
	  • Stromal edema
	  • Bowman's membrane scarring
	  • Epithelial edema/bullous keratopathy
		• At birth or young
		• "Polymorphous" picture
		• Vesicles, geographical or band-like opacities on Descemet's membrane ("tram-tracks")
		• May be associated with glaucoma (progressive synechial angle closure) and **Alport's** syndrome
			• Endothelium not visible
			• Stroma diffusely thickened and opacified

Treatment	• See below	• PKP in about 10%	• PKP needed **very early**

"The management of Fuch's endothelial dystrophy with cataract can be a difficult decision."
"There are two clinical problems which must be managed simultaneously, depending on the severity of each condition."
"Factors to consider include patient and ocular factors…."

Management of Fuch's Endothelial Dystrophy

1. **Patient factors — consider surgery early if**
   - Young age
   - High visual requirements
   - Poor vision in fellow eye

2. **Ocular factors**
   - Severity of cataract

- Severity of cornea decompensation:
  - History of blurring of vision in morning
  - Greater than 10% difference in corneal thickness between early morning and measurements later in the day
  - Severity of edema on clinical examination
  - Pachymetry > 650 μm corneal thickness
  - Endothelial cell count < 800 cells/mm²

Severity of corneal decompensation	Severity of cataract	Possible options
+	0	• Conservative treatment (lubricants, hypertonic saline, lower IOP, soft bandage contact lens)
+++	+++	• Combined cataract extraction and PKP (triple procedure)
+++	0	• PKP first • Cataract extraction later, after development of cataract
+++	+	• Triple procedure indicated • Alternatively PKP first, cataract extraction later but discuss with patient about advantages of triple procedure*
+	+++	• Cataract extraction first, PKP later • Alternatively, discuss with patient about advantages of triple procedure
0	+++	• Cataract extraction first • Corneal decompensation likely to develop, PKP later

*Disadvantages of individual procedures (PKP and cataract extraction in separate sittings):
- Two operations, increased cost and increased rehabilitation time
- Corneal graft more likely to fail
- Visibility poor during the second procedure
- IOL power difficult to calculate

*Fuch's endothelial dystrophy is one of the main indications for endothelial keratoplasty

Exam tips:
- **Remember there are no RIGHT or WRONG answers.**
- **First, be as conservative as possible. Give extremes of each scenario, then go to the more controversial middle ground.**
- **Opening statement is similar in all situations: "There are two clinical problems which must be managed simultaneously. Factors to consider include…." Then give your own scenario.**
- **See also management of neovascular glaucoma (page 69), bullous keratopathy (page 97) and glaucoma and cataract (page 25).**

KERATOCONUS

Overall yield: ✱✱✱✱ **Clinical exam:** ✱✱✱✱✱ **Viva:** ✱✱ **Essay:** ✱✱ **MCQ:** ✱✱✱

Q **Opening Question:** What are the Clinical Features of Keratoconus?

"Keratoconus is a noninflammatory ecstatic corneal condition."
"Characterized by central or paracentral stromal thinning, apical protrusion and irregular astigmatism." (**classical triad**)
"The clinical features can be early and subtle or late and gross."

Clinical Features of Keratoconus

1. **Early signs:**
   - Keratoscopy/Placido's disc (irregular rings)
   - Retinoscopy (scissoring reflex)
   - Direct fundoscopy (oil drop sign)
   - Vogt's striae
   - Prominent corneal nerves

2. **Late signs:**
   - Paracentral stromal thinning
   - Fleischer's ring
   - Corneal scarring
   - Munson's sign (bulging of lower lids when patient looks down)
   - Rizutti's sign (conical reflection off nasal cornea with slit lamp light from temporal side)

Q What are the Causes of Keratoconus?

Causes of Keratoconus

1. **Primary**
   - Idiopathic (prevalence: 400/100,000)
   - AD in 10%

2. **Secondary**
   - Systemic:
     - **C**hromosomal disorders (e.g. Down's syndrome)
     - **C**onnective tissue disorders (e.g. Marfan's syndrome, osteogenesis imperfecta)
     - **C**utaneous disorders (e.g. atopic dermatitis)
   - Ocular:
     - **C**ongenital ocular anomalies (e.g. aniridia, Leber's congenital amaurosis, retinitis pigmentosa)
     - **C**ontact lens wear

>
> **Exam tips:**
> - Remember the causes of CONES are the 5 "C"s!

Q What are the Histological Characteristics of Keratoconus?

Triad of

- Thinned stroma
- Epithelial iron deposit
- Breaks in Bowman's membrane layer (Descemet's membrane and endothelium are normal unless hydrops has developed)

Clinical approach to keratoconus

"On examination of this patient's anterior segment, there is evidence of keratoconus."

Look for

- *Classical signs:*
  - *Paracentral stromal thinning*
  - *Vogt's striae*
  - *Prominent corneal nerves*
  - *Fleischer's ring*
  - *Corneal scarring*
- *Secondary causes:*
  - *Down's syndrome, Turner's syndrome*
  - *Marfan's syndrome*
  - *Aniridia, ectopic lentis*

I'll like to

- *Evert lids to look for features of vernal keratoconjunctivitis*
- *Examine fundus to exclude RP*

Exam tips:
- Be very careful when you are asked to examine a young patient with an otherwise NORMAL SLIT LAMP EXAM (page 121) because the ocular findings of keratoconus can be subtle.
- Clue: A Placido's disc may be conveniently located next to the patient!

Q **When would You Consider Corneal Grafting for Keratoconus?**

1. **Conservative treatment first (usually good enough in 90% of patients):**
   - Spectacles
   - Special contact lens
   - Collagen cross-linking:
     - New technique in which photo-sensitizing agent (riboflavin) is applied to cornea and collagen cross-links are induced with UV-irradiation
     - Shown to retard keratoconus progression

2. **Indications for corneal grafting:**
   - Unable to achieve good vision with contact lens
   - Intolerant to contact lens wear
   - Scarring after acute hydrops

3. **Special preoperative and intraoperative factors to consider:**
   - Most cases are treated with lamellar keratoplasty these days
     - Lower risk of endothelial rejection
     - Young patients
   - Treat vernal keratoconjunctivitis aggressively
   - Large graft (but reduce graft over-sizing to reduce myopia)
   - Eccentric graft
   - Trephination:
     - Hard to fit trephine (may need hot probe to flatten cornea)
     - Shallow trephine (0.3 mm)

Causes of Prominent Corneal Nerves

1. **Ocular diseases:**
   - Keratoconus
   - Keratoconjunctivitis sicca
   - Fuch's endothelial dystrophy
   - Trauma
   - Congenital glaucoma

2. **Systemic diseases:**
   - Leprosy
   - Neurofibromatosis
   - Multiple endocrine neoplasia type IIb (medullary CA thyroid, parathyroid CA, pheochromocytoma)
   - Refsum's disease
   - Ichthyosis
   - Normal variant with increasing age

CRYSTALLINE KERATOPATHY AND MISCELLANEOUS KERATOPATHIES

Overall yield: ✪✪   **Clinical exam:** ✪✪   **Viva:** ✪   **Essay:** ✪   **MCQ:** ✪✪✪

Q **Opening Question:** What are the Causes of Crystalline Keratopathy?

Crystalline Keratopathy

1. **Infectious diseases**
   - Infectious crystalline keratopathy:
     - Occurs when there is **suboptimal** inflammatory response to organisms (e.g. post PKP)
     - Common organisms: *Streptococcus viridans, Staphylococcus epidermidis*)

2. **Noninfectious diseases**
   - Lipid deposit
     - Crystalline dystrophy of Schnyders
   - Mineral deposit:
     - Argyrosis (silver)
     - Band keratopathy (calcium)
   - Chrysiasis (gold)
   - Protein deposit:
     - Cystinosis
     - Dysproteinemia (multiple myeloma)
   - Medication deposit:
     - Topical ciprofloxacin
     - Amiodarone
     - Tamoxifen
     - Phenothiazines
     - Indomethacin
     - Chloroquine
   - Idiopathic:
     - Crystalline dystrophy of Bietti

 Clinical approach to vortex keratopathy

"On slit lamp examination, there are…."
"Grayish/brownish corneal epithelial deposits."
*"Radiating from a point **below** the pupillary axis."*
"The lesions are seen in both eyes."
"And are consistent with a diagnosis of vortex keratopathy."

Look for

- *Lens opacity (amiodarone, Fabry's disease)*
- *Bull's eye maculopathy (chloroquine), crystalline retinopathy (tamoxifen)*
- *Optic disc (tamoxifen)*

I'll like to
- *Ask patient for a history of:*
  - *Arthritis (indomethacin)*
  - *Breast CA (tamoxifen)*
  - *Cardiac diseases (amiodarone)*
  - *Connective tissue diseases (chloroquine)*
  - *Dementia, psychiatric diseases (chlorpromazine)*

Exam tips:
- **One of few differential diagnoses for NORMAL SLIT LAMP EXAM (page 121).**
- **The causes can be remembered as "ABCD."**

Q **Tell me about the Mucopolysaccharidosis.**

"Mucopolysaccharidoses are a group of systemic storage diseases due to deficiency of lysosomal enzymes."

"There are numerous specific types, each with its own **systemic** and **ocular** features."

"The systemic features include mental retardation, coarse facies, skeletal abnormalities and cardiac diseases."

"In general, the ocular features include **corneal** deposits, **retinal** degeneration and **optic** atrophy."

Type	Name	Cornea deposition	Retinal degeneration	Optic atrophy	Notes
1 H	Hurler	+++	+	+	All are AR **except** Hunter's (SLR)
1 S	Scheie	+++	+	+	Hurler and Scheie have the most severe corneal lesions
2	Hunter	−	++	+++	"Hunter" are **males** and have **clear** corneas
3	Sanfilippo	−	+++	+	
4	Morqio	+	−	+	4 and 6 no retinal degeneration
5	None				**5** became "**S**"cheie
6	Maroteaux — Lamy	+	−	+	

Q **Tell me about Wilson's Disease.**

"Wilson's disease is a metabolic systemic disease."

"Characterized by deficiency in alpha 2 globulin (**ceruloplasmin**)."

"Resulting in deposition of copper throughout the body."

Wilson's Disease

1. **Systemic features**
   - Liver (40%)
   - CNS (40%)
     - No mental retardation
     - Basal ganglia (flapping tremors)

- Spasticity, dysarthria, dysphagia
- Psychiatric problems
- Laboratory results:
  - **Normal** total serum copper
  - Low serum ceruloplasmin
  - High urine copper

2. **Ocular features**
   - Kayser Fleisher ring (KF ring):
     - 90% of all patients: Almost 100% if CNS involved

   - Deposition in **Descemet's membrane**
   - **Green "sunflower" cataract**
   - **Accommodation** difficulty (deposition in ciliary muscles)

3. **Treatment**
   - Decrease copper intake
   - Penicillamine (KF ring will **resolve** with treatment)

> **Exam tips:**
> - KF rings in one of few differential diagnoses for NORMAL SLIT LAMP EXAM (page 121).

SCLERITIS

Overall yield: ✪✪   Clinical exam: ✪   Viva: ✪✪✪   Essay: ✪   MCQ: ✪✪✪

Q Opening Question: What is Scleritis?

"Scleritis is an inflammatory disease of the sclera."
"It can be classified into…."

Scleritis

1. **Classification**
   - Anterior scleritis (Watson and Hayreh)
     - Non-necrotizing (**40%**):
       - Diffuse (benign disease)
       - Nodular (visual loss in 25%)
     - Necrotizing (**40%**):
       - With inflammation (visual loss in 75%: Mortality in 25%):
         - Veno-occlusive
         - Granulomatous
         - SINS
       - Without inflammation (scleromalacia perforans (benign))
     - Posterior scleritis (**20%**)

2. **Systemic associations (50%)**
   - Noninfective:
     - Rheumatoid arthritis (RA) (40%)
     - Systemic lupus erythematous, Wegener's granulomatous, polyarteritis nodosa, relapsing polychondritis
     - Surgically induced necrotizing scleritis (SINS)
   - Infective:
     - Herpes zoster
     - TB, syphilis

3. **Investigations**
   - CBC, ESR
   - VDRL, FTA
   - Collagen disease markers
   - CXR

4. **Treatment**
   - Treat associated systemic diseases
   - Treat associated ocular complications (glaucoma, cataract)
   - Treatment of scleritis depends on type and severity:
     - Anterior scleritis, non-necrotizing (NSAIDs)
     - Posterior scleritis (oral systemic steroids)
     - Anterior scleritis, necrotizing with inflammation (IV steroids and immunosuppressive agents)

Q What are the Clinical Features of Posterior Scleritis?

"Posterior scleritis is an inflammatory disease of the sclera posterior to the equator."
"It represents about 20% of all scleritis…."

Posterior Scleritis

1. **20% of all scleritis**
2. **20% associated with systemic diseases**
3. **80% associated with concomitant anterior scleritis**
4. **Visual prognosis is poor (80% develop visual loss)**
5. **Clinical presentation vary**

- 80% present as either disc swelling or exudative RD (important differential diagnosis of VKH)
- Other presentations:
  - Subretinal mass (more common in females)
  - Ring choroidal detachment (more common in males)
  - Vitritis
  - Macular edema, subretinal exudation, choroidal folds

Clinical approach to scleritis

"There is a yellowish necrotic nodule seen in the superior sclera."
"There is associated inflammation of the surrounding sclera and injection of scleral vessels."

Or

"There is marked thinning of the superior sclera with little inflammation seen."

Look for
• *Corneal peripheral thinning (important sign for RA, systemic lupus, Wegener's granulomatosis, polyarteritis nodosa)*
• *AC activity and keratitic precipitates*
• *Previous cataract or pterygium surgery (SINS)*
• *Bilateral disease (RA, systemic lupus, Wegener's granulomatosis, polyarteritis nodosa)*
• *Lid scarring (herpes zoster)*
• *Systemic features (RA, systemic lupus, Wegener's granulomatosis, polyarteritis nodosa)*

I'll like to
• *Check IOP (glaucoma in scleritis)*
• *Check fundus for optic disc swelling, choroidal folds, RD*
• *Examine patient systemically (RA, systemic lupus, Wegener's granulomatosis, polyarteritis nodosa)*

Notes

Differential diagnoses for a **NORMAL SLIT LAMP EXAM**

1. Cornea:
- Keratoconus
- Vortex keratopathy
- Microcystic epithelial corneal dystrophy
- Kayser–Fleischer ring
- Fuch's endothelial dystrophy

2. Iris:
- Rubeosis
- Atrophy
- Peripheral anterior synechiae

3. Lens:
- Phacodonesis
- Glankomflecken

4. Sclera:
- Scleritis

CORNEAL GRAFTS

Overall yield: ✪✪✪ **Clinical exam:** ✪✪✪✪✪ **Viva:** ✪✪ **Essay:** ✪✪ **MCQ:** ✪✪✪

Q Opening Question No. 1: Tell me about Corneal Grafts.

"Corneal graft is a surgical procedure in which diseased host cornea is replaced by healthy donor cornea."
"Broadly, corneal grafts can be either partial thickness/lamellar or full thickness/penetrating."
"The indications for full thickness corneal graft are…."
"Prior to the operation, the patient must be evaluated for…."

Exam tips:
- **This is a gift question! You should be able to talk for at least a few minutes without any interruption.**

Q Opening Question No. 2: What are the Indications for Penetrating Keratoplasty (PKP)?

"The indications for corneal grafts can be…."

Indications for PKP

1. **Optical**
   - Bullous keratopathy (pseudophakic and aphakic)
   - Keratoconus
   - Corneal dystrophy
   - Corneal inflammatory diseases — interstitial keratitis, HSV
   - Corneal traumatic scars
   - Failed grafts

2. **Tectonic**
   - Corneal perforation
   - Peripheral corneal thinning

3. **Therapeutic**
   - Infective keratitis

Q What are the Preoperative Factors and Manage Poor Prognostic Factors Prior to PKP?

1. **Evaluate patient's ocular condition and manage poor prognostic factors prior to PKP**
   - Factors (**Big 4** poor prognostic factors)
     - Ocular inflammation
     - Glaucoma
     - Corneal vascularization
     - Ocular surface abnormalities:
       · Associated lid abnormality (entropion, ectropion)
       · Tear film dysfunction and dry eyes
   - Other factors to consider:
     - Corneal hypoesthesia
   - Cornea irregularity
   - Pre-existing cataract (consider triple procedures)
   - Structural changes of AC (peripheral anterior synechiae, rubeosis)

2. **Assess visual potential**
   - Retinal and macular conditions (e.g. cystoid macular edema)
   - Amblyopia
   - Optic atrophy

   Topical antibiotics / steroids / cyclosporin A if necessary

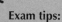

Exam tips:
• Remember the BIG 4 poor prognostic factors well.

Q **Opening Question No. 3:** How do You Perform a PKP?

Steps in PKP

1. **Preoperative preparation**
   • GA
   • Maumenee speculum
   • Superior and inferior rectus bridle suture with 4/O silk:
     • Flieringa ring if necessary (indications: Post vitrectomy, aphakia, trauma, children)
     • Overlay suture if necessary (7/0 silk at limbus)
   • Check recipient bed size with Weck trephine (usually 7.5 mm)

2. **Donor button**
   • Check corneoscleral disc
   • Harvest donor cornea button with Weck trephine on Troutman punch:
     • Approach from posterior endothelial side
     • Use trephine size 0.25–0.5 mm larger than recipient bed
   • Keep button moist with viscoelastic

3. **Recipient bed**
   • 3-point fixation (two from bridle suture, one with forceps)
   • Weck trephine imprint to check size and centration
     • Other types of trephine:
       · Baron Hessberg trephine and Hannah trephine (suction mechanism)

   • Set trephine to 0.4 mm depth
   • Enter into AC with blade
   • Complete incision with corneal scissors

4. **Fixation of graft**
   • Fill AC with viscoelastic
   • Place donor button on recipient bed
   • Four cardinal sutures with 10/0 nylon (at 12 o'clock first, followed by 6, 3 and then 9)
   • 16 interrupted sutures
     • Advantages of interrupted sutures:
       · Easier for beginners
       · Better for inflamed eyes and eyes with vascularization
   • Other suture techniques
     • Continuous suture:
       · Faster
       · Better astigmatism control
       · Not for cases where selective suture removal may be needed (e.g. infections)
     • Combined continuous and interrupted sutures

5. **End of operation**
   • Check water tightness and astigmatism with keratometer
   • Subconjunctival steroids/antibiotics

Notes
• "How do you check the corneoscleral disc?"
  • Container (name, date of harvest, etc.)
  • Media (clarity and color)
  • Corneal button (clarity, thickness, irregularity, surface damage)

Notes
• "Why is the donor button made larger than the recipient bed?"
  • Because donor button is punched from posterior endothelial surface
  • Tighter wound seal for graft
  • Increases convexity of button (less peripheral anterior synechiae postop)
  • More endothelial cells with larger button

"Storage media can be divided into…."

Storage Media

1. **Short term (days)**
   - Moist chamber:
     - Humidity 100%
     - Temp 4°C
     - Storage duration: **48 hours**
   - McCarey-Kaufman medium:
     - Standard tissue culture medium (TC199, 5% dextran, antibiotics)
     - Temp 4°C
     - Storage duration: **2–4 days**

2. **Intermediate term (weeks)**
   - Dexsol/Optisol/Ksol/Procell:
     - Standard tissue culture medium (TC 199) **plus** chondroitin sulphate, HCO3 buffer, amino acid, gentamicin

   - Temp 4°C
   - Storage duration: **1–2 weeks**
   - Organ culture:
     - Advantages: Decreased rejection rate? (Culture kills antigen-presenting cells)
     - Disadvantages: Increased infection rate?
     - Temp 37°C
     - Storage duration: **4 weeks**

3. **Long term (months)**
   - Cryopreservation:
     - Liquid nitrogen
     - Temp — 196°C
     - Storage duration: **1 year**
     - Disadvantages: Expensive and unpredictable results; usually not suitable for optical grafts

"The contraindications included patients with…."

Contraindications for Cornea Donation

1. **Systemic diseases**
   - Death from unknown cause
   - CNS diseases of unknown cause
     - Creutzfeld-Jakob disease, CMV encephalitis, slow virus diseases
   - Infections:
     - Congenital rubella, rabies, hepatitis, AIDS, Syphilis
     - Septicemia
   - Malignancies
     - Leukemias, lymphomas, disseminated cancer

2. **Ocular diseases**
   - Intraocular surgery

   - History of glaucoma and iritis
   - Intraocular tumors

3. **Age**
   - < 1 year old
     - Corneas are difficult to handle
     - Small diameter; friable
     - Very steep cornea (average K = 50D)
   - > 65 years
     - Low endothelial cell count

4. **Duration of death > 6 hours**

5. **Severe hemodilution: Affects accuracy of serological testing**

"The complications can be divided into complications specific to corneal grafts and general complications of intraocular surgery."
"They can occur in the early or late postoperative period…."

Complication of Corneal Grafts

1. **Early postoperative:**
   - Glaucoma or hypotony
   - Persistent epithelial defect
   - Endophthalmitis
   - Wound leak
   - Recurrence of primary disease

2. **Late postoperative:**
   - Rejection
   - Infective keratitis
   - Recurrence of disease
   - Astigmatism
   - Persistent iritis
   - Late endothelial failure

3. **Other complications of intraocular surgery:**
   - Cataract
   - RD
   - Expulsive hemorrhage
   - Retrocorneal membrane
   - CME

 Q **What are the Causes of Graft Failure?**

"Graft failure can be divided into early failure and late failure."

Graft Failure

1. **Early failure (< 72 hours):**
   - Primary donor cornea failure
     - Unrecognized ocular disease
     - Low endothelial cell count
     - Storage problems
   - Surgical and postoperative trauma:
     - Handing
     - Trephination
     - Intraoperative damage
   - Recurrence of disease process (e.g. infective keratitis)
   - Others:
     - Glaucoma
     - Infective keratitis

2. **Late failure (> 72 hours):**
   - Rejection (30% of late graft failures)
   - Glaucoma
   - Persistent epithelial defect
   - Infective keratitis
   - Recurrence of disease process
   - Late endothelial failure

Exam tips:
- **Do not confuse graft failure with graft rejection (which is one of the causes of graft failure and may or may not lead to failure).**

Q **What are the Factors Which Affect Graft Survival?**

"The factors which affect graft survival can be divided into…."

Graft Survival

1. **Factors associated with higher risk of graft rejection:**
   - Young age
   - Blood group incompatibility (Collaborative Corneal Transplant Study)
   - Repeat grafts
   - Size of graft (large graft)
   - Position of graft (eccentric graft)
   - Presence of peripheral anterior synechiae
   - Exposed sutures
   - Deep stromal **vascularization**

2. **Other factors associated with graft failure:**
   - Preexisting glaucoma and high **IOP**
   - **Ocular surface** (lids, tears)
   - Intraocular **inflammation** (iritis)

Exam tips:
- **Remember the BIG 4 poor prognostic factors!**

Brightbill's Classification

GRADE I (Excellent)
- **Keratoconus**
- **Lattice and granular dystrophy**
- Traumatic leukoma
- Superficial stromal scars

GRADE II (Good)
- **Bullous keratopathy**
- **Fuch's dystrophy**
- **Macular dystrophy**
- Small vascularized scars
- Interstitial keratitis
- Failed Grade I PKP
- Combined PKP and cataract op

GRADE III (Fair)
- **Active bacterial keratitis**
- **Vascularized cornea**

- Active HSV keratitis
- Congenital hereditary endothelial dystrophy
- Failed Grade II PKP

GRADE IV (Guarded)
- **Active fungal keratitis**
- **Congenital glaucoma**
- **Pediatric grafts**
- Mild keratoconjunctivitis sicca
- Mild chemical burns
- Corneal blood staining
- Corneal staphylomas
- Failed Grade III PKP

GRADE V (Poor)
- Severe keratoconjunctivitis sicca (Stevens Johnson ocular cicatrical pemphigoid, chemical and thermal burns)

Exam tips:
- Just remember the ones in BOLD!

Q Tell me about Graft Rejection.

"Graft rejection is a type 4 immune reaction."
"It can be divided into epithelial, subepithelial, stromal and endothelial rejection."

Graft Rejection

1. **Pathophysiological basis of rejection:**
   - **Type 4** immunological reaction
   - Divided into: Epithelial, subepithelial, stromal and endothelial rejection
   - Immunological phenomenon

2. **Risk factors:**
   - Age (young age)
   - Repeat grafts
   - Size of graft (large grafts)
   - Position of graft (eccentric graft)
   - Peripheral anterior synechiae
   - Exposed sutures
   - Deep stromal vascularization

3. **Clinical features:**
   - Two weeks onwards (if less than two weeks, consider other diagnosis)
   - Epithelial rejection:
     - Epithelial rejection line (advancing lymphocytes, replaced by epithelial cells from recipient)

   - Usually low grade, asymptomatic, eye is quiet
   - Subepithelial rejection:
     - Nummular white infiltrates (Krachmer's spots)
     - Mild AC activity
   - Stromal rejection:
     - Most important of the 4 types
     - Symptoms:
       - Decreased VA
       - Redness
       - Pain
     - Signs:
       - Limbal injection
       - AC activity
       - Keratic precipitates
       - Endothelial rejection line (Khodadoust line)
       - Stromal edema
   - Endothelial rejection:
     - Combination of stromal and endothelial rejection

Notes

- "What is the evidence that rejection is an immune phenomenon?"
  - Rejection of 2nd graft from same donor begins after shorter interval and progresses more rapidly
  - Brief period of latency (2 weeks) before rejection
  - Rejection correlates with amount of antigen introduced in graft
  - Neonatally thymectomized animals reject grafts with difficulty

Notes

- "What are the problems of large grafts?"
  - Increased risk of rejection (nearer vessels)
  - Increase IOP (more peripheral anterior synechiae)
  - Large epithelial defect (limbal stem cell failure)

 Clinical approach to corneal grafts

"This patient has a corneal graft…."
"The graft has interrupted sutures…."

Look for

- *Type of graft (important in modern context)*
  - *Anterior lamellar graft*
    - *Interface usually visible (may have fine debris)*
- *Endothelial graft:*
  - *Posterior lamella (look for the edge)*
  - *Venting incisions (aid egress of fluid from graft-host interface)*
  - *Temporal scleral tunnel incision*
  - *PIs (prevent pupil block during air tamponade)*
- *Age of graft: Interface scarring, sutures*
- *Pseudophakic/aphakic (pseudophakic or aphakic bullous keratopathy)*
- *Rejection:*
  - *Hazy graft/local edema*
  - *Keratic precipitates, AC cells, Khodadoust line*
  - *Peripheral anterior synechiae*
  - *Stromal vascularization*
- *Other eye for corneal dystrophies, Keratoconus, (**underlying disease**)*
- *Peripheral anterior synechiae*

I'll like to

- *Check IOP*
- *Assess with Placido disc*

Q What is the Role of Cyclosporin A in Corneal Grafts?

1. **Indications (high risk of graft rejection):**
   - Young patient
   - Repeat grafts
   - Large grafts/sclerokeratoplasty
   - Deep stromal vascularization
   - Limbal allografts (chemical injury, SJS)
   - Post-graft rejection
2. **Investigations prior to treatment**
   - Blood tests:
     - CBC
     - Renal function tests and uric acid levels
     - Fasting blood glucose and HB A1C
     - Liver function tests
     - Hepatitis B screen and serology for hepatitis C, herpes zoster, CMV and HIV
   - Urine tests
   - CXR
   - ECG
3. **Treatment regime:**
   - Cyclosporin A (neoral) 5 mg/kg/day in two divided doses
   - Treatment continued for at least one year
   - Dosage gradually tapered after three months
4. **Monitoring during treatment:**
   - BP, height and weight
   - CBC, renal function, liver function
   - CXR, ECG
   - Serum cyclosporin level
   - Co-management with renal transplant physician

Q Tell me about Lamellar Keratoplasty.

"Lamellar keratoplasty is a partial thickness corneal graft."

Lamellar Keratoplasty

1. **Indications**
   - Partial thickness corneal diseases:
     - Superficial corneal dystrophies (Reis-Buckler)
     - Superficial corneal scars
     - Recurrent pterygium
     - Corneal thinning (Terrien's marginal degeneration)
     - Corneal perforation
     - Congenital lesions (limbal dermoid)
     - Superficial tumors
     - Endothelial dystrophies/endothelial failure
2. **Advantages**
   - Anterior lamellar keratoplasty:
     - Minimal donor tissue requirements
     - No intraocular entry
     - Faster wound healing and rehabilitation
     - Lower risk of rejection and less use of topical steroids
   - Endothelial keratoplasty (DSAEK — Descemet's Stripping Automated Endothelial Keratoplasty):
     - Reduced astigmatism
     - Smaller wound — lower risk of wound rupture
     - Replaceable and repeatable
     - Reduced risk of rejection (controversial)
3. **Disadvantages**
   - Interface scarring
   - Technically more difficult
   - Not suitable when residual lamella (Descemet's/endothelium in anterior lamellar keratoplasty, anterior stroma in endothelial keratoplasty) is not clear/intact
4. **Complications**
   - Anterior lamellar keratoplasty:
     - Intraoperative perforation
     - Astigmatism
     - Double anterior chamber
     - Interface haze/scarring
   - Endothelial keratoplasty:
     - Donor dislocation
     - Primary endothelial failure

BASICS IN CONTACT LENS

Overall yield: ✪✪✪   **Clinical exam:**   **Viva:** ✪✪✪   **Essay:** ✪✪   **MCQ:** ✪✪

Q **Opening Question:** What are the Indications for Contact Lens in Ophthalmology?

"The indications can be divided into…."

Indications for Contact Lens

1. **Refractive (most common)**
2. **Therapeutic (see below)**
3. **Cosmetic:**
   - Corneal scar
   - Leukocoria
   - Phthsis bulbi
4. **Diagnostic and surgical (goniolens, fundus contact lens)**

Q What are the Therapeutic Indications for Contact Lens?

Therapeutic Indications for Contact Lens

1. **Optical**
   - Uniocular aphakia
   - Irregular astigmatism — keratoconus
2. **Pain relief**
   - Bullous keratopathy
   - Corneal abrasions
   - Post-photorefractive keratectomy
3. **Promote corneal healing**
   - Recurrent corneal erosion
   - Persistent epithelial defect
   - Thygeson's keratitis
   - Superior limbic keratoconjunctivitis
   - Filamentary keratitis
4. **Protect cornea**
   - Exposure keratopathy
   - Entropion, trichiasis
   - Post-ptosis operation or "Post-op ptosis"
5. **Perforated corneas**
   - Descemetocele
6. **Pharmaceutical delivery device**

Exam tips:
- One "O" and five "P"s!

Q What are the Materials Used for Contact Lens?

"The ideal material for contact lens should be…."
"Currently, (the) materials include…."

Ideal Material

1. **Optically clear**
2. **High oxygen transmission**
   - Water soluble
   - Thin
   - Related to Dk/L, where Dk = Permeability, L = thickness

3. **Comfortable**
   - Soft
   - Surface wettability
4. **Low complication rate**
5. **Durable**
   - High tensile strength
   - Resistant to deformation, tear
6. **Ease of sterilization**

Current Contact Lens Material

1. **Hard — PMMA (polymethylmethacrylate)**

2. **Soft — hydrogel (HEMA)**
   - High water content — extended wear soft contact lens (EWSCL)
   - Low water content — daily wear soft contact lens (DWSCL)
   - Silicone hydrogels — high gas permeability, for extended wear
3. **Semi-flexible/rigid gas permeable (RGP)**
   - CAB (cellulose acetate butyrate)
   - Silicone
   - Polycon (90% PMMA and 10% silicone)

Q **Tell me about Contact Lens. What are the Advantages and Disadvantages?**

"Soft contact lens can be broadly divided into extended wear (EWSCL) or daily wear (DWSCL)."
"They are made of hydrogel, with varying water contents…."

Soft Contact Lens

1. **Advantages of soft CL:**
   - Comfortable
   - Greater stability
   - Ease of fitting
   - Ease of adaptation
   - Rarely get overwear syndrome
   - Lack of spectacle blur
2. **Disadvantages:**
   - Poorer VA in eyes with astigmatism

   - Higher risk of complications
   - Durability low
3. **Indications for DWSCL:**
   - First time wearer
   - Part time wearer
   - Failed extended wear
4. **Indications for EWSCL:**
   - Infants, children and elderly
   - Lack of manual dexterity
   - Therapeutic indications

Q **What are the Pathophysiological Changes to the Eye with Contact Lens Wear?**

"The pathophysiological changes included…."

Pathophysiological Changes to the Eye

1. **Desiccation**
2. **Microtrauma**

3. **Hypoxia**
4. **Hypersensitivity/toxicity**
5. **Endothelial blebbing (transient)**

Q **What are the Complications of Contact Lens?**

"Contact lens complication can be divided into blinding and nonblinding complication."

Complications of Contact Lens Wear

1. **Blinding**
   - Infective keratitis
   - Corneal scarring
   - Corneal warping (rarely)
2. **Nonblinding (Note: Related to the four pathophysiological changes!)**
   - Related to desiccation
     - Dry eye syndrome

   - Related to microtrauma:
     - Punctate epithelial erosions
     - Corneal abrasion
     - Superior limbic keratoconjunctivitis
   - Related to hypoxia:
     - Corneal edema
     - Epithelial microcysts, acute overwear syndrome (rupture of cysts)
     - Corneal vascularization

- Related to hypersensitivity/toxicity:
  - Giant papillary conjunctivitis
  - Allergic conjunctivitis (disinfectant, preservative — thiomersal)
  - Sterile infiltrates

3. **Contact lens changes**
   - Distortion, breakage
   - Deposits:
     - Minerals — iron, calcium
     - Organic — mucin, lipid, protein
     - Microorganisms — bacteria, fungi

Q | **Tell me about Giant Papillary Conjunctivitis.**

"GPC is one of the common contact lens complication…."
"Secondary to hypersensitivity."
"GPC presents in different stages…."

GPC

1. **Stages**
   - Stage 1: Preclinical GPC (symptoms only)
   - Stage 2: Macropapillae (0.3 mm–1 mm)
   - Stage 3: Giant papillae (> 1 mm)
   - Stage 4: Subconjunctival scarring

2. **Zones**
   - Zone I: Forniceal
   - Zone II: Tarsal
   - Zone II: To lid margin

3. **Etiology**
   - Contact lens wear:
     - 30% of patients with EWSCL
     - 15% of patients with DWSCL
     - 1–5% of patients with RGP
   - Hypersensitivity (asthma, hay fever)
   - Trauma (foreign body and prosthesis)

4. **Management**
   - Stage 1 and 2:
     - Lens hygiene
     - Decrease wearing time
     - Reevaluate fit and material/change to RGP if needed
     - Topical antihistamines and mast cell stabilizers
     - Topic steroids if necessary
   - Stage 3 and 4:
     - Consider discontinuation of contact lens wear

Q | **How do You Fit Contact Lens?**

Contact Lens Fitting

1. **History**
   - Visual requirements, ocular diseases

2. **Fitting procedure for soft contact lens**
   - Base curve — inversely proportional to the keratometry (K) reading:
     - Take mean K + 1 (aim for flatter contact lens)
     - Choose from three standard curves available (8.1, 8.4, 8.7 mm)
   - Refraction
   - Corneal diameter (13, 13.5, 14 mm)
   - Ocular examination:
     - Palpebral aperture and tightness
     - SLE
     - Fundus exam
   - Select trial lens (base curve/refraction/corneal diameter e.g. 8.4/–4.0D/13.5)
   - Assess fit (with fluorescein staining):
     - Tightness (too flat or too steep)
     - Centering
     - Mobility
     - Aim for three-point touch
   - Over-refract with contact lens on (e.g. If –1.5D gives VA of 20/20)
   - Prescribe final fit (e.g. 8.4/–5.5D/13.5)

3. **Fitting procedure for hard contact lens**
   - Base curve:
     - Take mean K (do not need to add 1)
     - Choose from different individual curves (7.2 to 8.5)
   - Refraction (choose from different powers for each base curve)
   - Corneal diameter (8.8, 9.2, 9.6 mm)

REFRACTIVE SURGERY

Overall yield: ✪✪✪✪✪ **Clinical exam: Viva:** ✪✪✪✪ **Essay:** ✪✪✪✪ **MCQ:** ✪✪✪✪

Q **Opening Question:** What are the Different Types of Refractive Surgery Available?

"Refractive surgery is a procedure to **alter the refractive status** of the eye."
"This usually involves procedure on the **cornea** or the **lens.**"
"They can be broadly divided into **incisional** procedures, **laser** procedures or **intraocular** surgical procedures."

Correction of Myopia

1. **Incisional procedures**
   - RK (radial keratotomy)
     - Up to –5D
     - PERK (prospective evaluation of RK) study showed that 40% had hyperopic shift of 1D or more after 10 years
     - Obsolete procedure
     - Disadvantages of RK:
       · Weakened cornea
       · Diurnal variation in refraction
       · Hyperopic shift
   - Epikeratoplasty
     - Remove corneal epithelium and create peripheral annular keratotomy incision
     - Frozen donor corneal lenticule fixed to recipient cornea
     - Current indications (not many left with advances in PRK and LASIK):
       · Childhood aphakia
       · Keratoconus
       · Extremely high myopia
   - Keratomileusis
     - Cornea sliced off with microkeratome
     - Cornea cap then frozen, shaped and reapplied to corneal bed
   - ALK (automated lamellar keratoplasty)
     - Cornea cap sliced off with automated microkeratome
     - Second pass of microkeratome to cut a corneal disc from stromal bed
     - Cornea cap is then reapplied to cornea bed

2. **Laser procedures**
   - PRK (photorefractive keratectomy)
     - Up to –6D

- LASIK (laser in-situ keratomileusis)
  - Modification of ALK, using laser for the second pass
  - Up to –15D
  - Variants:
    · Epi-LASIK: "Bladeless LASIK": Epithelial sheet cleaved off surface (no flap)
    · LASEK: Surface epithelial sheet loosened with alcohol
    · Wavefront optimized ablations: Reduce spherical aberration — reduce night vision problems, glare and halos
    · Wavefront guided ablations: Customized ablation guided by individual wavefront map

3. **Intraocular surgery**
   - ICSR (intracorneal stromal ring)
     - PMMA half rings are threaded into peripheral mid stroma to effect a flattening of the cornea
     - Up to –6D
   - **High myopia procedures (> –12D)**
     - Clear lens extraction (with IOL)
   - AC phakic IOL implantation
     - Conventional four-point fixated AC IOL
     - Iris-fixated phakic IOL
     - Suffers from complications of ACIOLs:
       · Glaucoma
       · Iris chafing/uveitis
       · Hyphema
       · **Corneal** endothelial damage
   - PC phakic IOL implantation
     - Sulcus fixated phakic IOL
     - Silicon injectable IOL (implantable collamer lens)

- Complications:
  - Glaucoma (angle closure, hence need for PI)
  - Iris chafing/uveitis
  - Hyphema
  - **Cataract**
- Scleral sling:
  - Up to 18–22D
  - Use donor sclera/synthetic materials to sling around globe

Exam tips:
- **Extremely common and important essay or viva topic. Keep up with the latest refractive surgery trends.**

Q **What are the Options in the Correction of Hyperopia?**

Hyperopia

1. **Hexagonal keratotomy**
2. **Epikeratoplasty**
3. **ALK**
4. **PRK and LASIK**
5. **Radial intrastromal thermokeratoplasty**
   - Small coagulation burns applied to cornea stroma with retractable cautery probe

6. **Laser thermokeratoplasty**
   - Small coagulation burns applied to cornea stroma with holmium laser
7. **AC phakic IOL**

Q **What are the Options in the Correction of Astigmatism?**

Astigmatism

1. **AK (Astigmatic keratotomy)**
   - Preoperatively need to have keratometer readings, corneal topography and pachymetry
   - Procedure:
     - Guarded diamond knife
     - 95% corneal depth cut
     - 45 degrees at the steep axis
   - 6–8 mm optical zone
   - Each cut corrects 1 to 1.5D of astigmatism
2. **PARK (Photoastigmatic refractive keratectomy) and LASIK**
3. **Toric IOL**
   - Plate haptic silicon design IOL after lens removal
   - Need precise axis orientation

Q **Tell me about PRK.**

"PRK is photorefractive keratectomy and is a form of refractive surgery."

PRK

1. **Procedure**
   - 193 nm argon fluoride excimer laser used to ablate cornea
   - Every 10 micron = –1D of myopia
   - Three types of ablation:
     - Wide area ablation
     - Scanning slit
     - "Flying spot"
2. **Indications and limitations**
   - PRK works well for low and moderate myopia and astigmatism

- For myopia < –6D
  - 80–90% see 20/40 or better
  - 70–80% predictability
  - 1% significant corneal haze
  - 1–5% loss of BCVA
- High myopia > –6D
  - 50–75% see 20/40 or better
  - 30–70% predictability
  - 5–15% corneal haze
  - Up to 20% loss of BCVA
  - More regression
  - Higher retreatment rate

3. **Advantages and disadvantages of PRK (see below)**

"LASIK stands for **L**aser **I**n-situ **K**eratomileusis and is a form of refractive surgery."

LASIK

1. **Procedure:**
   - Microkeratome creates corneal flap that is hinged, either nasally or superiorly
   - Flap is reflected
   - Excimer laser ablates stroma of cornea for refractive correction
   - Flap is replaced without sutures
   - Femtosecond laser
     - Newer technique for creating flaps using multiple extremely short (femtosecond) pulses of IR light
     - Pattern of pulses programmable
     - Theoretical advantages:
       · Lower risk of flap complications
       · Fewer higher order aberrations induced
     - Possible disadvantages
       · Irregularity/haze at interface
       · Cost
       · Longer operating time

2. **Indications and limitations:**
   - Maximum refractive errors that can be treated are dependent on central corneal thickness
   - Contraindications:
     - Thin corneas and ectatic disorders (keratoconus) — **absolute** contraindication
     - Wound healing problems (e.g. connective tissue disease, diabetes)
     - Corneal infections (HSV)
     - Pregnancy (unstable refraction)
     - Glaucoma (relative contraindication — high pressure applied during procedure)
     - Dry eye and ocular surface problems
   - Current limits:
     - Myopia up to –5D
     - Hyperopia up to –5D
     - Astigmatism up to 4D

   - Compound myopic and hyperopic astigmatism

3. **Advantages of LASIK (five distinct advantages):**
   - Better predictability
   - More stability
   - Minimal pain
   - Rapid visual rehabilitation (< 24 hrs)
   - Low risk of corneal haze/scarring and therefore, less steroids needed

4. **Disadvantages:**
   - Expensive and complex microkeratome required, in addition to an excimer laser
   - More technical and surgical expertise required with steep learning curve
   - Risk of visually threatening complications
   - Risk of flap complications (see below) and reduced residual stromal thickness because of need for tissue for flap

5. **Complications:**
   - Flap complications:
     - Free flaps/incomplete flaps/button hole flaps
     - Flap striae/dislodged flaps
     - Flap melts
     - Flap striae
   - Interface complications:
     - Epithelial ingrowth
     - Interface debris
     - Interface haze
     - Diffuse lamellar keratitis ("Sands of Sahara")
   - Induced irregular astigmatism
   - Decentration of ablation zone
   - Night vision problems (hence aspheric corrections)
   - Bacterial keratitis
   - Progressive ectasia of cornea

	PRK	LASIK
Predictability/Accuracy	• Up to –6D	• Up to –15D
Stability	• Up to –6D	• Up to –15D
Pain and rehabilitation	• Pain from epithelial defect (1–2 days) • Prolonged visual rehabilitation (up to 1 week)	• Minimal pain • Rapid visual rehabilitation (< 24 hrs)

(Continued)

	PRK	LASIK
Corneal haze	• Up to 10% (destruction of Bowman's layer) • Poor contrast sensitivity • Halos • Glare	• Minimal haze
Complications	• Rare	• Uncommon
Irregular astigmatism	• 1%	• 3–10%
Training and equipment	• Short training period • Less expensive equipment	• Steep learning curve • More expensive equipment
Retreatment	• Easier	• More difficult

Q What is Corneal Astigmatism?

"An optical aberration resulting from **variation** in the refractive power of the cornea due to an asymmetry in its curvature."

Classification

1. **Regular**
   - Steepest and flattest meridian are 90° from each other
   - Subdivided into "with the rule" and "against the rule"
   - Blurred retinal images can be improved with an appropriate cylindrical correction

2. **Oblique**
   - Steepest and flattest meridians are not at 90° from each other

3. **Irregular**
   - Amount of astigmatism changes along a given meridian and varies from meridian to meridian
   - Secondary to irregular corneal surface

Further Classification

4. **Simple myopic astigmatism**
   - Emmetropic in one meridian and myopic in other

5. **Compound myopic astigmatism**
   - Both steepest and flattest meridians focused in front of retina

6. **Simple hyperopic astigmatism**

7. **Compound hyperopic astigmatism**

8. **Mixed astigmatism**
   - One meridian focused in front of retina, one behind

Causes

1. **Idiopathic**

2. **Secondary to ocular diseases**
   - Developmental — keratoconus
   - Degeneration — pellucid marginal degeneration, Terrien's degeneration
   - Infection — scar formation
   - Inflammation — peripheral ulcerative keratitis (RA, Mooren's ulcer)
   - Traumatic — scar formation

3. **Iatrogenic**
   - Large incision cataract surgery
   - Penetrating keratoplasty

Assessment of Astigmatism

1. **Refraction**

2. **Keratometry**

3. **Corneal topography**
   - Placido disc
   - Computerized videokeratometry
   - Elevation based systems
   - Orbscan:
     - One of the commonest systems used
     - Combination of Placido and elevation based systems
     - Generates four maps:
       - Anterior float (anterior elevation)
       - Posterior float (posterior elevation)
       - Keratometry
       - Pachymetry

- Indications:
  - Assessment of regular and irregular astigmatism
  - Diagnosis of "forme fruste" keratoconus (important in pre-keratorefractive surgery assessment)

- Signs:
  - Inferior-superior asymmetry
  - Inferior steepening
  - Elevated anterior and posterior float
  - Inferior thinning
  - Inter-eye asymmetry

Q What are the Options in the Management of Corneal Astigmatism?

1. **Glasses**
2. **Contact lens**
3. **Photorefractive keratectomy**
4. **Surgery — cuts in steep incision**
   - Transverse and arcuate keratotomy

- Semiradial incision
- Trapezoidal keratotomy

MISCELLANEOUS CORNEAL PROCEDURES

Q Opening Question: When and How do You Perform a Corneal Biopsy?

1. **Indications:**
   - Infective keratitis (culture negative, not responding to treatment)
   - Amoebic keratitis
   - Carcinoma intraepithelial neoplasia

2. **Procedure:**
   - Stop antibiotic for 24–48 hours
   - Topical anesthesia
   - Debride slough
   - Avoid visual axis
   - Choose between lesion and good cornea
   - Use a dermatological trephine with 2, 3 or 4 mm diameter to mark tissue
   - Lamellar dissection of tissue with blade
   - Divide tissue for histology and culture

Q When and How do You Perform Corneal Gluing?

1. **Composition:**
   - Corneal glue made of isobutyl cyanoacrylate (histoacryl)

2. **Indications:**
   - Small perforation < 1 mm in size

3. **Procedure:**
   - Topical anesthesia
   - Debride slough and necrotic tissue
   - Dry cornea
   - Apply glue onto cellophane plastic disc
   - Apply glue and cellophane disc on perforation — leave to dry
   - Apply bandage contact lens

Q When do You Perform a Conjunctival Flap?

1. **Indications:**
   - POOR visual potential
   - Chronic epithelial/stromal ulcer after resolution of active infective disease
   - Neurotrophic ulcer
   - Chemical injury
   - Bullous keratopathy
   - Descematocoele

2. **Problems with conjunctival flap:**
   - Temporary treatment
   - No view of cornea
   - Low drug penetration
   - Postoperative complication (button hole, epithelial cyst, retraction of flap, bleeding, ptosis)

SURGICAL RETINA

TOPIC 1

THE RETINA

Overall yield: ✪✪✪✪✪ **Clinical exam:** **Viva:** ✪✪✪✪ **Essay:** ✪✪ **MCQ:** ✪✪✪✪

Q Opening Question No. 1: What is the Anatomy of the Retina?

"The retina is the innermost layer of the globe…."
"It is divided into the inner neurosensory layer and the outer retinal pigment epithelium."

Gross Anatomy of the Retina

1. **Neurosensory retina and RPE**
   - Classic 10 layers:
     - RPE
     - Outer segment of photoreceptor
     - Outer limiting membrane
     - Outer nuclear layer (nuclei of **photoreceptor**)
     - Outer plexiform layer (Henle's layer, synapse between photoreceptor and bipolar cells)
     - Inner nuclear layer (nuclei of **bipolar** cells, plus nuclei of horizontal, amacrine, Muller's cells)
     - Inner plexiform layer (synapse between bipolar cells and ganglion cells)
     - **Ganglion** cell layer
     - Nerve fiber layer
     - Inner limiting membrane

   - Ora serrata:
     - Anterior limit of retina (8 mm from nasal limbus, but 8.5 mm from temporal limbus)
     - Vitreous base firmly adherent to ora serrata

2. **Bruch's membrane**
   - Separates RPE from choriocapillaris
   - Classic five layers:
     - Basement membrane of RPE
     - Inner collagen layer
     - Middle elastic layer
     - Outer collagen layer
     - Basement membrane of choriocapillaris

3. **Choroid**
   - Separates retina from sclera
   - Classic three layers:
     - Choriocapillaris
     - Middle vascular layer
     - Outer vascular layer

Exam tips:
- **Remember there are 10 layers in the retina, 5 in Bruch's membrane and 3 in the choroid.**

Q Opening Question No. 2: Tell me about the Rods and Cones.

Rods and Cones

1. **Rods**
   - 120 million; 50 μm long
   - Nucleus
   - Inner segment:
     - Inner (myoid) contains Golgi apparatus

   - Outer (ellipsoid) contains mitochondria
   - Outer segment:
     - Composed of 1,000 stacked discs
     - Discs separate from cell membrane
     - Discs have visual pigments
     - Renewal of outer segment

- Discs formed at proximal end (i.e. near inner segment) and shed at distal end (next to RPE)
- Old discs phagocytosed by RPE cells
- Rate of shedding: 1–5 per hour
- Regeneration over 14 days
- Shedding maximal in early **light** cycle, when functionally less active

2. **Cones**
   - 6 million (i.e. only 5% of rods) and 25 μm long (i.e. half as long as rods)

- Nucleus
- Inner segment
- Outer segment:
  - Stacked disc connected to cell membrane
  - Renewal of outer segment:
    - Diffuse renewal (no proximal to distal direction)
    - Regeneration over 9 months
    - Shedding maximal in early **dark** cycle, when functionally less active

Q What are the Visual Pigments?

Visual Pigments

1. **Outer segment discs made up of lipid bilayer membrane**
2. **Visual pigments contained in lipid bilayer membrane**
3. **Visual pigments made up of chromophore plus protein (opsin)**
4. **Chromophore:**
   - Linked to opsin via Schiff base reaction
   - **11-*cis* retinal** is chromophore in all four types of visual pigments
   - Chromophore aligned parallel to plane of lipid bilayer (to increase light capture)
5. **Four types of visual pigments (based on different absorption characteristics):**
   - Rods — contains rhodopsin (max absorption: 500 nm)

- Blue cone — contains short wavelength sensitive/blue sensitive iodopsin (max: 440 nm)
- Green cone — contains medium wavelength sensitive/green sensitive iodopsin (max: 535 nm)
- Red cone — contains long wavelength sensitive/red sensitive iodopsin (max: 570 nm)

6. **Opsin in rods called rhodopsin:**
   - Transmembranous protein
   - N terminus exposed to intradisc space
   - C terminus exposed to interdisc (cytoplasmic) space

Q What is the Visual Cycle?

Visual Cycle

1. **In the dark:**
   - Outer segment cell membranes allow entry of sodium ions
   - Inner segment actively secretes sodium out via sodium potassium ATPase pump → **dark current** (electric current flows from inner to outer segment)
2. **In the light (bleaching):**
   - Light causes change in visual pigments
   - 11-*cis* retinal converted to **all-trans-retinal**

- All-trans-retinal converted to all-trans-**retinol**
- All-trans-retinal transported out of photoreceptor into RPE cells
- Intermediate retinal (metarhodopsin II) causes a series of reactions which blocks sodium channels in outer segment → decreased intracellar sodium → graded **hyperpolarization** (From − 40 mV to − 70 mV) → reduced neurotransmitter release

Q What is the Vitamin A Cycle?

Vitamin A Cycle

1. **Vitamin A occur in four forms:**
   - Acid (retinoic acid)

- Aldehyde (retinal)
- Alcohol (retinol)
- Ester (retinyl ester)

2. **Three sources of vitamin A**
   - From **diet and liver**:
     - Vitamin A stored in liver as retinyl ester
     - Hydrolyzed to retinol → combined with serum retinol binding protein → delivered to RPE →
     - Stored as retinyl ester
   - From fragments of rod outer segments during **shedding and phagocytosis**
   - From rod outer segments during **bleaching**
   - During bleaching → **all-trans-retinal** released from opsin → converted to all-trans-retinol in outer segment
   - All-trans-retinol transported to RPE → converted back to 11-*cis* **retinol** by isomerase
   - 11-*cis* retinol transported back to outer segment → converted to **11-*cis* retinol** by reductase → combined with opsin to form rhodopsin again

---

Q | Tell me about the Bipolar Cells.

"Bipolar cells are first-order neurons of the visual pathway."
"They are located in…."

Bipolar Cells

1. **Anatomy:**
   - 30 million
   - Located in inner nuclear layer
   - First-order neurons
   - Account for "b" wave of ERG
   - Synapses:
     - Single or multiple dendrites synapse with cones and rods (and other cells)
     - Single axon synapse with ganglion cell (2nd order)
     - In fovea (single cone synapse with single bipolar cell and then with single ganglion cell)
   - In periphery (100 rods synapse with single bipolar cell)
2. **Five types**
   - Rod bipolar cells
   - Invaginating:
     - Midget
     - Diffuse
   - Flat:
     - Midget
     - Diffuse

Q | Tell me about the Ganglion Cells in the Retina.

"Ganglion cells are second-order neurons along the visual pathway."
"They are located in…."

Ganglion Cells

1. **Anatomy**
   - 1 million (ratio of rods: cones: ganglion cells = **120:6:1**)
   - Located in ganglion cell layer:
     - Macula (more than one layer of ganglion cells)
     - Fovea (piled eight layers high)
     - Foveola (absent)
   - Second-order neurons
   - Synapse (connect bipolar cells to lateral geniculate body)
2. **Functions**
   - At fovea:
     - Cone: ganglion cell ratio is **1:1**
   - **PARVO** cellular pathway to lamella **1–4** in lateral geniculate body
   - Responsible for visual sensation of "**What do I see?**"
   - At periphery:
     - Rod: ganglion cell ratio may be up to **10,000:1**
     - **MAGNO** cellular pathway to lamella **5–6** in lateral geniculate body
     - Responsible for visual sensation of "**Where do I see it?**"

"RPE is a single layer of cells interposed between Bruch's membrane/choroid and the neurosensory layer."

RPE

1. **Anatomy**
   - 6 million (like cones!)
   - Single layer of cuboidal epithelium
   - Base (in contact with Bruch's membrane, extensive basal infoldings)
   - Apex (in contact with neurosensory layer, extensive apical microvilli)
   - Side (zona occludens for blood retinal barrier)
   - Melanin granules (absorb light)

2. **Functions**
   - Physical:
     - Outer blood retinal barrier
     - Adhesion to neurosensory retina:
       - Secretion of mucopolysaccharides
     - Active transport of water from subretinal space via **ocular dipole**
     - Embryogenesis (development of photoreceptors)
   - Optical:
     - Absorption of stray light
   - Metabolic:
     - Vitamin A cycle (uptake, transport, storage, metabolism, re-isomerization of vitamin A)
     - Transportation of materials to and from retina
     - Phagocytosis (recognition, ingestion and phagocytosis of shed outer segment)
     - Detoxification

THE VITREOUS

Overall yield: ✸ ✸   **Clinical exam:**   **Viva:** ✸ ✸   **Essay:** ✸   **MCQ:** ✸ ✸

Q **Opening Question:** Tell me about the Anatomy of the Vitreous.

Vitreous

1. **Gross anatomy**
   - Transparent viscoelastic gel
   - Located behind lens and in front of retina
   - 4 ml (80% of volume of globe) and 4 g
   - Shape is a sphere with anterior depression (hyaloid fossa):
     - Central Cloquet's canal
     - Intermediate zone
     - Vitreous cortex
   - Various named regions:
     - Hyaloideocapsular ligament (of Weiger):
       - Annular region 2 mm wide and 8 mm in diameter where vitreous is attached to posterior lens capsule
     - Berger's space:
       - Center of hyaloideocapsular ligament; potential space behind posterior capsule
     - Cloquet's canal:
       - Arises from Berger's space and courses posteriorly through central vitreous

   - Area of Martegiani:
     - Posterior funnel shaped region of Cloquet's canal; clinically seen as Weis ring with posterior vitreous detachment occurs

2. **Microscopic anatomy**
   - Water content: 98–99.7%
   - PH: 7.5
   - Refractive index: 1.33 (less than aqueous)
   - > 90% of visible light transmitted through vitreous
   - Acellular, normal vitreous cells restricted to cortical layers
   - Main constituent:
     - **Type II collagen fibers**, which are entrapped in **hyaluronic acid (HA)** molecules
   - Collagen provides solid structure to vitreous, which is "inflated" and "stabilized" by HA:
     - If collagen is removed → vitreous becomes viscous solution
     - If HA is removed → gel shrinks
   - Large domains of HA spread apart collagen fibers to minimize light scattering

Exam tips:
- **The three most important sections here are the functions, attachments and embryology. You may want to "skip" the rest!**

Q What are the Functions of the Vitreous?

"The vitreous has several functions…."

Functions of the Vitreous

1. **Mechanical function**
   - Prevents globe from collapsing
   - Viscoelastic property of HA-collagen interaction

   - Shock absorbing function for lens and retina during eye movement and physical activity
   - Blunt trauma: Direct force is dissipated within vitreous
   - Prevents retinal detachment

- Majority of retinal breaks not associated with RD: Sealed by post-vitreous cortex
- "Simple" RD: Intact, albeit detached post-vitreous cortex → requires only SB or internal tamponade operations (e.g. pneumatic retinopexy), retinal breaks will be sealed by intact vitreous cortex
- "Complex" RD: Derangement of post-vitreous cortex → more difficult to repair, increased risk of proliferative vitreoretinopathy

2. **Metabolic functions**
   - Lens clarity and retinal function dependent on presence of normal vitreous
   - Oxygenation of interocular tissues
   - Metabolic repository:
     - Presence of glucose, galactose, mannose, fructose and amino acid
     - Provides nutrients to retina in emergency situations (e.g. ischemia)
   - Waste depository:
     - Physical depository for lactic acid, which is toxic to retina

- Vitreous ascorbic acid scavenger for free radicals from lens and retina metabolism
- HA acts as an "anionic shield" against potentially destructive electrons from ionizing radiation
- Movement of water and solutes within eye
  - Transvitreous diffusion and bulk flow across retina involved in maintaining retinal attachment

3. **Optical functions**
   - Refractive index: 1.33 (same as aqueous)
   - Transmits 90% of light between 300–1,400 nm
   - Optical transparency achieved by:
     - HA-collagen interaction: Large HA molecules separating collagen fibers
     - Lack of macromolecular solutes: Molecular sieve as a barrier to influx

4. **Role in accommodation**
   - Supporting role to ciliary body: Vitreous may push lens forward during accommodation (however, vitrectomized eyes can still accommodate)

Q **What are the Attachments of the Vitreous?**

"The attachments can be physiological or pathological."

Attachment of Vitreous

1. **Physiological attachments**
   - The vitreous is adjacent to retina posteriorly and behind ciliary body and lens anteriorly
   - Areas of attachment:
     - Ora serrata (via the vitreous base at pars plana)
     - Post lens capsule (via the hyaloideocapsular ligament of Weiger)
     - Optic disc margins (via Cloquet's canal)
     - Retinal vessels (via vitreoretinovascular bands)
     - Macula (via "attachment plaques")
   - At all sites, interface with adjacent tissues consists of a complex formed by **vitreous cortex and basal membrane (BM)** of adjacent cells
   - Only region not adjacent to basal laminae is peripheral annulus of anterior vitreous cortex
     - Directly exposed to zonules and aqueous humor of posterior chamber (important in malignant glaucoma pathogenesis where

aqueous actually accumulates in this space!)
- Anterior to ora serrata, cortex attaches to BM of ciliary body
- Posterior to ora serrata, cortex attaches to BM of Muller cells of the retina (i.e. internal limiting membrane or ILM)
  - Complex of post-vitreous cortex and ILM acts as a "molecular sieve," preventing cell infiltration (when this is breached, formation of epiretinal membrane)
  - ILM is **thin** over macula but vitreous attachment is strong (pathogenesis of macular hole)
  - ILM is **absent** over optic disc (increased frequency of neovascularization at optic disc)

2. **Pathological attachments:**
   - New vessels
   - Lattice and other retinal degenerations

Exam tips:
- **This is a rather complex but fairly important topic for the pathogenesis of most disorders.**

Zonules

1. Referred to as "tertiary vitreous"
2. Resemble collagen fibrils in terms of diameter:
   - More tightly packed
   - Resist collagenase digestion
   - Solubilized by alpha-chymotrypsin (basis of its use in ICCE)
   - Have amino acid composition that resembles elastin
3. Arise from ciliary processes to insert onto lens capsule via two bundles
   - Orbiculo-anterocapsular bundle
   - Orbiculo-posterocapsular bundle
     - Between the two the canal of Hannover
     - Between orbiculo-posterocapsular bundle and anterior vitreous cortex is canal of Petit

Q What is the Embryology of the Vitreous?

"There are classically three overlapping phases of vitreous development."

Embryology of Vitreous

1. **Primary vitreous (vascular vitreous)**
   - 4th week of gestation: Early vitreous forms in space between lens plate and optic vesicle
   - 5th week: Optic fissure fuses, vitreous becomes closed compartment
   - 6th week: **Hyaloid** artery develops and reaches post pole of lens vesicle
   - Primary vitreous atrophies during development of secondary vitreous, by 7th month, hyaloid artery no longer carries blood and is resorbed at birth
2. **Secondary vitreous (avascular vitreous)**
   - 6th week: Secondary vitreous formation begins between the retina and posterior branches of hyaloid vessels
   - Essentially **acellular**, this consists of extracellular matrix of type II collagen, with little HA at this stage
   - Demarcation line between primary and secondary vitreous becomes walls of Cloquet's canal
3. **Tertiary vitreous (zonules)**
   - Begins at 6th month, product of ciliary epithelium
4. **Anomalies of hyaloid vessel regression**
   - Mittendorf's dot:
     - Post lens surface
     - Site of anastomosis between hyaloid artery and tunica vasculosa lentis

- Bergmeister's papillae:
  - Posterior portion of hyaloid artery with associated glial tissues
- Vitreous cysts:
  - Benign lesions with abnormal regression of either anterior or post hyaloid vascular system
- Persistent fetal vasculature (formerly known as Persistent hyperplastic primary vitreous (PHPV)):
  - Anterior or posterior manifestations
  - Abnormal regression and hyperplasia of primary vitreous
  - Adherent to post lens capsule and extends laterally to ciliary processes
  - 90% unilateral (although fellow eyes may have Mittendorf's dot)
  - Usually retina not involved (posterior PFV is less common)
  - Important differential diagnosis of leukocoria
  - Signs:
    - Persistent pupillary membrane
    - Iridohyaloid vessels: Curve around pupillary margin causing atypical "colobomas' 'brittle star'" posterior capsular opacity
    - Mittendorf's dot
    - Persistant hyaloid vessel
    - Muscae volitantes
    - Bergmeister's papilla
    - Congenital non-adherence of the retina/ congential retinal detachment (rare and severe form)
    - Microphthalmia

Comparison Between Asteroid Hyalosis and Synchisis Scintillans

	Asteroid hyalosis	Synchisis scintillans
Etiology	• Vitreous fibril degeneration of unknown cause • Prevalence: 0.5% of population	• Chronic vitreous hemorrhage
Biochemical structure	• Calcium soaps	• Cholesterol crystals
Clinical features	• Yellow-white spherical opacities • Absolute acoustic shadowing on B-scan	• Flat, refractile bodies, golden-brown
Associations	• Intimately associated with vitreous gel, move with vitreous displacement	• Freely mobile, associated with liquid vitreous, settles in dependent portion of eye

Q **What are the Changes in the Vitreous with Age?**

"There are two distinct phases in the development of the vitreous...."

Vitreous Changes with Age

1. **Development of vitreous from childhood to adult**
   - Development not complete until eye reaches adult size
   - Human embryonal vitreous is dense and scatters light (collagen and HA concentration low at birth)
   - With age, increasing concentration of collagen and HA:
     - HA separates collagen fibrils → vitreous becomes less dense and optically more transparent
     - HA concentration reaches adult levels by 12 years of age
     - Total collagen content also does not change after 20–30 years of age

2. **Posterior vitreous detachment**
   - During childhood, vitreous is homogeneous and collagen fibrils not seen

- In adult, alteration of HA-collagen interaction causes dissociation of the two components:
  - Collagen fibrils aggregate with each other → macroscopic fibers seen clinically in adult vitreous coursing antero posteriorly
  - Pooling and redistribution of HA in areas adjacent to collagen → "liquid" vitreous in between fibers
  - Central vitreous first to liquefy
  - Reduction in size of vitreous → posterior vitreous cortex detaches
  - Escape of liquid vitreous into subhyaloid space leads to posterior vitreous detachment (PVD)
  - Abnormalities in retinal adhesions lead to retinal traction (pathogenesis of macular pucker/ holes)

Exam tips:
- Alternate question is "What is the pathogenesis of posterior vitreous detachment?"

RETINAL BREAKS AND DEGENERATIONS

Overall yield: ✪✪✪ **Clinical exam:** ✪✪ **Viva:** ✪✪✪✪ **Essay:** ✪✪ **MCQ:** ✪✪✪✪

Q Opening Question: Tell me about Retinal Breaks.

"A retinal break is a full-thickness defect in the neurosensory retina."

Retinal Breaks Classification:

1. **Hole:**
   - Atrophic
   - Operculated

2. **Tear**

Q When do You Need to Treat Retinal Breaks?

"Not all retinal breaks need to be treated."
"Treatment depends on the characteristics of the break, the type of eye and the type of patient."

Indications for Treatment of Retinal Break

1. **Type of break:**
   - Acute, **symptomatic** (absolute indication)
   - Associated with subclinical RD
   - U-shaped tear (absolute indication)
   - Large (relative indication)
   - Superotemporal or posterior location (relative indication)
   - Absent pigments (relative indication)

2. **Type of eye:**
   - Only eye
   - Fellow eye has history of RD

   - Aphakic or pseudophakic eye
   - High myopia
   - Vitreoretinopathy (e.g. Wagner's syndrome)

3. **Type of patient:**
   - Family history of RD
   - Systemic conditions (Marfan's, Stickler's, Ehlers-Danlos syndrome)
   - No access to health care
   - Not compliant to follow-up
   - High risk occupation

Q Tell me about Retinal Degenerations.

"Retinal degenerations can be broadly divided into benign degenerations and those associated with higher risks of RD."

Retinal Degenerations

1. **Benign degenerations:**
   - Retinal hyperplasia/hypertrophy
   - Microcystoid changes

   - Snowflakes
   - Pavingstone degenerations
   - Peripheral drusens

2. **Degenerations with increased risks of RD:**
   - Lattice degenerations (see below)
   - Acquired retinoschisis (see below)

   - White with pressure and white without pressure (associated with giant retinal tear)
   - Cystic retinal tufts

Q **When do You Need to Treat Retinal Degenerations?**

Indications for Treatment of Retinal Degenerations

1. White without pressure — fellow eye with giant retinal tear
2. Retinoschisis — 2-layer retinal break plus risk factors
3. Lattice degeneration:
   - Associated with retinal breaks
   - Associated with other risk factors (type of eye, type of patient)

Q **Tell me about Lattice Degeneration.**

"Lattice degeneration is a common retinal degeneration."

Lattice Degeneration

1. **Epidemiology**
   - 8–10% of general population (but 20–40% of RD)
   - Higher frequency in myopia, Marfan's syndrome, Ehlers-Danlos syndrome
2. **Pathology**
   - Discontinuity of internal limiting membrane
   - Atrophy of inner layers of retina
   - Overlying pocket of liquefied vitreous
   - Adherence of vitreous to edge of lattice (posterior edge)
   - Sclerosis of retinal vessels
3. **Clinical features**
   - Well defined areas of retinal thinning
   - Circumferentially orientated
   - Location:
     - Between equator and ora serrata
     - Temporal
     - Superior

Q **How do You Distinguish Acquired Retinoschisis from Retinal Detachment?**

"Acquired retinoschisis is a retinal degeneration in which…."
"The retina is split into two layers, an outer choroidal layer and an inner vitreous layer…."
"The typical type involves a split in the plexiform layer, while the reticular type involves a split in the nerve fiber layer."

Acquired Retinoschisis

	Retinal detachment	Acquired retinoschisis
High risk group	• Myopia	• Hypermetropia
Location	• Superior temporal	• Inferior temporal
Scotoma	• Relative	• Absolute
Pigments	• Present	• Absent
Surface	• Corrugated	• Smooth
Shifting fluid	• May be present	• Absent
Reaction to photocoagulation	• No reaction	• Present

> **Exam tips:**
> • The typical type is split in the plexiform layer while the reticular type is split in the nerve fiber layer.

Q **What is Proliferative Vitreoretinopathy?**

"Proliferative vitreoretinopathy (PVR) is the commonest cause of late failure after RD operation."

Proliferative Vitreoretinopathy

1. **Pathology**
   • Retinal tear or detachment causes break in inner limiting membrane and blood retinal barrier
   • RPE cells migrate into vitreous
   • RPE cells proliferate and transform into myofibroblasts
   • Further stimulus for migration and proliferation from blood derived products
   • RPE cells release transforming growth factors (TGF) which stimulates fibrosis and collagen production
   • Membranes contract (in anteroposterior and tangential directions) and this leads to tractional RD

2. **Risk factors**
   • RD factors:
     • Retinal break (large and multiple)
     • Associated vitreous hemorrhage and inflammation
     • Re-detachment
   • Iatrogenic factors:
     • Excessive cryotherapy or laser photocoagulation
     • Use of viscoelastic, gas or silicone oil
     • Iris trauma

3. **Classification (know the differences between the Retina Society and Silicone Study grading schemes)**
   • Grade A
     • Vitreous haze or pigment clumps

   • Grade B
     • Wrinkling of inner retina
     • Retinal stiffness
     • Vessel tortuosity
     • Rolled edge of retinal break
     • Decreased vitreous mobility
   • Grade C
     • Full thickness retinal folds:
       · Focal
       · Diffuse
       · Circumferential
       · Subretinal
       · Anterior
     • Defined as either anterior or posterior and by number of clock hours

4. **Treatment**
   • Surgery usually required:
     • Pneumoretinopexy/scleral buckling (grade B and below)
     • Vitrectomy usually required
   • Pharmacological adjuncts: 5FU, low molecular weight heparin (not shown to be effective)
   • Timing of surgery:
     • Balance between threat to macula (if still attached) and easier and more complete removal of mature membranes
     • In general, if macula attached and chance for preservation of useful vision → early surgery
     • If macular chronically detached, better to await membrane maturation (4–8 weeks) before surgery

Q **What is the Silicone Study?**

"The Silicone study was randomized trial to compare the use of silicone oil (SO) vs gas in the treatment of PVR."

Silicone Study (*Arch Ophthalmol*, 1992;110:770 and 780)

1. **Aim:**
   - Study effect of SO vs gas in treatment of PVR
   - Cases had rhegmatogenous RD and silicone study PVR grade C-3 and above
   - Report 1: SO vs SF_6
   - Report 2: SO vs C_3F_8

2. **Conclusions:**
   - SO more effective than SF_6
   - SO and C_3F_8 equally effective in maintaining retinal attachment
   - Hypotony higher in C_3F_8
   - Keratopathy same between SO and C_3F_8
   - Re-detachment occurs in 20% of eyes after SO removal

RETINAL DETACHMENT SURGERY

Overall yield: ✪✪✪✪ **Clinical exam:** **Viva:** ✪✪✪✪ **Essay:** ✪✪✪ **MCQ:** ✪✪✪✪

Q Opening Question: What are the Principles of Retinal Detachment Surgery?

"The principles of RD surgery are…."

Principles of RD Surgery

1. **Find all retinal breaks**
   - Indirect ophthalmoscopy with scleral indentation
   - Based on Lincoff's rule (see below)
2. **Seal all retinal breaks**
   - Cryopexy OR
   - Laser photocoagulation
3. **Drain subretinal fluid (SRF) if necessary**
4. **Relieve vitreoretinal traction**
   - Scleral buckle OR
   - Vitrectomy OR
   - Pneumatic retinopexy

Exam tips:
- **These principles are shown step-by-step in the scleral buckles section (page 158)**

Q What are Lincoff's Rules?

"Lincoff's rules are a set of guidelines on finding the retinal break based on the configuration of the RD."
- Based on retrospective analysis of 1,000 cases of RD.
- Only applicable to primary Rhegmatogenous RD (96% of cases conformed to these rules).

Lincoff's Rules (*Arch Ophthalmol* 1971;85:565–69)

1. **"Lateral" RD (inferior RD with SRF higher on one side of the disc) (98%)**
   - Break is at one and a half clock hours from higher side of RD
2. **"Superior" RD (SRF crosses the vertical midline above disc) (93%)**
   - Break is superior, within a triangle with its apex at 12 o'clock at ora serrata and base at 11 and 1 o'clock at equator
3. **"Inferior" RD (inferior RD with equal SRF on both sides of disc) (95%)**
   - Break is inferior, at 6 o'clock position
4. **"Inferior bullous" RD**
   - Break is on higher side of RD, above horizontal meridian, with SRF tracking inferiorly

What is Cryotherapy?

"Cryotherapy is the treatment technique involving the use of cold temperature."

Cryotherapy

1. **Mechanism of action**
   - Freezing temperature causes conversion of liquids to solids, and intracellular and extracellular water to ice
   - This leads to tissue death and a sterile inflammatory reaction

2. **Cryoprobe**
   - Probe temperature is between –40°C (carbon dioxide) or –70°C (liquid nitrogen), temperature at tissue around –10°C
   - Thermal energy is absorbed by rapid expansion of carbon dioxide and liquid nitrogen into gaseous state (Jules-Thomson effect)
   - Expansion occurs at gas tip with an exhaust system drawing away gas
   - An insulation compartment limits freezing to tip of probe
   - Heater wire in probe defrosts tip after each freeze
   - Retinal adhesion takes about two weeks to gain strength (slower than laser retinopexy)

3. **Indications in ophthalmology:**
   - **A**dhesion (retinal breaks)
     - "When would you prefer to use cryopexy instead of laser photocoagulation?"
       - Small pupil
       - Peripheral retina which cannot be treated adequately with lasers
       - Opaque media
   - **B**lood vessels (PDR new vessels, telangiectasia of Coat's disease)
     - "When would you prefer to use cryopexy for PDR?" (same as for retinal breaks)
   - Small pupil
   - Peripheral retina which cannot be treated adequately with lasers
   - Opaque media
   - **C**iliary body (cyclodestructive procedures for glaucoma)
   - **C**ataract extraction (ICCE)
   - **D**estruction (lid and intraocular tumors, trichiasis)

4. **Procedure:**
   - Check cryoprobe by freezing and unfreezing a few times
   - Place probe over scleral area with indirect ophthalmoscopic view of retinal break
   - Initiate freezing
   - Observe for whitening of retina
   - Spray water on cryoprobe and wait for complete melting of ice-ball before removing from sclera
   - Thaw and repeat again

5. **Complications:**
   - Early:
     - Pain and chemosis
     - Conjunctival fibrosis (increase risk of trabeculectomy failure)
     - Vitritis
     - CME
   - Late:
     - PVR
     - ERM
     - Diplopia from muscle injury
     - Scleral necrosis
     - Depigmentation (cutaneous application)

Exam tips:
- **The indications for cryotherapy are "ABCD."**

When and How do You Perform Subretinal Fluid (SRF) Drainage?

"SRF drainage is not an essential part of RD surgery."
"This is because in most cases, SRF will usually be absorbed spontaneously with adequate support and sealing of the retinal breaks."
"SRF drainage can be divided into internal or external drainage."

SRF Drainage

1. **Indications**
   - RD is:
     - Bullous (unable to appose retina for adequate retinopexy)
     - Long-standing (viscid SRF)
     - Immobile because of PVR
     - Inferior (usually bullous, long-standing and breaks cannot be localized)
   - Break cannot be localized or sealed
   - Patient factors:
     - Elderly (less efficiency of RPE pump)
     - Preexisting glaucoma
     - Undergone recent cataract surgery
     - Thin sclera

2. **Procedure**
   - Choose site of drainage
   - Cauterize site of drainage
   - Incise sclera radially until choroid can be seen
   - Cauterize lips of incision, pre-place 5/0 vicryl sutures to lips
   - Use either 27G needle or endolaser to puncture choroid at an oblique angle:
     - Controlled SRF drainage with cotton tips and finger
     - "Milk out" viscid SRF if necessary
   - Check for flattening of retina:
     - Check for hypotony (have syringe of air or saline on standby)
     - Suture lips with 5/0 vicryl

3. **Complications**
   - Hypotony (commonest complication):
     - Choroidal folds
     - Macular and disc edema
     - Corneal edema
   - Suprachoroidal hemorrhage (most dangerous complication)
   - Iatrogenic break formation
   - Retinal prolapse and incarceration
   - Vitreous prolapse
   - Postoperative endophthalmus

Notes
- "Where would you choose your site of drainage?"
  - Above or below horizontal recti (avoid vortex veins near the vertical recti)
  - Between ora and equator
  - Temporal retina (usually more accessible)
  - Away from break (less risk of vitreous incarceration)
  - At the point where RD is most bullous
  - In the bed of the scleral buckle

Q **Tell me about Scleral Buckles.**

"Scleral buckles (SB) are devices to relieve vitreoretinal traction in RD surgery."
"They can be divided into…."

Scleral Buckles

1. **Classification:**
   - Radial
   - Segmental circumferential
   - Encirclage circumferential

2. **Materials**
   - Silicon:
     - Tires
       - Provide even indentation, low risk of infection, extrusion or migration
     - Sponges
       - Imbibe fluid postoperatively to increase tension, but more complications
   - Band
     - Usually for encirclage
   - Hydrogels:
     - Soft and elastic, nontoxic and nonpyogenic, imbibe fluid postoperatively to increase tension but more expensive than silicon
     - No longer in use due to high risk of long-term complications — continued swelling leads to mass effect, diplopia, infections
   - Gelatin
     - Temporary (lasts 3 to 6 months)

3. **Factors affecting choice of SB:**
    - Retinal break (size, number and location)
    - Distribution of SRF
    - Amount of vitreous traction and PVR
    - Phakic status
    - Available eye volume
    - State of sclera

4. **Indications for radial SB**
    - Usually in two situations:
        - Large U-shaped tears with "fishmouthing"
        - Posterior breaks

5. **Indications for segmental SB**
    - "Standard" buckles for most RD:
        - Small — medium size breaks in single location
        - Multiple small — medium size breaks in one or two quadrants

6. **Indications for encirclage SB**
    - Used for more "complicated RD" (although some surgeons use this routinely):
    - Large breaks and multiple breaks in three or more quadrants
    - Extensive RD without detectable breaks
    - Mild PVR
    - Aphakic RD
    - Lattice degeneration in three or more quadrants
    - Excessive drainage of SRF
    - Failed segmental buckle without apparent reason

7. **Procedure:**
    - GA or LA
    - Conjunctival peritomy — 360° or limited peritomy

- Dissect tenons and isolate recti with squint hook
- Sling recti with 5/0 silk suture
- Position buckle beneath recti
- Localized all breaks with indirect ophthalmoscopy and scleral indentation (Principle No. 1)
- Seal all breaks with cryopexy or indirect laser (Principle No. 2)
- Decide whether to perform SRF drainage (Principle No. 3)
- Relieve vitreoretinal traction by suturing SB with 8/0 nylon (Principle No. 4)
- Check for position of buckle and check pulsation of central retinal artery (to exclude CRAO)
- Close conjunctiva with 8/0 vicryl

8. **Complications**
    - Intraoperative:
        - Scleral perforation
        - Rectus muscle trauma
        - Complications of SRF drainage
        - Conjunctival buttonholing, tears
        - Complications of gas/SO tamponade
    - Postoperative:
        - Fish-mouthing (large breaks, high buckles) and posterior slippage (GRT)
        - Extrusion, exposure
        - Refractive changes: myopia, astigmatism
        - Anterior segment ischemia
        - Diplopia/motility problems
        - Glaucoma (vortex vein compression)

Exam tips:
- **The principles of RD surgery (page 155) are shown in the procedures section.**

Q **What are the Indications for Vitrectomy in Retinal Detachment?**

"The indication for vitrectomy can be divided into uncomplicated RD and complicated RD."

Indications for Vitrectomy in RD

1. **Rhegmatogenous RD**
    - Uncomplicated:
        - Posterior breaks and macular holes
        - Multiple breaks in different meridians
        - Associated vitreous hemorrhage
        - Controversial (high myopes, pseudophakics, bullous superior RD with no breaks seen)
    - Complicated RD:
        - Severe proliferative vitreoretinopathy grade C or more
        - Giant retinal tear

2. **Tractional RD threatening fovea**

"Pneumoretinopexy is a form of RD surgery."
"It is indicated for…."

Pneumoretinopexy

1. **Principles:**
   - Works by intravitreal injection of an **expansile volume** of gas (100% concentration)
     - 0.6 ml of 100% SF_6 will give 1.2 ml after full expansion
     - 0.3 ml of 100% C_3F_8 will give 1.2 ml after full expansion
   - The retinal break is sealed with tamponade from buoyancy and surface tension of gas (see intraocular gas, page 161)

2. **Indications:**
   - Retinal breaks in superior 8 o'clock hours
   - Not indicated when there is:
     - Preexisting glaucoma
     - Grade C PVR
     - Hazy media
     - Unable to move or travel by air

3. **Procedure:**
   - Injection site: Pars plana
   - Aim to inject gas into cortical vitreous (prevent sub-hyaloid gas), forming single large bubble (avoid fish-eggs)
   - If macula threatened: Steamroller technique (position patient such that gas bubble tamponades macula first, then slowly reposition bubble over break)

4. **Advantages:**
   - No hospitalization
   - No complications of SB
   - Minimal tissue trauma
   - Shown to be as effective as SB (~80% reattachment rate with single procedure in both)

5. **Disadvantages and complications:**
   - Failure of retinal attachment
   - New retinal tears/breaks (up to 20%)
   - Risk of glaucoma and CRAO
   - Vitreous hemorrhage and vitreous incarceration
   - Gas can migrate into subretinal space with extension of RD

Complications of RD Surgery

1. **Early:**
   - Missed breaks and re-detachment (commonest cause of **EARLY** failure)
   - Acute ACG (forward displacement and congestion of ciliary body)
   - Anterior segment ischemia
   - Vitritis (usually from cryopexy)
   - Choroidal detachment (hypotony usually from SRF drainage)
   - Endophthalmitis (SRF drain)

2. **Late:**
   - PVR (commonest cause of **LATE** failure)
   - Induced refractive error
   - Diplopia
   - Scleral buckle problems (infection, dislocation and extrusion)
   - CME
   - ERM

VITRECTOMY AND VITREOUS REPLACEMENT

Overall yield: ✪✪✪   **Clinical exam:**   **Viva:** ✪✪✪   **Essay:** ✪✪   **MCQ:** ✪✪✪✪

Q Opening Question: What are the Indications for Vitrectomy?

"Vitrectomy can be used for either therapeutic or diagnostic purposes."
"Common indications may include…."

Indications for Vitrectomy

1. **Complicated retinal detachments**
   - Rhegmatogenous RD
     - Uncomplicated RD:
       - Posterior breaks and macular holes
       - Multiple breaks in different meridians
       - Associated vitreous hemorrhage
       - Controversial (high myopes, pseudophakics, bullous superior RD with no breaks seen)
     - Complicated RD:
       - Severe proliferative vitreoretinopathy grade C or more
       - Giant retinal tear
   - Tractional RD threatening fovea

2. **Advanced diabetic retinopathy (see page 192)**

3. **Other proliferative vitreoretinopathies**

4. **Severe ocular trauma and intraocular foreign body (IOFB):**
   - Associated with endophthalmitis
   - IOFB impacted on retina
   - No view of IOFB (e.g. vitreous hemorrhage)
   - Large, nonmagnetic or organic IOFB

5. **Macular diseases:**
   - Epiretinal membrane (ERM)
   - Macular hole

6. **Complications of anterior segment surgery:**
   - Postoperative endophthalmitis
   - Dropped nucleus
   - Massive expulsive hemorrhage
   - Malignant glaucoma

7. **Chronic posterior segment inflammation/vitritis:**
   - Diagnostic vitrectomy

Recent Developments in Vitrectomy Techniques

1. **Vitrectomy instrumentation**
   - 23G and 25G vitrectomy:
     - Self-sealing sclerostomies — faster recovery
     - Better fuildics (smaller bore — lower likelihood of aspirating retina)
   - Chandelier illumination: Self-retaining illumination allowing bimanual surgery

2. **Chemical vitrectomy**
   - Vitrase: Bovine hyaluronidase
     - Shown to be safe and effective in clearing vitreous hemorrhage in two multinational RCTs with > 1,100 patients

Complications of Vitrectomy

Intraoperative	Postoperative
• Retinal break	• Retinal break
• Suction near mobile retina	• Intraocular hemorrhage
• Intraocular hemorrhage	• Choroidal hemorrhage
• Suprachoroidal hemorrhage	• Vitreous hemorrhage
• Vitreous hemorrhage	• Cataract
• Cataract	• Glaucoma
• Lens trauma with instruments	• Cornea
• Raised IOP	• Recurrent corneal erosion
• Infusion bottle too high	• Filamentary keratitis
• Decreased IOP	• Bullous keratopathy
• Infusion bottle too low	• Phthsis bulbi
• Miosis of pupils	• Endophthalmitis
• Subretinal infusion	• Failure of surgery

Q What are Vitreous Substitutes?

"They are substances injected into the vitreous cavity during a vitrectomy."
"The main purpose is either for volume replacement or as a tamponade."
"The common vitreous substitutes include…."

Vitreous Substitutes

1. **Ideal substitute (important):**
   • Clear/transparent
   • Inert/nontoxic
   • Low viscosity
   • Immiscible with H_2O
   • Durable/slowly absorbed

2. **Classification:**
   • Intraocular gas
   • Saline
   • Silicone oil
   • Heavy liquids

Exam tips:
• The ideal substitute has a LIST of properties that can be used for ALL the individual substitutes and therefore is well worth to be remembered.

Q Tell me about Intraocular Gases.

"Intraocular gases are common vitreous substitutes…."
"They can be divided into…."
"The common indications are for either volume replacement (nonexpansile volume) or as a tamponade (expansile volume)…."

Intraocular Gas

1. **Classification:**
   • Nonexpansile
     • Air, helium, argon, nitrogen, xenon
   • Expansile
     • Sulphur hexafloride (SF_6), perfluoreopropane (C_3F_8), C_2F_6, C_4F_{10}

2. **Biomechanical properties**
   • Physical properties:
     • Properties of ideal substitute (page 161)
       · Clear/transparent
       · Inert/nontoxic
       · Low viscosity

- Immiscible with water
- Durable/slowly absorbed **PLUS**
- High surface tension
  - Bubble of gas does not enter retinal break and prevents fluid from entering break
- High buoyancy
  - 10 times greater force than SO
  - Force maximal at apex of angle
- Dynamic properties
  - Three phases:
    - Expansion
      - Oxygen, carbon dioxide diffuses in
- Maximum at 6–8 hours (therefore be careful of CRAO during this time)
- Equilibrium
  - Nitrogen last to diffuse
  - Maximal expansion when gas diffusion in = diffusion out
- Dissolution
  - Exponential decline
  - Depends on size and water solubility
  - First order kinetics — bubble has useful ARC of contact for approximately 25% of total duration of gas in eye

3. **Comparison of air, SF_6, C_3F_8**

Gas	Duration	Time of maximal expansion rate	Time to maximal expansion	Expansion volume	Nonexpansile concentration
Air	5 days	NA	NA	×1	NA
SF_6	2 weeks	6–8 hours	24–48 hours	×2	**20%**
C_2F_6	3 weeks	6–8 hours	48–72 hours	×3	**18%**
C_3F_8	2 months	6–8 hours (same as SF_6)	72–96 hours	×4	**15%**

4. **Indications for SF_6 or C_3F_8**
   - Volume **replacement** after vitrectomy (nonexpansile volume)
     - Indications for vitrectomy (see page 160)
   - **Tamponade** retina (expansile volume):
     - Adjunct to RD surgery (posterior breaks or macular holes)
     - Adjunct to DRF drainage
     - Selected giant retinal tear
     - Flatten radial folds on a high buckle
     - Pneumoretinopexy (use 100% gas without vitrectomy; see page 159)

5. **Complications:**
   - Glaucoma and CRAO
     - Especially during maximum rate of expansion (6–8 hours after operation)
   - Cataract (posterior subcapsular "feathery" cataract)
   - Bullous keratopathy
   - New/enlarged breaks
   - Subretinal seepage
   - Dislocation of IOLs
   - PVR

Q **Tell me about Silicone Oil.**

"Silicone oil is a vitreous substitute."
"It has the following properties…."

Silicone Oil (SO)

1. **Properties:**
   - Properties of ideal substitute (page 161)
     - Clear/transparent
     - Inert/nontoxic
     - Low viscosity
     - Immiscible with water
       - Surface tension of SO however lower than gases — tendency to emulsify
     - Durable/not absorbed **PLUS**
   - Refractive index close to vitreous:
     - Acts as plus lens in aphakic eyes
     - Acts as minus lens in phakic eyes
   - High viscosity
     - 1,000–30,000 centistokes (water = 1 centistoke)
   - Lighter than water (0.93G)
     - Heavy silicone oil (denser than water) occasionally used for inferior detachments

2. **Indications:**
   - Long-lasting volume replacement following vitrectomy
   - Common indications:
     - PVR
     - Giant retinal tear
     - Intraoperative control of vitreous hemorrhage
     - Elderly patient who cannot posture
     - One-eyed patient who needs immediate good vision postoperation
     - Patient who needs to travel by air

3. **Advantages**
   - "What are the advantages of SO over intraocular gases?"
   - Intraoperative advantages:
     - Better intraoperative visualization
     - Easier retinopexy
     - Control of hemorrhage and effusion
   - Postoperative advantages:
     - Longer-lasting tamponade
     - Posturing less critical
     - Better immediate VA

- Air travel not contraindicated
- Lower risk of hypotony
- Control over timing of repeat surgery

4. **Complications**
   - Glaucoma:
     - ACG (from pupil block, therefore inferior iridectomy (Ando) is usually needed)
     - Delayed OAG (from emulsification)
     - Hypotony (not common)
   - Cataract
   - Filamentary keratitis, band keratopathy
   - Emulsification of SO:
     - Uveitis
     - Subretinal seepage
     - Subconjunctival cyst formation
     - Retinal toxicity? (ERG and EOG detected abnormalities)
   - ERM/retro-silicone proliferation:
     - Accumulation of growth factors, inflammatory debris at lower meniscus of bubble
     - Cause of recurrent epiretinal proliferation
   - Recurrent RD (25–40%)

Q **What are Heavy Liquids?**

"Heavy liquids are vitreous substitutes used as intraoperative tools."
"They are essentially extension of perfluorocarbon gases with seven or more carbon atoms (and therefore **liquid** at room and body temperature)."

Heavy Liquids

1. **Properties**
   - Properties of the ideal substitute (page 161):
     - Clear/transparent
     - Inert/nontoxic (with short-term use)
     - Low viscosity (0.8–8 centistokes)
     - Immiscible with water
     - Durable/slowly absorbed **PLUS**
   - High specific gravity (2G, two times more than water or SO)
   - High tamponade force (4G, like gas and 10 times more than SO)

2. **Examples**
   - Perfluorodecalin ($C_{10}F_{18}$)
   - Perfluoro-N-octane (C_8F_{18})

3. **Indications**
   - Intraoperative tool for complicated VR surgery (not for prolonged tamponade):
     - PVR
     - Giant retinal tear
     - Subluxed/dislocated lens
     - IOFB
     - Subretinal macular hem
     - Traumatic RD

MEDICAL RETINA

THE MACULA

Overall yield: ✪✪✪   **Clinical exam:**   **Viva:** ✪✪✪   **Essay:**   **MCQ:** ✪✪✪

Q   Opening Question: What is the Anatomy of the Macula?

"The macula is an area in the posterior pole of the fundus…."

Anatomy of the Macula

1. **Macula**
   - Location: Area bounded by temporal arcades, **4 mm** temporal, **0.8 mm** inferior to optic disc
   - Size: 5 mm in diameter/**3.5** disc diameter/18° of visual angle
   - Histologically,
     - >**1 layer** of ganglion cells
     - **Xanthophyll** pigments

2. **Fovea**
   - Location: Depression inside macula
   - Size: 1.5 mm in diameter/**1** disc diameter/5° of visual angle
   - Histologically,
     - **6–8 layers** of ganglion cells
     - Tall RPE cells

   - Thick internal limiting membrane

3. **Foveola**
   - Location: Central floor of fovea
   - Size: 0.35 mm in diameter/**0.2** disc diameter/0.54 minutes of visual angle
   - Histologically,
     - Thinnest part of retina
     - **No** ganglion cells or rods
     - Only **cones**: 150,000/mm²

4. **Foveal avascular zone (FAZ)**
   - Location: Area bounded by fovea and foveola
   - Histologically (accounts for "darkness" in FFA),
     - Avascular
     - Tall RPE cells with increased melanin
     - Increased xanthophyll pigments

Q   How do You Evaluate Macular Function?

"The macula can be assessed **clinically** and with appropriate **tests**…."

Macular Function

1. **Clinical**
   - VA
   - Color vision and pupil (should be normal unless the macular is extensively damaged)
   - Binocular ophthalmoscopy and slit lamp biomicroscopy (with 78D or 90D lens)
   - Confrontational VF and light projection

2. **Ancillary tests**
   - **Amsler grid:**
     - Screening test for macular function
     - Evaluates **20°** of visual angle (macular subtends only 18°)

   - Standard chart with 10 cm large square and 5 mm small square
   - Chart should be read at **1/3** of meter (small **square** subtends **1°**)
   - Seven charts in total:
     - Chart 1: Standard chart
     - Chart 2: Diagonal lines to help central fixation, when central scotoma is present
     - Chart 3: Standard chart, but red lines on black background, for color scotoma
     - Chart 4: No lines, only dots, reveals only scotoma

- Chart 5: Parallel horizontal lines, to show metamorphopsia
- Chart 6: Similar to Chart 5, but with finer horizontal lines in the central area
- Chart 7: Similar to Chart 1, but with finer lines in central area
- **Photostress test:**
  - Principle of the **dark adaptation test** (evaluate recovery time of photoreceptors to re-synthesize visual pigments)
  - Procedure:
    - Snellen VA assessed
    - Patient fixates on torch light for 10 seconds
    - Photostress recovery time = time taken to read Snellen letters one line above the pre-test level (normal: 30 seconds)
    - Compare with other eye
- **Flying corpuscle test:**
  - Principle of the **entoptic phenomenon** (subjective perception of white blood cells moving in perifoveal capillaries)
  - Procedure:
    - Patient asked to look into blue light of entoptoscope

- Patient should see 15 or more white blood cells in entire area
- Abnormal macular function:
  - No corpuscles/decreased number of corpuscles
  - Slow speed of corpuscles
  - No corpuscles in a specific area
- **Laser interferometer:**
  - Principle of **interference**
  - Two coherent light beams creates fringe pattern (black and bright bands) by process of interference
  - Fringe pattern in different orientations and progressively finer gratings are used to estimate VA and macular function
- **Potential acuity meter:**
  - Projection of a miniature Snellen acuity chart into retina, through a clear area of cataract or other media opacities
  - Usually best for VA <20/200

Exam tips:
- An alternate question may be, "How do you assess the macular function in a patient with a dense cataract?"
- Remember to talk about the clinical examination first (what you would normally do in your daily practice), before going on to the more esoteric tests.

FUNDAL FLUORESCEIN ANGIOGRAPHY

Overall yield: ✪✪✪   **Clinical exam:** ✪   **Viva:** ✪✪✪   **Essay:**   **MCQ:** ✪✪

Q Opening Question: What are the Clinical Uses of Fluorescein?

Clinical Uses of Fluorescein

1. **Lacrimal system**
   - Tear break-up time (dry eyes)
   - Jones test: Dye disappearance test (blockage of lacrimal system)
2. **Cornea**
   - Detect epithelial defect (corneal abrasion, superficial punctate keratopathy)

   - Siedal's test (wound leak)
   - Contact lens fitting (assess contact lens fit)
3. **Anterior chamber**
   - Detect iris neovascularization
   - Applanation tonometry
4. **Retina**
   - FFA

Exam tips:
- **Fundal fluorescein angiography (FFA) is NOT the only use of fluorescein!**

Q What are the Principles of Fundal Fluorescein Angiography (FFA)?

"Fundal fluorescein angiography is based on two principles...."
"The principle of **fluorescence**, which is the ability of...."
"And the principle of the **blood-retinal barrier**, which consists of...."

Principles of FFA

1. **Fluorescence**
   - Fluorescence: Ability of a substance to emit light energy of a **longer** wavelength (emission wavelength) when stimulated by light of a **shorter** wavelength (excitation wavelength)
   - Fluorescein:
     - Excitation wavelength peak: 490 nm (blue)
     - Emission wavelength peak: 530 nm (green)
   - Basic FFA:
     - White light from retinal camera passes through a blue excitation filter, which allows only **blue light** to enter eye
   - Interaction of blue light with fluorescein molecules in blood vessels, with emission of yellow-green light (fluorescence)
   - Yellow-green and reflected blue light travel out of retina to camera, passes through blue interference filter, allowing only **yellow-green light** to be imaged onto film

2. Blood-retinal barrier (BRB)

- Inner blood-retinal barrier: Tight junctions of **retinal capillary endothelial cells**
- Outer blood-retinal barrier: Tight junction of **RPE**
- When fluorescein is injected into blood stream, **inner BRB** prevents leakage of fluorescein and allows retinal vessels to be seen
- On the other hand, there is leakage of free fluorescein from choroidal vessels, but **outer BRB** prevents free fluorescein from traveling across RPE into sensory retina
- Therefore, leakage of fluorescein from either retinal vessel or RPE is abnormal

---

Notes
- "What is autofluorescence?"
  - Ability of a substance to emit yellow-green light when stimulated by blue light in the **absence of fluorescein**
  - Classic example: Drusens

Notes
- "What is pseudofluorescence?"
  - Ability of substance to emit yellow-green light when stimulated by blue light in the **presence of mismatched filters**

Q What are the Indications for FFA?

"FFA is useful as an aid in the **diagnosis** and **management** of various posterior segment diseases."

Indications for FFA

1. **Aid in diagnosis of:**
   - Macular diseases:
     - AMD, central serous retinopathy, CME
   - Retinal vascular diseases:
     - Neovascularization in DR, CRVO, BRVO, retinal telangiectasia
   - Inflammatory retinal/choroidal diseases:
     - Posterior uveitis, CMV retinitis
   - Optic nerve disorders:
     - Disc drusens, papilledema, optic neuritis
   - Tumors:
     - Choroidal hemangiomas
2. **Aid in laser treatment of:**
   - CNV, central serous retinopathy, DM maculopathy, CRVO and BRVO

Q What are the Side Effects of FFA?

"FFA is usually a safe procedure with few side effects."

1. **Mild and more common side effects:**
   - Nausea and vomiting
   - Yellow discoloration of skin, urine and tears
   - Pain at injection site (especially if there is extravasation)
   - Rashes
2. **Serious but rare side effects:**
   - Anaphylactic shock
   - Airway spasm
   - Collapse and death

Q. Tell me about the Normal FFA. What Abnormalities can FFA Detect?

"The abnormalities are either related to hyperfluorescence or hypofluorescence...."

Results of FFA

1. **Normal FFA**
   - Phase 1: Pre-arterial phase/choroidal filling
     - Arm-retina time: 9–12 seconds
   - Phase 2: Arterial phase
     - One second after Phase 1
   - Phase 3: Arteriovenous phase/capillary phase
     - Complete filling of arterioles and capillaries
     - Early venous filling (lamellar flow)
   - Phase 4: Venous phase
     - Complete venous filling
     - Recirculation of dye
     - Intensity of fluorescence decreases

2. **Cause of hyperfluorescence**
   - **Window defect** (transmission of dye from choroid):
     - Atrophy or destruction of RPE cells (e.g. AMD), RPE tear
     - Occurs early in FFA
   - **Pooling** (increase in **intensity** of hyperfluorescence but not in size):
     - Dye in sub-RPE space (e.g. pigment epithelial detachment)
     - Dye in sub-retinal space (e.g. exudative RD)

   - Occurs early in FFA
   - **Leakage** (increase in **size and intensity** of hyperfluorescence) from:
     - Choroidal vessels occur early (e.g. choroidal neovascularization)
     - Retinal vessels occur late (e.g. NVD in DR)
     - Optic nerve head occurs late (e.g. papilledema)
   - **Staining** (dye in tissue):
     - Retinal scars, sclera, abnormal vessels
     - Occurs late

3. **Cause of hypofluorescence**
   - **Masking** (blockage of dye transmission from choroid):
     - Retinal hemorrhages
     - Edema and hard exudates
     - Pigments (melanin and xanthophyll)
     - Lipofuscin (e.g. Best disease)
   - **Filling defect** (delay of filling or occlusion of vessels):
     - Retinal ischemia (e.g. CRVO, DR)
     - Choroidal ischemia (e.g. HPT retinopathy)
     - Retinal atrophy (e.g. myopia)

Q **Tell me about Indocyanine Green (ICG) Angiography.**

"ICG is a complementary test to the FFA in the **diagnosis** and **management** of various posterior segment diseases."

Indocyanine Green Angiography

1. **Advantages over FFA**
    - ICG is highly bound to plasma proteins (**98**%) as compared with FFA (**80**%)
        - Choroidal circulation is more easily seen
    - ICG has maximum absorption at **805 nm** and fluorescence at **835 nm**
        - Wavelength of ICG can penetrate RPE and macular xanthophyll better

2. **Indications**
    - AMD:
        - Occult and recurrent CNV
        - PED
        - Submacular hemorrhage
    - Inflammatory choroidal diseases:
        - White dot syndromes
        - Vogt-Koyanagi-Harada syndrome
    - Tumors:
        - Choroidal melanoma

OPTICAL COHERENCE TOMOGRAPHY

Overall yield: ✸✸   **Clinical exam:** ✸   **Viva:** ✸✸   **Essay:**   **MCQ:** ✸✸

Q Opening Question: What is Optical Coherence Tomography?

"OCT is a low coherence interferometry which allows non-contact in vivo imaging of ocular tissues at a high resolution."

OCT

1. **Principle**
   - Works as an "optical ultrasound," by using light reflections to provide cross-sectional images

2. **Types**
   - Time domain OCT:
     - Mirrors used to scan tissue and provide cross-sectional image of optic nerve
     - Acquires images at 400 axial scans/second
       - Artifacts from eye movement
     - Axial resolution of 10 μm
     - More widely used

   - Frequency domain OCT:
     - Spectral/Fourier domain OCT
     - Mirrors not used, all wavelengths of returning light analyzed simultaneously
     - Acquires images at 20,000 axial scans/second
       - Less artifacts and improved quality of images
     - Axial resolution 5 μm
     - More expensive

Q What are the Applications of Optical Coherence Tomography in Ophthalmology?

"OCT is widely used in ophthalmology…."
"It is used to image the macula both the anterior and posterior segment."

Applications of OCT

1. **Posterior segment**
   - Macula:
     - CSME
     - AMD and PCV: Macular edema, PED
     - CSR
     - CME
     - ERM and VMT
     - Macular hole
     - RPE atrophy
     - Maculoschisis

   - RNFL:
     - Reduced in:
       - Glaucoma
       - High myopia
     - Increased in:
       - Swollen disc

2. **Anterior segment**
   - AC angles: Open or closed
   - Mechanisms of angle closure: Pupil block, angle crowding, bulky lens

ELECTROPHYSIOLOGY

Overall yield: ✪✪✪   **Clinical exam:**   **Viva:** ✪✪✪   **Essay:**   **MCQ:** ✪✪✪

Q **Opening Question:** What is the Electroretinogram, Electrooculogram and Visual Evoked Potential?

- **ERG** = Measure of electrical mass response of the **retina**, reflecting electrical activity of **photoreceptor and bipolar cells**
- **EOG** = Measure of electrical mass response of the **eye**, reflecting the metabolic activity of the **RPE**

- **VEP** = Measure of electrical response of the **occipital visual cortex** to stimulation of the retina with either light or pattern stimulus, reflecting activity of the **entire visual system** (from retina, especially macula to cortex)

Exam tips:
- **A clear definition of the three main types of electrophysiological tests is important.**

Q **Tell me about the Principles of Electroretinography.**

Electroretinography (ERG)

1. **Anatomical basis**
   - Rods
     - Distribution:
       - 120 million
       - Absent in foveola, increase to peak density **15°** from foveola center, then decrease slightly towards periphery
     - Sensitivity:
       - Maximal in **scotopic** conditions
       - Maximal to **blue green** light
       - Unable to follow flicker greater than 8 to 10 cycles/second (longer refractory period)
   - Cones
     - Distribution:
       - 6 million
       - Peak density in **foveola**, decrease in density 15° from foveola center, lowest density in peripheral retina
       - However, majority of cones lie **outside** fovea (therefore localized disease of the fovea will still result in a normal cone ERG

and abnormal cone ERG implies widespread retinal disorder)
     - Sensitivity:
       - Maximal in **photopic** conditions
       - Maximal to **green-yellow** light
       - Able to follow **flicker** greater than 8 to 10 cycles/second

2. **Normal ERG waveform**
   - A-wave:
     - Negative waveform
     - Photoreceptor hyper-polarization when exposed to light stimulus
     - Reflects **photoreceptor** function
   - B-wave:
     - Positive waveform
     - Midretinal cells, initiated by bipolar cells, magnified by Müller cells
     - Reflects **Müller cells** and bipolar cells
   - C-wave:
     - Occasionally present
     - Reflects **RPE** cells

- Oscillatory potential:
  - Wavelets on rising B-wave

- Interaction between Amacrine and Interplexiform cells
- Reflects primarily **cone** function

Q What are the Types of ERG and How do You Use/Apply Each of Them?

Types of ERG

1. **Equipment**
   - Stimulator:
     - Ganzfeld stimulator, diffuse illumination of entire retina
   - Electrodes:
     - Active electrode (contact lens electrode, gold foil lid electrode)
     - Reference electrode (forehead)
     - Ground electrode (earlobe)
   - Amplification and display system

2. **ERG waveform measurement**
   - Amplitude:
     - **Trough** of "A-wave" to the **peak** of "B-wave" (microvolts)
     - Reflects efficiency of the retina in producing an electrical signal, dependent on pupil size, refractive error, fundal pigmentation and age
   - Implicit latency:
     - **Time** of stimulus to peak of B-wave (milliseconds)

3. **Types of ERG**
   - **Maximal response ERG:**
     - Reflects a combination of **cone and rod functions**
     - Dark adaptation
     - Bright flash stimulus

- **Dark adapted ERG:**
  - Reflects **rod** function
  - Dark adaptation (for 20 to 30 minutes)
  - Low intensity blue flash or low intensity white flash stimulus
  - Absent/minimal A-wave
- **Light adapted ERG:**
  - Reflects **cone** function
  - Light adaptation (for 10 minutes)
  - Bright flash stimulus
  - Waveform amplitude is about 30% smaller
- **Flicker ERG:**
  - Reflects **cone** function
  - Light adaptation
  - Flicker 30 Hz stimulus
- **Focal ERG (FERG):**
  - ERG evoked by a small focal stimulus
  - Retina is bleached by background light
  - Focal stimulus applied on to retina
  - Usually only **cone** function at **macula** can be assessed easily
- **Pattern ERG (PERG):**
  - Reflects **ganglion** cell layer function
  - Stimulus is a pattern reversal checkerboard
  - May have applications in **glaucoma** and **optic nerve disease**

Q Tell me about the Electrooculogram.

Electrooculogram (EOG)

1. **Principle**
   - Measures standing potential between electrically **positive cornea** and **negative retina/RPE**
   - Exposure to light causes a **rise** in standing potential (apical portion of RPE cells depolarize, giving rise to a positive wave seen on the EOG)

2. **Procedure**
   - Electrodes are placed on medial and lateral canthal area on either side of eye
   - The eye is made to perform saccades between two points about 30° apart
   - The electrodes pick up **voltage differences** between front and back of the eye as it rotates back and forth

- Amplitude of voltage is recorded

3. **Interpretation**
   - Amplitude swings increase with light exposure and decrease in darkness:
     - The swings are expressed as light peak to dark trough ratio **(Arden ratio)**
     - Normal ratio = 1.65
   - Abnormal ratio reflects widespread **RPE abnormality:**
     - EOG generally parallels ERG readings in assessing **rod** function. However, EOG cannot assess cone function well
     - Most useful in **Best's disease** (EOG light rise is absent but ERG is normal)

Visual Evoked Potential (VEP)

1. **Principle**
   - Measures the potentials generated at **occipital lobe** by visual stimuli
   - Primarily the **foveal areas** are represented at superficial part of occipital lobe where the potential is measured
   - Abnormalities of the VEP are caused by lesions anywhere between photoreceptor and occipital lobe

2. **Procedure**
   - Stimulus:
     - Flash (variable response, useful in opaque media)
     - Pattern reversal (reversing checks or stripes, generates maximal cortical activity)
     - Amplitude of voltage is recorded

3. **Interpretation**
   - Waveform:
     - Extremely variable in size and shape. Amplitude may vary
     - Relatively constant positive waveform occurs at 100 millisecond (**P100 wave**)
     - The P100 latency is therefore the most useful clinical indicator

4. **Clinical indications**
   - VEP acuity (decrease checkerboard size until VEP approaches zero)
   - Optic nerve disease (increased latency/decreased amplitude to flash or pattern VEP)
   - Fovea or macular disease (increased latency/decreased amplitude to pattern VEP)
   - Amblyopia (increased latency/decreased amplitude to pattern VEP)
   - Malingering (should be normal)

AGE-RELATED MACULAR DEGENERATION

Overall yield: ✪✪✪✪✪   **Clinical exam:** ✪✪✪✪   **Viva:** ✪✪✪   **Essay:** ✪✪✪   **MCQ:** ✪✪✪✪

Q Opening Question: What is Age-Related Macular Degeneration (AMD)?

"Age-related macular degeneration refers to a spectrum of disease associated with…."
"The pathogenesis is poorly understood, but the risk factors include…."
"There are two classic forms of AMD…."

Age-Related Macular Degeneration

1. **Definition**
   - Spectrum of disease
   - Visual loss, RPE changes, drusens, geographical atrophy of retina, choroidal neovascularization (CNV)
   - Usually in persons aged 50 years or above
   - Drusens alone without visual loss is not considered AMD

2. **Pathogenesis**
   - Multifactorial etiology:
     - Genetic predisposition, racial patterns
     - Environmental risk factors:
       - Smoking
       - HPT, cardiovascular disease
       - UV exposure
   - Initial changes include RPE dysfunction, followed by deposition of drusens, thickening of Bruch's membrane and RPE atrophy

   - Later, PED occurs and CNV follows (sequence here is unclear)

3. **Classification**
   - Early AMD:
     - Drusens
     - +/– RPE changes
   - Late AMD:
     - Geographic atrophy (dry AMD):
       - Extensive RPE atrophy
     - Exudative AMD (wet AMD):
       - Classic/occult CNV
       - Pigment epithelial detachment
       - Subretinal hemorrhage
       - Vitreous hemorrhage
       - Disciform scar
       - Massive exudation (intra/subretinal)

Exam tips:
- **The definition of AMD is important but usually poorly answered.**

Q What are Drusens?

"Drusens are lipid-like materials deposited in...."

Drusens

1. Definition and pathology
- Lipid-like/lipofuscin material deposited in Bruch's membrane (between basement membrane of RPE and inner collagen layer)

2. Types
- Hard drusens
- Soft drusens
- Confluent drusens
- Calcified drusens

- Nodular drusens (younger onset, may have family history)

3. Risk of AMD
- Size of drusens
- Type of drusens:
  - Hard drusens → nonexudative AMD
  - Soft/confluent drusens → exudative AMD
- Family history of AMD
- Fellow eye has AMD

Q What are the Causes of CNV?

"The commonest cause of CNV is AMD, but other causes include...."

CNV

1. Definition
- Proliferation of fibrovascular lesions from choriocapillaris through defects in Bruch's membrane into subretinal space

2. Causes
- Degenerative:
  - AMD
  - Pathological myopia
- Others (optic disc drusen, angioid streaks)
- Inflammatory disease:
  - POHS (presumed ocular histoplasmosis syndrome)
  - Posterior uveitis (toxoplasmosis, Vogt-Koyanagi-Harada syndrome)
- Traumatic (choroidal rupture, laser photocoagulation)
- Tumor (choroidal nevus, choroidal hemangioma)

Exam tips:
- There are a number of possible scenarios. If drusens are seen, it is important to exclude CNV. If a disciform scar is seen, it is important to not only consider AMD, but myopic degeneration and trauma as well.

Clinical approach to AMD/subretinal hemorrhage

"On examination of this patient's fundus...."
"The most obvious lesion is at the macula where a large subretinal hemorrhage/disciform scar about 2 disc diameter in size is seen."

Look for
- Drusens (AMD)
- Tessellated fundus, peripapillary atrophy (myopic degeneration)
- Rare causes of CNV:
  - Optic disc drusen, angioid streaks, choroidal nevus
  - Iatrogenic (excessive laser photocoagulation)
- Other eye:
  - Bilateral drusens, disciform scar (Likely CNV)
  - Normal fellow eye (likely PCV)

(Continued)

I'll like to
- *Check VA*
- *Perform a FFA to delineate site of leakage from CNV, and ICG to determine presence of polyps*

Q **What are the FFA Changes in AMD?**

FFA Changes in AMD

1. **Early AMD**
   - Drusens:
     - Autofluorescence on red-free photograph
     - Staining
     - Can be hypo- or hyperfluorescent
   - RPE atrophy:
     - Window defects

2. **Late AMD**
   - Geographic atrophy:
     - Window defects
   - Exudative AMD:
     - Pigment epithelial detachment (PED):
       - Pooling
       - RPE tear: Window defects, hypofluorescence (masking)
     - CNV:
       - Leaking
       - Hemorrhage: Blocked fluorescence

   - Scars: Staining

3. **MPS definition ("How is classic and occult CNV defined in MPS?")**
   - **"Classic" CNV** — well defined CNV occurring early in the course of FFA:
     - Extrafoveal (> 200 microns from foveola/FAZ)
     - Juxtafoveal (< 200 microns from foveola/FAZ but not involving center itself)
     - Subfoveal (encroaching into center of foveola/FAZ)
   - **"Occult" CNV** — 2 basic patterns:
     - Fibrovascular PED (irregular elevation of RPE fills more slowly than classic CNV)
     - Late leakage of undetermined source (region of hyperfluorescence at the level of RPE, best appreciated in late phases, without the features of classic CNV in the early phases)

Notes

Classification of occult CNV by ICG (*Ophthalmology* 1996;103:2054–2060)
- Hot spots (< 1 DD):
  - Second most common
  - Can be treated by laser
- Plaques (> 1 DD):
  - Most common
  - Poor natural history
- Combination of hot spots and plaques:
  - Rare

Q **What are the Results of the Macular Photocoagulation Study (MPS)?**

"The MPS is a multicenter randomized clinical trial to evaluate the effectiveness of...."

MPS

1. **Hypothesis: "Is argon laser photocoagulation effective in preventing severe visual loss in eye with...."**
   - Extrafoveal CNV (*Arch Ophthalmol* 1982;100:192–198)
   - Juxtafoveal CNV (*Arch Ophthalmol* 1990;108:825–831)
   - Subfoveal CNV (*Arch Ophthalmol* 1991;109:1220–1231)

2. **Treatment**
   - Argon laser photocoagulation vs no treatment

3. **Outcome**
   - SVL (severe visual loss) defined as loss of six lines or more of VA
4. **Results**
   - Extrafoveal: 45% SVL (laser) vs 64% SVL (no laser) at 5 years
   - Juxtafoveal: 47% SVL (laser) vs 58% SVL (no laser) at 3 years

- Subfoveal:
  - No prior laser: 20% SVL (laser) vs 37% SVL (no laser) at 2 years
  - Recurrent CNV: 9% SVL (laser) vs 37% SVL (no laser) at 2 years
5. **Conclusion**
   - Laser beneficial in all types of classic CNV
   - SVL occurs in both treated and untreated cases
   - Risk of immediate decrease in VA following treatment

Notes

Relative indications for PDT
- PCV
- Myopic CNV
- Small classic CNV
- CNV associated with POHS
- Chronic CSR
- Hemangiomas
- When anti-VEGF contraindicated

Q **What is the Role of PDT in Exudative AMD?**

"Verteporfin is an intravenous photosensitizer which is activated by a diode laser source...."
"With the introduction of anti-VEGF, the use of PDT is less common...."

1. **Mechanism of action**
   - Selectively damages CNV by:
     - Preferential localization to CNV (complexes with LDL and CNV has increased LDL receptors)
     - Irradiation confined to CNV
   - Light activation causes free radical release, endothelial cell damage and thrombus formation
2. **Clinical trials**
   - Treatment of AMD with photodynamic therapy (TAP) study
     - Inclusion criteria:
       - Subfoveal, classic/predominantly classic CNV, ≤ 5400 μm
       - VA between 6/12 and 6/60
     - Treatment groups: PDT vs placebo
     - Main outcome measures: Stable (<15 logMAR letters lost) or improved vision
     - Results:
       - Stable/improved vision at 12 months: 61% treated, 46% placebo (*Arch Ophthalmol* 1999;117:1161–1173)
       - Stable/improved vision at 24 months: 53% treated, 38% placebo (*Arch Ophthalmol* 2001;119:198–207)

   - Results better for pure classic CNV compared to predominantly classic CNV
   - Verteporfin also shown to be effective in:
     - Pure occult CNV: Verteporfin in Photodynamic Therapy (VIP) study
     - Minimally classic CNV: Verteporfin in Minimally Classic CNV (VIM) study
     - CNV associated with pathological myopia: VIP study
3. **Treatment regime**
   - Intravenous verteporfin (6 mg/kg body weight) infused over 10 minutes
   - After five minutes, lesion treated with diode laser for 83 seconds
   - Patient reviewed every three months, treatment repeated if there is persistent or new leakage
4. **Complications**
   - Ocular:
     - Hemorrhage from CNV
     - RPE rip
   - Systemic:
     - Pain at injection site
     - Photosensitivity
     - Low back pain

"Anti-VEGF is the established treatment for exudative AMD…."
"The optimal treatment regime is still being evaluated…."

1. **Mechanism of VEGF**
   - VEGF is an important mediator in the pathogenesis of exudative AMD
   - It stimulates angiogenesis and the development of CNV, and also promotes vascular leakage

2. **Anti-VEGF antibodies used in the treatment of exudative AMD**
   - Ranibizumab (Lucentis): Recombinant, humanized murine antigen-binding fragment. Approved by the FDA for the treatment of exudative AMD
   - Bevacizumab (Avastin): Humanized, full-length monoclonal antibody. Off-label use in the treatment of exudative AMD
   - Pegaptanib (Macugen): Aptamer that binds and inhibits only the extracellular isoforms of VEGF

3. **Which lesions should be treated?**
   - All major CNV subtypes (predominantly classic, minimally classic, occult) in subfoveal and juxtafoveal location
   - "Active" disease:
     - Retinal thickening
     - Intraretinal/subretinal hemorrhage
     - New/persistent leakage on FFA
     - Enlargement of CNV size on FFA
     - Worsening VA
   - Any baseline VA

   - Serous PED, retinal angiomatous proliferation (RAP), PCV: Can be considered for treatment but detailed evidence not available

4. **Treatment regime**
   - Loading dose of monthly injections for 3 months (ANCHOR and MARINA trials)
   - Maintenance dose (controversial):
     - Monthly: MARINA and ANCHOR trials (evidence for best VA outcomes)
     - 3-Monthly: Initial VA improvement not maintained
     - Individualized
   - Can be combined with PDT or IVTA (combination therapy)

5. **Outcomes (ANCHOR and MARINA)**
   - Gain of 15+ ETDRS letters: 33–40% 0.5 mg Lucentis vs 4–9% sham
   - Loss of < 15 ETDRS letters: ~ 95% 0.5 mg Lucentis vs 62–64% sham

6. **Complications**
   - Ocular:
     - Retinal detachment
     - Vitreous hemorrhage
     - Uveitis
     - Endophthalmitis
     - RPE rip
   - Systemic (uncommon):
     - Stroke, myocardial infarction

Notes
- "What is the natural history of exudative AMD if left untreated?"
  - Four lines lost over 24 months
  - Three lines lost over 12 months
  - Two lines lost over 6 months
  - One line lost over 3 months

"Management of AMD must be individualized to the patient and depends on the **type** and **severity** of AMD and the amount of **visual disability** and **visual requirements** of the patient."
"If the patient has the nonexudative type of AMD, there is no…." "On the other hand, if the patient has exudative type of AMD, I will consider….."

Management of AMD

1. **Early AMD and geographic atrophy**
   - No effective curative treatment
   - Stop smoking
   - High levels of antioxidants (Vit C, Vit E, Vit A), zinc and copper reduce progression to advanced AMD and vision loss: Age-Related Eye Disease Study (AREDS)
     - High levels of beta-carotene increases risk of lung cancer in smokers
   - Reassure patient that total blindness rarely occurs
   - Follow-up patient with Amsler grid monitoring
   - Monitor fellow eye
   - Low vision aid if necessary

2. **Exudative AMD**
   - FFA to detect and localize CNV
   - Treatment would depend on:
     - Location of CNV
     - Duration of symptoms
     - Presence of "active" disease
     - Presence of scarring
   - Extrafoveal CNV: Direct laser
   - Juxtafoveal and subfoveal CNV:
     - Offer monthly injections of intravitreal anti-VEGF for at least three months
     - Offer combination therapy with PDT if PCV is present
   - No proven benefit in treating disciform scar. Long-term follow-up required
   - **20%** risk to fellow eye in three years

Exam tips:
- Give a short concise answer, be as conservative as possible, and lead the examiner to ask you about a topic you know well.

Notes
- "How do you monitor a patient with exudative AMD?"
  - Visual symptoms
  - Visual acuity
  - New hemorrhages/exudation
  - OCT
  - Repeat FFA/ICG when new signs/symptoms occur

Q How do you Administer an Intravitreal Injection?

"I would administer intravitreal injections under aseptic conditions...."

1. Topical anesthesia
2. Clean and drape patient
3. Lid speculum
4. ½ strength iodine to sterilize eye
5. (Optional) Subconjunctival lignocaine
6. Measure and mark injection site with calipers:
   - Pseudophakic: 3 mm behind limbus
   - Phakic: 4 mm behind limbus
7. Administer intravitreal injection at marked injection site with 27G–30G needle
8. Withdraw needle and apply pressure at injection site with sterile cotton bud
9. Check that patient has at least "Counting Fingers" vision post-injection
10. (Optional) Check IOP
11. Prescribe topical antibiotics for a week after the injection
12. Warn the patient of risk of:
    - Endophthalmitis: Red eyes, pain, blurring of vision
    - Retinal detachment: Floaters, flashes, visual field defects

Q What is Polypoidal Choroidal Vasculopathy (PCV)?

"PCV is an abnormality of the inner choroidal vessels…."
"It typically affects darker-skinned races such as Asians and African Americans…."

1. **Pathogenesis**
   - Etiology is idiopathic, but similar genetic mutations are associated with PCV and AMD
   - Dilated network consisting of multiple terminal aneurysmal protuberances in a polypoidal configuration
   - Predilection for macular and peripapillary areas

2. **Signs**
   - Orange nodules may be visible
   - Serosanguinous maculopathy
   - Vitreous hemorrhage and massive subretinal/sub-RPE bleeds more common than CNV associated with AMD

3. **ICG findings**
   - Large choroidal vascular network associated with localized terminal polyp-like bulbs
   - "Bunch of grapes"

4. **Treatment**
   - Extrafoveal: Direct laser
   - Juxtafoveal and subfoveal:
     - PDT
     - Anti-VEGF
     - Combination therapy

Q What is Retinal Angiomatous Proliferation (RAP)?

"RAP is an uncommon cause of exudative AMD, in which the abnormal vessels arise from the retinal vasculature rather than the choriocapillaris."

1. **Pathogenesis**
   - Etiology is idiopathic but thought to be age-related
   - Angiomatous proliferation originates from the retina and extends posteriorly into the subretinal space, eventually intersecting, in some cases, with choroidal new vessels

2. **Signs**
   - Similar to AMD
   - Patients tend to be older than patients with CNV

3. **Stages**
   - Stage I: Intraretinal neovascularization
   - Stage II: Subretinal neovascularization
   - Stage III: CNV

4. **Angiography**
   - FFA: Indistinct leaking simulating occult CNV
   - ICG: Hot spot in mid or late frames
     - CSLO-ICGA: Hot spot appears after, instead of before, retinal artery filling

5. **Treatment**
   - Anti-VEGF
   - PDT with adjunctive triamcinolone/anecortave may be successful
   - Conventional laser photocoagulation often disappointing
   - Experimental: Surgical excision of feeder artery and draining vein

6. **Prognosis**
   - Aggressive course and poorer prognosis

TOPIC 6

OTHER MACULAR DISEASES

Overall yield: ✸✸✸✸✸ **Clinical exam:** ✸✸✸✸ **Viva:** ✸✸✸ **Essay:** ✸✸✸ **MCQ:** ✸✸✸✸

Q **Opening Question:** Tell me about Pathological Myopia.

"Degenerative or pathological myopia is defined as a progressive form of severe myopia."
"Usually in patients with axial length of > **26 mm**."
"It may be an isolated anomaly or associated with…."

Pathological Myopia

1. **Associations**
   - **Ocular:**
     - ROP
     - Congenital glaucoma
     - Albinism, congenital stationary night blindness
     - Ectopic lentis
     - RP
     - Wagner's syndrome
   - **Systemic association:**
     - Marfan's, Stickler's, Ehlers-Danlos syndrome
     - Down's syndrome
     - Alport's syndrome

2. **Problems**
   - Higher risk of *nuclear sclerosis* cataract and POAG
   - Myopic macular degeneration, CNV, macular hole
   - Retinal breaks and RD

  Clinical approach to myopic fundus

"On examination of this patient's fundus…."

Describe
- Tessellated fundus, chorioretinal atrophy
- Tilted disc, peripapillary atrophy
- Posterior staphyloma
- Lacquer cracks
- CNV
- Foster Fuch's spots (old subretinal hemorrhage and pigmentation)
- Related complications
  - Macular changes
  - Macular hole
  - Lattice degeneration, retinal breaks, RD

I'll like to
- Examine the anterior segment for cataract
- Check the IOP for POAG

Exam tips:
- Also refer to "What are the potential problems with high myopia?" (page 27).

Q How does Atropine Affect Myopia Progression?

"Atropine has been shown to be effective in reducing myopia progression."
"It is generally well-tolerated, but the ocular and systemic side effects
may be bothersome in some children."

Atropine and Myopia Progression

- Atropine reduces childhood myopia progression and axial elongation
  - Atropine in the Treatment of Myopia (ATOM) study (*Ophthalmology* 2006;113:2285–2291)
- After cessation of treatment, eyes treated with atropine demonstrated higher rates of myopia progression compared with eyes treated with placebo
  - However, the absolute myopia progression after three years was significantly lower in the atropine group compared with placebo

- Side effects of atropine:
  - Ocular:
    - Poor near vision
    - Photophobia
    - Conjunctival irritation
    - Long-term side effects of pupillary dilatation (e.g. retinal phototoxicity, early cataract formation) unknown
  - Systemic (rare):
    - Hypotension, arrhythmias
    - Dry mouth, abdominal distension
    - Respiratory depression
    - Confusion, hallucinations, drowsiness

Q What is an Epiretinal Membrane?

"Epiretinal membrane (ERM) is a common acquired maculopathy...."
"It may be idiopathic or associated with...."

Epiretinal Membrane

1. **Pathogenesis**
   - Histology: Fibro-cellular layer with varying degrees of cellularity (retinal glial cells, astrocytes, hyalocytes, fibrocytes, myofibrocytes)
   - Pathogenesis: **PVD** → vitreomacular traction → dehiscence of internal limiting membrane at the macular → migration and proliferation of cells → epiretinal membrane → contraction of membrane → macular pucker

2. **Classification**
   - Idiopathic:
     - Age-related
     - Up to 20% bilateral
   - Secondary associations:
     - Vascular disease (diabetic retinopathy, CRVO)
     - Inflammatory disease (posterior uveitis)
     - Trauma
     - Retinal surgery (RD surgery, laser photocoagulation, cryotherapy)

Clinical approach to ERM

"On examination of this patient's fundus, the most obvious lesion is at the macula...."
"There is a translucent membrane seen, associated with tortuosity of surrounding retinal vessels."
"This patient has an epiretinal membrane...."
"On examination of the rest of the retina, there is evidence/no evidence of:"

Look for
- *Diabetic retinopathy*
- *Retinal vein occlusion*
- *Retinal detachment*
- *Photocoagulation or cryotherapy scars*
- *Retinitis pigmentosa*
- *Choroiditis (POHS, white dot syndromes)*

I'll like to
- *Examine fellow eye — bilateral in 20%*

I'll like to ask for this patient's
- *VA*
- *Duration of poor vision*
- *Visual requirements*

Q **How Would You Manage a Patient with ERM?**

"The management must be individualized...."
"Factors to consider are...."

Management of ERM

1. **Factors affecting management:**
   - Patient factors:
     - Age of patient
     - Duration of visual loss
     - Visual requirements
   - Ocular factors:
     - VA
     - Well-defined ERM edge
     - Associated CME

2. **Indications for surgery (vitrectomy and membrane peeling) include:**
   - High visual requirements (occupation, young age)
   - Duration of visual loss < 6 months
   - VA < 20/60
   - Well-defined ERM edge
   - No associated CME

3. **Complications of surgery:**
   - Recurrence of ERM
   - Progression of cataract
   - Iatrogenic breaks/RD
   - VH
   - Endophthalmitis

"Macular holes are common acquired maculopathies…."
"They can be idiopathic or associated with…."

Macular Hole

1. **Pathogenesis:**
   - Pathogenesis: Cellular infiltration of internal limiting membrane/posterior hyaloid face of vitreous → tangential vitreomacular traction → occult macular hole → secondary contraction → fully developed macular hole → **PVD**

2. **Classification:**
   - Idiopathic:
     - Age-related
     - Post-menopausal women
     - Up to 20% bilateral
   - Secondary associations:
     - High myopia
     - Trauma
     - Solar retinopathy

3. **Stages (Gass's macular hole classification):**
   - Stage 1a (**impending** macular hole):
     - Absent foveal reflex
       - Yellow spot seen at foveola (xanthophyll), intrafoveal cyst
   - Stage 1b (**occult** macular hole):
     - Centrifugal displacement of foveolar retina and xanthophylls
     - Characterized by yellow ring
     - Decrease in visual acuity and metamorphopsia
     - ~ 50% of Stage 1 holes resolve spontaneously
   - Stage 2 (**early** macular hole)
     - Enlargement of yellow ring
     - <400 micron in size
   - Stage 3 (**fully** developed macular hole):
     - Punched out area surrounded by rim of subretinal fluid
     - Yellow deposits within hole
     - >400 micron in size
   - Stage 4 (macular hole associated with **PVD**):
     - >400 micron in size
     - Associated with PVD

Clinical approach to macular hole

"There is a full thickness round punched out defect sees at the fovea."
"With a rim of subretinal fluid surrounding the lesion."

Look for
- ERM
- Myopic fundus
- Retinal detachment
- Weiss ring (PVD)

I'll like to
- Examine the fellow eye — bilateral in 20%

I'll like to ask patient for
- A history of trauma or solar exposure
- VA (If < 20/200 → usually means Stage 3 or 4 hole)
- Duration of decreased VA

Exam tips:
- The pathogenesis and management of the macular hole and epiretinal membrane are almost identical but the pathogenesis sequence is different. PVD occurs early in the course of epiretinal membrane, but is a late event in the macular hole.

> **Notes**
> - Why macular?
>   - Macula is thin
>   - Macula is avascular
>   - Increased vitreoretinal traction at this location

> **Notes**
> Diagnostic tests for macular hole:
> - Watzke-Allen test
> - Laser beam aiming test
> - OCT
> - FFA

Q How Would You Manage this Patient with a Macular Hole?

"The management must be individualized...."
"Factors to consider are...."

Management of Macular Hole

1. **Factors affecting management:**
   - Patient factors:
     - Age of patient
     - Duration of visual loss
     - Visual requirements
   - Ocular factors:
     - VA
     - Etiology of macular hole
     - Stage of macular hole
     - Associated RD

2. **Macular hole not associated with RD:**
   - Full thickness macular hole:
     - **Conservative treatment if:**
       - Elderly
       - > 1 year duration of visual loss
       - Low visual need

     - Good VA in fellow eye
   - Surgical treatment if:
     - Young
     - Recent onset of visual loss
     - High visual needs
     - Poor VA in fellow eye
       - Principles of surgery: Vitrectomy/gas exchange/laser/posture
   - **Partial thickness** macular hole:
     - Conservative treatment will usually suffice
       - Follow up patient with Amsler grid monitoring

3. **Macular hole associated with RD:**
   - Need to look for peripheral retinal breaks
   - Not common in idiopathic type of macular hole (usually traumatic and myopic types)

Q What is Central Serous Retinopathy (CSR)?

"Central serous retinopathy is a common acquired macular disorder...."
"High risk groups include...."

Central Serous Retinopathy (CSR)

1. **Pathogenesis:**
   - Choroidal vascular abnormalities (including increased permeability of choriocapillaris) and RPE pump dysfunction/reversal of RPE pump → breakdown of outer blood retinal barrier → accumulation of subretinal fluid → CSR

2. **Classification:**
   - Idiopathic:
     - Young
     - Males
     - Type-A personality, psychiatric disorders
     - High serum epinephrine level
     - Associated with steroid consumption

3. **Secondary associations:**
   - Optic disc pit
   - Optic disc coloboma
4. **Choroidal tumor clinical presentation:**
   - Patient presents with blurred vision, relative scotoma, **micropsia** and metamorphopsia
   - VA moderately reduced (20/30 to 20/40), correctable with **weak plus lens**
   - Serous RD
     - "Blister"-like localized detachment
   - May be associated with:
     - PED
     - Subretinal precipitates
     - RPE atrophic changes
     - "Pseudo" RP changes
     - CNV
5. **FFA:**
   - Classic "**smoke stack**" pattern (10–20% of cases)
   - "**Ink blot**" pattern (80–90% of cases)
   - Others:
     - PED
     - RPE window defect
     - Extramacular RPE atrophic tract

- RPE window defect in fellow eye (indicates previous subclinical CSR in that eye)
6. **Management:**
   - Prognosis:
     - 60% spontaneous resolution in three months
     - 80% spontaneous resolution in six months
     - Near 100% within one year
     - Minority will have chronic course with decreased VA
   - Recurrence:
     - 40% of all cases
   - "What are indications for laser photocoagulation?"
     - High visual requirements
     - Persistent leakage beyond six months
     - Recurrent CSR with decreased VA after each attack
     - Fellow eye with CSR associated with decreased VA
   - "Does laser work?"
     - Laser **speeds up** resolution, but does not alter:
       · Final VA
       · Recurrence rate
       · Risk of chronicity

Q **Tell me about Cystoid Macular Edema.**

"Cystoid macular edema is a condition in which fluid accumulates within the retina (outer plexiform and inner nuclear layers) in the macula region."

Cystoid Macular Edema

1. **Pathogenesis:**
   - Breakdown of the blood-retinal barrier → leakage of fluid → formation of cystoid spaces
   - Inflammatory mediators and mechanical factors may play a role
2. **Investigations:**
   - OCT: Intraretinal thickening with cystoid spaces
   - FFA: "Petaloid" pattern of leakage in macula
3. **Causes and treatment:**
   - Retinal vascular disease (DR, CRVO etc)
     - Treatment: Laser photocoagulation (not for CRVO), intravitreal anti-VEGF and steroids

- Intraocular inflammation
  - Treatment: Immunosuppression, acetazolamide
- Post-surgery (Irvine-Gass)
  - Treatment: Acetazolamide, steroids (topical), NSAIDS (oral and topical), vitrectomy
- Drug-induced (adrenaline, latanoprost)
  - Treatment: Cessation of medication
- Vitreomacular traction and ERM
  - Treatment: Vitrectomy and relief of traction
- Others: Retinal dystrophies, tumors

DIABETIC RETINOPATHY

Overall yield: ✹ ✹ ✹   **Clinical exam:** ✹ ✹ ✹ ✹ ✹   **Viva:** ✹ ✹ ✹   **Essay:** ✹ ✹   **MCQ:** ✹ ✹ ✹

Q **Opening Question No. 1:** What are the Ocular Manifestations of DM?

"Diabetic retinopathy (DR) is the most important and common ocular complication."
"Other ocular manifestations can be classified into…."

Ocular Manifestations of DM

1. **Anterior segment:**
   - Cornea:
     - Corneal hypoesthesia (risk of neurotrophic keratitis)
     - Decrease corneal healing (risk of recurrent corneal erosion)
   - Iris and pupils:
     - Ectropion uvea
     - Increase pigment at angles
     - Difficulty in dilating pupils
     - Argyll Robertson pupils
   - Glaucoma:
     - POAG and neovascular glaucoma
   - Lens:
     - Cataract

2. **Posterior segment:**
   - DR
   - Retinal vascular occlusions
   - Asteroid hyalosis
   - Lipemia retinalis

3. **Neurological manifestations:**
   - CN palsies (classically pupil sparing III CN palsy)
   - Anterior ischemic optic neuropathy

4. **Others:**
   - Xanthelasma
   - Orbital mucormycosis

Exam tips:
- Listen carefully to the question; this question is related to "ocular manifestations of DM," not "ocular features of DR" (see next question).

Q **Opening Question No. 2:** What are the Ocular Features of DR?

DETAILED ANSWER

Diabetic Retinopathy

1. **Nonproliferative retinopathy (NPDR)**
   - Mild NPDR
     - Microaneurysm (one or more)
   - Moderate NPDR
     - Microaneurysm
     - Retinal hemorrhages (dot and blot)
     - Hard exudates
     - Cotton wool spots (CWS)
   - Venous beading
   - Arteriolar narrowing
   - Intra-retinal microvascular abnormalities (IRMA)
   - Severe NPDR (= preproliferative DR):
     - All of above plus any one of the following three (the famous **4:2:1** rule in ETDRS):
       - Blot hemorrhages in four quadrants

- Venous beading in two quadrants
- IRMA in one quadrant

2. Proliferative retinopathy (PDR)
- Early PDR:
  - New vessels at disc or within 1 DD of disc (NVD) or elsewhere (NVE)
- High risk PDR:
  - NVD greater than 1/4 disc diameter
  - NVD less than 1/4 disc diameter with vitreous hemorrhage
  - NVE greater than 1/2 disc diameter with vitreous hemorrhage

3. Macular edema
- Early macular edema:
  - Retinal thickening or hard exudates within 1 disc diameter from fovea
- Clinically significant macular edema (CSME):
  - Retinal thickening or edema less than 500 micron from fovea
  - Hard exudates less than 500 micron from fovea associated with retinal thickening
  - Retinal thickening greater than 1,500 micron in size, any part of which lies within 1,500 micron from fovea

VIVA ANSWER
"Diabetic retinopathy (DR) can be divided into two stages."
"And can occur with or without macular edema."

Diabetic Retinopathy

1. Nonproliferative retinopathy (NPDR)
- Microaneurysms, dot and blot hemorrhages, hard exudates
- Pre-proliferative stage (CWS, venous beading, arteriolar narrowing and IRMA)

2. Proliferative retinopathy (PDR)
- New vessels at the disc (NVD) or elsewhere (NVE)
- Vitreous hemorrhage, tractional RD and neovascular glaucoma

3. Maculopathy
- Exudative maculopathy
- Edematous maculopathy
- Ischemic maculopathy

Exam tips:
- The latest convention uses "nonproliferative vs proliferative" and NOT "background vs proliferative."
- The DETAILED answer is based on definitions used by DRS and ETDRS (page 189).
- The VIVA answer ignores these research definitions and is more useful from a clinical perspective.

 Clinical approach to diabetic retinopathy

"On examination of this patient's fundus, there are…"
"Diffuse dot and blot hemorrhages seen in four quadrants."
"Associated with scattered hard exudates, cotton wool spots and venous tortuosity."

Look for
- *Disc new vessels (NVD)*
- *New vessels at arcades (NVE)*
- *Macular edema and thickening*
  (I'll like to confirm the macular edema by further examination using a 78D lens at the slit lamp)

"This patient has: Mild NPDR, severe NPDR or proliferative DR and/or CSME."

(Continued)

(Continued)

I'll like to

- *Check fellow eye*
- *Examine anterior segment for cataract and rubeosis iridis*
- *Check IOP and perform gonioscopy (rubeosis at angles)*
- *Ask for associated risk factors for progression (DM control, DM complications like nephropathy and neuropathy and HPT)*

Follow-up question: "How would you manage this patient?" (page 188)

Q   When is FFA Useful in the Diagnosis of DR?

"FFA is not routinely indicated in the diagnosis of DR and macular edema."

Indications for FFA

1. **Diagnosis:**
   - Ischemic maculopathy
   - Areas of capillary nonperfusion
   - Differentiate new vessels from IRMA

2. **Aid in treatment:**
   - Delineate fovea and fovea avascular zone
   - Delineate area of leakage

Notes

- "What are the causes of visual loss from diabetic retinopathy?"
  - Diabetic macular edema
  - Ischemic maculopathy
  - Consequences of neovascularization (VH, TRD)

Q   What are the Risk Factors for Developing Retinopathy in a Patient with DM?

Risk Factors for Developing DR

1. Increased duration of DM
2. Poor metabolic control
3. Hypertension
4. Nephropathy
5. Pregnancy
6. Others: Smoking, obesity, hyperlipidemia, anemia

MANAGEMENT OF DIABETIC RETINOPATHY

Overall yield: ✹✹✹✹✹ Clinical exam: ✹✹✹✹✹ Viva: ✹✹✹✹✹ Essay: ✹✹✹ MCQ: ✹✹✹✹✹

Q Opening Question No. 1: How do You Manage a Patient with DR?

DETAILED ANSWER

Summary of DRS and ETDRS Definitions and Treatment

Definition	Criteria	Treatment
Mild NPDR	• 1 microaneurysm	• Observe (ETDRS)
Moderate NPDR	• Microaneurysm, hard exudates, hemorrhages, cotton wool spots, etc (not meeting criteria below)	• Observe (ETDRS)
Severe NPDR (Preproliferative)	• Blot hemorrhages in four quadrants • Venous bead in two quadrants • IRMA in one quadrant	• PRP (ETDRS)
Early PDR	• NVD or NVE (not fulfilling criteria below)	• PRP (ETDRS)
High risk PDR	• NVD > ¼ disc diameter • NVD < ¼ disc diameter with VH • NVE > ½ disc diameter with VH	• PRP (DRS)
Advanced PDR and VH	• High risk PDR with tractional RD involving macular or with VH	• Early vitrectomy for Type I DM (DRVS)
Macular edema	• Retinal thickening or **hard exudates** within 1 disc diameter from fovea	• Observed at 6-monthly intervals (ETDRS)
CSME	• Retinal edema < 500 micron from fovea • Hard exudates < 500 micron from fovea with adjacent retinal thickening • Retinal edema > 1,500 micron, any part of which is within 1,500 micron from fovea	• Focal/grid laser (ETDRS)

Exam tips:
• The DETAILED answer is for your information, based on treatment guidelines used by DRS and ETDRS. It is not wise to start talking about the multicenter studies at this stage.
• The VIVA answer ignores these research definitions, summarizes the main problems and gives the examiner the impression that you know the issues, have thought through the results of the trials, and are now applying it for patients in your clinical practice!

VIVA ANSWER

"The management of DR involves an assessment of the risk of progression...."
"Management depends on the stage of DR and the presence or absence of macular edema."

Management of DR

1. **Assess risk of progression of disease and control high risk factors**
   - Joint management with family physician or endocrinologists
   - Ensure good DM control
   - Treat associated systemic disease (e.g. HPT, DM, hyperlipidemia)

2. **Mild NPDR**
   - Follow-up patient and watch for progression and macular edema

3. **Severe NPDR**
   - Follow up patient very closely
   - In my practice, I would consider **scatter PRP** if:
     - Patient is a young insulin dependent diabetic (IDDM)
     - Patient has poor DM control with associated DM complications (nephropathy)
     - Fellow eye is blind from DR
     - Family history of blindness from DR
     - Poor patient compliance to follow-up

   - Prior to cataract operation or pregnancy

4. **Proliferative DR**
   - I would consider this an ocular emergency
   - I would perform full PRP immediately with 2,000–3,000 laser shots over 2–3 sittings
   - Watch patient very closely

5. **Macular edema**
   - I would perform macular laser (focal / grid) if there is clinically significant macular edema
   - I would follow-up the patient at 4-month intervals, and would repeat the macular laser if the edema is not resolved
   - In cases of persistent macular edema despite multiple laser attempts, I would consider administering intravitreal anti-VEGF or corticosteroids
   - If the macular edema is secondary to vitreomacular traction, I would offer the patient vitrectomy to relieve the traction

---

Q **What are the Major Clinical Trials in the Management of Diabetic Retinopathy?**

DRS (Diabetic Retinopathy Study) (*Ophthalmology* 1981;88:583–600 *Ophthalmology* 1987;94:739–760)

1. **Aim:** Assess effect of PRP on **PDR**. Determine if PRP reduces the incidence of severe visual loss (VA < 5/200)
2. **Inclusion criteria:** PDR in both eyes (1,758 patients)
3. **Treatment:** PRP in one eye vs no treatment in other eye
4. **Outcome:** SVL (severe visual loss) defined as VA < 5/200 on two follow-up visits
5. **Results:**
   - **50% decrease in rates of SVL** in treated eyes as compared with controls at five years
   - Eyes that benefited most from PRP were **high-risk PDR**
   - Complication of Argon laser (10% decrease in VA by one or more lines)
6. **Conclusion: Early PRP** recommended for **high risk PDR**

ETDRS (Early Treatment Diabetic Retinopathy Study) (*Arch Ophthalmol* 1985;88:583–600 *Ophthalmology* 1991;98:757; *Ophthalmology* 1991;98:766–785)

1. **Aims:**
   - Assess effect of PRP on DR and less than high-risk PDR
   - Assess effect of aspirin on preventing the progression of DR
   - Assess effect of macular laser on diabetic macular edema
2. **Inclusion criteria:** Mild DR to PDR (not meeting criteria for high-risk PDR) with or without macular edema in both eyes (3,711 patients). VA ≥ 20/200
3. **Treatment:**
   - PRP in one eye vs no treatment in other eye until high-risk PDR developed
   - Grid laser vs no treatment for macular edema
   - Aspirin vs placebo
4. **Outcome: MVL** (moderate visual loss) defined as doubling of visual angle, drop of 15 or more letters or three or more Snellen acuity lines

5. **Results:**
   - Efficacy of laser treatment on CSME — **50% decrease in rates of MVL** in treated eyes
   - Optimal timing of PRP:
     - PRP recommended for severe NPDR and early PDR (decreases incidence of developing high risk PDR)
     - Follow-up for mild or moderate NPDR
   - Aspirin treatment:
     - No effect on rates of progression
     - No effect on VA
     - No increased risk of VH
     - Not contraindicated for use in cardiovascular or medical conditions

DRVS (Diabetic Retinopathy Vitrectomy Study) (*Arch Ophthalmol* 1985;103:1644–1652; *Ophthalmology* 1988;95:1307–1320)

1. **Aim:** Assess effect of early vitrectomy on **advanced PDR and vitreous hemorrhage (VH)**

2. **Treatment:** Early vitrectomy vs late vitrectomy (1 year)

3. **Inclusion criteria:** VH or advanced PDR with useful vision (VA < 5/200)

4. **Outcome:** Percentages of eyes with 20/40 VA at 2 and 4 years

5. **Results:**
   - VH (in Type I DM, 36% recovered to 20/40 for early vitrectomy vs only 12% for late vitrectomy)
   - Advanced PDR with useful vision (44% recovered to 20/40 for early vitrectomy vs 28% for late vitrectomy)

6. **Conclusion: Early vitrectomy** recommended for vitreous hemorrhage and advanced PDR in **Type I DM**

DCCT (Diabetic Control and Complications Trial) (*New Engl J Med* 1993;329:977–986; *New Engl J Med* 2000;342:381–389)

1. **Aim:**
   - Primary prevention: Assess effect of tight glycemic control on **DM complications (nephropathy, neuropathy and DR)**
   - Secondary prevention: Assess effect of tight glycemic control on rate of progression of DM complications (nephropathy, neuropathy and DR)

2. **Treatment:** Tight glycemic control vs normal control

3. **Inclusion criteria:** Type I DM

4. **Outcome:**
   - Rates of onset or progressive DR from baseline
   - Rates of progression to high risk PDR
   - Rates of laser treatment

5. **Results:**
   - **Tight control delays onset and progression of DR**, neuropathy and nephropathy
   - Tight control lowers the onset of DR in the primary prevention group by 50% at five years
   - Tight control decreases the rate of progression of DR in the secondary prevention group by 50%
   - ~50% decrease in the development of severe NPDR, PDR and the need for PRP
   - Early worsening of DR in the first year of tight glycemic control. At least three years needed to demonstrate the beneficial effect of tight control
   - However, tight control increases severe hypoglycemia events by 2–3 times, and there is a 33% increased risk of becoming overweight

UKPDS (United Kingdom Prospective Diabetes Study)

1. **Aim:**
   - Assess effect of intensive glycemic control on the risk of microvascular complications of DM (including DR)
   - Assess effect of BP control in hypertensive patients on the risk of microvascular complications of DM (including DR)

2. **Treatment:**
   - Diet control vs intensive treatment with hypoglycemic agents
   - Tight vs less tight BP control

3. **Inclusion criteria:** Type 2 DM, with and without hypertension

4. **Outcome:** Progression of DR and other microvascular and macrovascular complications of DM

5. **Results:**
   - Intensive glycemic control slows the progression of DR and reduces the risk of other microvascular complications of DM
   - Tight BP control slows progression of DR and reduces the risk of other microvascular and macrovascular complications of DM

Exam tips:
- You must be fairly comfortable with the five major studies in DR over the past three decades.

Q What are the Indications for Laser PRP in Your Practice?

"While the DRS and ETDRS defined the ideal indications for PRP...."
"In my practice, I would consider PRP in the following patients if...."

Indications for PRP

1. **PRP for high-risk PDR**
2. **Consider PRP in cases of less than high-risk PDR:**
   - Early PDR (any NVD or NVE)
   - Severe NPDR
   - Ischemic NPDR (FFA indicates ischemia)
   - In my practice, I would consider **scatter PRP** for these cases, especially if:
     - Patient is a young insulin dependent diabetic (IDDM)

- Patient has poor DM control with associated DM complications (nephropathy)
- Fellow eye is blind from DR
- Family history of blindness from DR
- Poor patient compliance to follow-up
- Prior to cataract operation or pregnancy

Exam tips:
- This is an opportunity to show that you have developed your own approach based on practice guidelines.

Q How do You Perform PRP?

"I would elect to perform fractionated PRP with an aim of between 2,000–3,000 laser shots in patients with PDR, divided over 2 to 3 laser sessions."

Procedure for PRP

1. **I would use the following:**
   - Contact lens: Mainster wide field
   - Laser type: Argon blue-green laser
   - Laser settings: 200 µm size, 0.18 s, 0.18 W
2. **I would first instill topical LA, position patient, fixation target**

3. **The laser is then performed:**
   - Mark vascular arcades with two rows of laser
   - Start on inferior fundus
   - Avoid disc, macular, vessels, fibrovascular membranes and areas with vitreoretinal traction
   - Target: Gray-white burns
4. **Follow-up patient within next week for top-up PRP**

Q What are the Signs that DR is Less Active Post-PRP?

Post-PRP Changes

1. **Regression of new vessels and increased fibrosis**
2. **Vessel attenuation**
3. **Resolution of retinal hemorrhages**
4. **Disc pallor**

Complications

1. **Early:**
   - Iris burns
   - Macular burns
   - Retinal tears
   - VH
   - CME
   - Choroidal detachment
   - Malignant glaucoma

2. **Late:**
   - Loss of VA of one line (11%) and two lines (3%)
   - VF defects
   - Deterioration of night vision and color vision
   - Tractional RD
   - ERM
   - CNV

Q How does PRP Work?

Mechanisms of PRP

1. **Decrease retinal demand for oxygen**
   - PRP destroys healthy peripheral retina, allowing diseased retinal vessels to deliver limited oxygen to remaining central retina

2. **Decrease release of angiogenic factors**
   - PRP decreases amount of hypoxic retina and therefore less angiogenic factors are released

3. **Mechanical inhibition of NV formation**
   - Scars contain new vessel growth

Q What are the Indications for Vitrectomy in DR?

"The common indications for vitrectomy include...."

Indications for Vitrectomy

1. **Common:**
   - Tractional RD involving macula
   - Combined tractional and rhegmatogenous RD
   - Persistent VH (more than 6 months for NIDDM, 3 months for IDDM)

2. **Less common:**
   - Progressive fibrovascular proliferation (especially anterior hyaloid fibrovascular proliferation)

   - Rubeosis with VH (preventing adequate PRP)
   - Dense premacular VH
   - Ghost cell glaucoma
   - Macular edema with macular traction
   - Significant recurrent VH despite maximal PRP

RETINAL ARTERY OCCLUSION

Overall yield: ✪✪✪   **Clinical exam:**   **Viva:** ✪✪✪   **Essay:** ✪✪   **MCQ:** ✪✪

Q **Opening Question No. 1:** What are the Causes of Retinal Artery Occlusion?

"Retinal artery occlusion can be caused by systemic or ocular conditions...."

Retinal Artery Occlusion

1. **Systemic**
   - Carotid emboli (most common cause of **BRAO**):
     - Cholesterol emboli (small size, causes Hollenhorst plaques in retinal arterioles)
     - Fibrinoplatelet emboli (medium size, causes transient ischemic attacks/amaurosis fugax)
     - Calcific emboli (large, causes CRAO or BRAO)
   - Cardiac emboli (most common cause in **young** patient with either BRAO or CRAO):
     - Thrombus (from myocardial infarct or mitral valve stenosis)
     - Calcific (from aortic valve)
     - Bacteria (from endocarditis)
     - Myxomatous (from atrial myxoma) – very rare

   - Vasculitis:
     - Giant cell arteritis
     - Systemic lupus, polyarteritis nodosa and others
   - Coagulation disorders: Protein C/S deficiencies, antithrombin-III deficiency, anti-phospholipid syndrome

2. **Ocular**
   - Raised IOP:
     - Retrobulbar hemorrhage during retrobulbar anesthesia
     - Orbital tumor, orbital inflammatory disease
     - RD surgery
     - Neurosurgery

> **Exam tips:**
> - **As a general rule, CRAO is caused by atherosclerosis of the carotid and retinal arteries, while BRAO is caused by an emboli.**

Q How do You Manage a Patient with CRAO?

"CRAO is an ocular emergency...."
"The acute treatment is aimed at restoring normal circulation as far as possible...."

Management of CRAO

1. **Clinical features:**
   - Acute decrease in VA (10% **bilateral**)
   - RAPD

   - "Cherry red spot" in white retina
     - Macular sparing due to macular perfusion from cilioretinal artery (20% of population)

- Isolated cilioretinal artery occlusion leads to macular infarct (rare)
- Attenuated retinal arterioles
- Optic disc pallor

2. **Acute management:**
   - Patient should lie flat
   - Patient given carbogen (mixture of 5% carbon dioxide and 95% oxygen)
   - Ocular massage for 15 minutes
   - Intravenous Diamox
   - Anterior chamber paracentesis
   - Other treatment options:
     - Intra-arterial fibrinolysis

- EAGLE study (*Graefe's Archive of Clinical and Experimental Ophthalmology* 2006; 244L:950–956): terminated due to adverse events)
- Retrobulbar tolazoline (to decrease retrobulbar resistance to flow)

3. **Manage systemic disease:**
   - **Mortality in 20%** over 5 years
     - Investigate and treat systemic disease
   - **Iris neovascularization in 20%** within 3 months (lower risk than CRVO)
     - But neovascular glaucoma <5%

Notes
- "What are the causes of "cherry red spot" in the macula?"
  - Acquired
    - CRAO
    - Macular hole
    - Commotio retinae
    - Drug (quinine toxicity)
  - Congenital
    - Niemann-Pick disease
    - Tay Sach's disease
    - Gangliosidoses

RETINAL VEIN OCCLUSION

Overall yield: ✹✹✹✹✹ **Clinical exam:** ✹✹✹✹✹ **Viva:** ✹✹✹ **Essay:** ✹✹ **MCQ:** ✹✹

Q Opening Question No. 1: What are the Causes of Vitreous Hemorrhage?

1. **Trauma is an important cause of VH**
2. **The most common nontraumatic causes are…**
   - Proliferative DR (50%)
   - BRVO/CRVO (10%)
   - RD, tears (10%)
   - CNV with breakthrough bleed (10%)
   - PVD (10%)

3. **Other less common causes include…**
   - Vascular diseases with ischemia
     - HPT, ocular ischemic syndrome
     - Eales disease
     - ROP/familial exudative vitreoretinopathy
     - Retinal telangiectasia
   - Inflammatory diseases with ischemia
   - Blood dyscrasias

Q Opening Question No. 2: What are the Features of Branch Retinal Vein Occlusion (BRVO)?

"BRVO is a common retinal vascular disease."
"The risk factors include…."

Branch Retinal Vein Occlusion

1. **Risk factors**
   - Systemic:
     - Age
     - HPT
     - Blood dyscrasias
   - Ocular:
     - Vasculitis (Behcet's syndrome, sarcoidosis)

2. **Classification**
   - Main BRVO:
     - At disc
     - Away from disc
   - Macular BRVO
   - Peripheral BRVO

3. **Sites (usually at AV crossing)**
   - Superotemporal (50%)
   - Inferotemporal (30%)
   - Hemispherical (15%)
   - Supero/inferonasal (5%)

4. **Clinical features**
   - Acute:
     - Dilated and tortuous veins, retinal hemorrhages, VH, cotton wool spots, disc swelling
   - Subacute:
     - Vascular sheathing and collaterals, CME
   - Chronic:
     - Pigmentary changes ("pseudo" retinitis pigmentosa), macular RPE changes and epiretinal membrane

5. **Prognosis and complications**
   - 50% of patients will have uncomplicated BRVO and recover to VA 20/40 or better
   - In the other 50%, one or more complications:
     - Macular edema (most common cause of persistent poor VA)

- Macular ischemia
- Combined macular edema and macular ischemia

- Neovascularization (40% of ischemic BRVO): 10% NVD; 20–30% NVE

Q Opening Question No. 3: What are the Features of Central Retinal Vein Occlusion (CRVO)?

"CRVO is a common retinal vascular disease."
"The risk factors include…."

Central Retinal Vein Occlusion

1. **Risk factors**
   - Systemic:
     - Age
     - HPT
     - Blood dyscrasias
   - Ocular:
     - Raised IOP
     - Hypermetropia
     - Congenital anomaly of central retinal vein
     - Vasculitis (Behcet's syndrome, sarcoidosis, AIDS, systemic lupus)

2. **Classification and clinical features**

	Ischemic	Nonischemic
Frequency	75%	25%
VA	20/400 or worse (90%)	Better than 20/400 (90%)
RAPD	Marked	Slight
VF defect	Common	Rare
Fundus findings	Extensive hemorrhages and cotton wool spots	Less extensive hemorrhages, few cotton wool spots
FFA	Widespread capillary non-perfusion	Good perfusion
ERG	Reduced "b"-wave amplitude Reduced "b:a" wave ratio	Normal
Prognosis	50% develop rubeosis and neovascular glaucoma in 3 months (**100 day glaucoma**) VA improves in 1/3, stable in 1/3, and deteriorates in 1/3	3% develop rubeosis and neovascular glaucoma while 50% return to VA of 20/40 or better Conversion to ischemic CRVO: 34% in 3 years

Exam tips:
- **The differentiation between ischemic and nonischemic CRVO is important.**

Clinical approach to BRVO/CRVO

"On examination of this patient's fundus, there are…."
"Flame-shaped hemorrhages seen along the superotemporal vascular arcade."
"Associated with scattered hard exudates, cotton wool spots, vessel tortuosity and dilatation."

Look for
- *Disc swelling*
- *Cup disc ratio (glaucoma can lead to CRVO and vice versa)*

- *New vessels (NVD, NVE)*
- *Macular edema*
  (I'd like to confirm the edema using a 78D lens at the slit lamp)
- *Treatment (PRP scars and ERM)*

I'll like to
- *Check fellow eye (10% bilateral)*
- *Check IOP and perform gonioscopy (new vessels at the angle)*
- *For CRVO:*
  - *Undilated SLE for new vessels on the iris*
  - *Check RAPD*
- *Ask for VA*
- *Ask whether patient has a history of DM, HPT, hyperlipidemia*
- *Check BP*
- *Conduct the following investigations:*
  - *CBC (polycythemia and hyperviscosity), blood sugar levels, lipids*
  - *FFA (after 3 months)*

Exam tips:
- **Be careful here, "old" BRVO or CRVO can have features similar to RP ("pseudo" RP).**

Q How do You Manage BRVO/CRVO?

"The management of BRVO/CRVO must be individualized…."
"The factors to consider are the patient's VA and whether there are associated complications like macular edema or neovascularization…."
"The prognosis for CRVO is poor…."

Management of BRVO

1. **Investigate and treat associated systemic disease (e.g. HPT, DM, hyperlipidemia)**

2. **Ocular management**
   - Two main **complications** are: Macular edema and neovascularization at disc
   - Wait for hemorrhage to clear (3 months)
   - Perform OCT and FFA at 3 months
   - If macular edema is present and VA < 20/40:
     - **Grid laser photocoagulation**
     - Intravitreal anti-VEGF if grid laser treatment failure or in eyes with extensive macular hemorrhage (BRAVO Study: Ophthalmology 2010; Epub)
     - Consider intravitreal anti-VEGF as primary treatment if VA > 20/40
     - If 5 disc diameter of nonperfusion is seen → **close follow-up** to look for neovascularization or **sector PRP**
   - Once new vessels are seen → **sector PRP** is indicated
   - Other treatment modalities:
     - IVTA: Does not improve VA in macular edema from BRVO and there are significant side effects of raised IOP and cataract (SCORE Study: *Arch Ophthalmol* 2009:127:1115–1128)
     - Dexamethasone implant: Improves VA in macular edema from BRVO, but side effects of raised IOP and cataract TPPV with AV sheathotomy

Management of CRVO

1. **Investigate and treat associated systemic disease (e.g. HPT, DM, hyperlipidemia)**

2. **Ocular management**
   - Two main **complications** are: Macular edema and neovascular glaucoma
   - Need to differentiate between ischemic/ non-ischemic CRVO
   - Wait for hemorrhage to clear (3 months)
   - Perform OCT and FFA at 3 months:
     - If **nonischemic** → **no treatment** is needed, prognosis is good (50% 20/40 of better VA)
     - If **ischemic** → prognosis is poor (50% neovascular glaucoma in 3 months), **close follow-up** is needed to look for new vessels at iris; or **full PRP**
     - Once new vessels at iris are seen → **full PRP** is indicated
   - If macular edema is present and VA < 20/40:
     - Intravitreal anti-VEGF (CRUISE Study: *Ophthalmology* 2010; Epub)
   - IVTA: Improves VA in macular edema secondary to non-ischemic CRVO, but significant side effects are raised IOP and cataracts (SCORE study)
   - **No benefit** in treating macular edema in CRVO with grid laser
- Other treatment modalities:
   - Dexamethasone implant: Improves VA but significant side effects are raised IOP and cataracts
   - Laser-induced chorioretinal venular anastomosis (Central Retinal Vein Bypass Study: *Ophthalmology* 2010; in press):
- May improve VA in non-ischemic CRVO
- Complicated by CNV and vitreous hemorrhage
- Radial optic neurotomy and retinal vein cannulation with tPA infusion

---

Q	**What are the Main Findings of the Branch Vein Occlusion Study (BVOS)? The Central Vein Occlusion Study (CVOS)?**

	BVOS	**CVOS**
Macular edema	Is argon grid laser useful in improving VA in eyes with BRVO and macular edema with VA ≤ 20/40?	Is argon grid laser useful in preserving or improving VA in eyes with CRVO and macular edema with VA ≤ 20/50?
	Conclusion: **Yes** Gain of at least two lines of VA from baseline When should laser be performed? Not answered in the study	Conclusion: **No** Treatment clearly reduced FFA evidence of macular edema but no difference in final VA
Neovascularization	Can peripheral argon sector PRP prevent 1. Neovascularization? 2. VH?	Can prophylactic argon PRP in ischemic CRVO prevent two clock hours of iris or angle neovascularization? Or is it more appropriate to start PRP only when new vessels are seen?
	Conclusion: **Yes** PRP prevents neovascularization and VH When should laser be performed? Should be started **after** development of neovascularization	Conclusion: 1. **No**, PRP does not prevent iris or angle neovascularization 2. Regression is faster in untreated eyes 3. Therefore, PRP should be started **after** development of iris or angle neovascularization
Recommendations	1. FFA when hemorrhage clears (3 months) 2. If macular edema and VA < 20/40 seen → grid laser 3. If 5 disc diameter of nonperfusion, follow-up closely for new vessels 4. Once new vessels are seen → sector PRP is indicated	1. If 10 disc diameter of nonperfusion, careful observation with undilated SLE and gonioscopy 2. PRP indicated only after neovascularization develops 3. No benefit for treatment of macular edema

Exam tips:
- **One of the more common clinical trials asked in exams. Refer to BVOS (*Am J Ophthalmol* 1984;98:271–282; *Arch Ophthalmol* 1986;194:34–41) and CVOS (*Ophthalmol* 1995;102:1425–1433).**

Exam tips:
- **Refer to BRAVO and CRUISE (Ophthalmology 2010; Epub).**

Q **What are the Main Findings of the BRAVO and CRUISE Studies?**

	BRAVO	CRUISE
Aim	To assess efficacy and safety of 0.3 mg or 0.5mg ranibizumab in patients with macular edema following BRVO	To assess efficacy and safety of 0.3 mg or 0.5mg ranibizumab in patients with macular edema following CRVO
Design	Prospective randomized multicenter studies	
Inclusion criteria	1. Macular edema involving foveal center secondary to BRVO/CRVO 2. Central foveal thickness ≥250μm 3. BCVA <20/40	
Treatment groups	Monthly intraocular injections of 0.3mg or 0.5mg ranibizumab, or sham injections	
Outcome measures	1. Mean change from baseline BCVA at month 6 2. Gain of 3 lines (15 letters) of BCVA at month 6 　Central foveal thickness at month 6	
Results	Mean change in baseline BCVA at month 6: • 0.3mg ranibizumab: 16.6 letters • 0.5mg ranibizumab: 18.3 letters • Sham: 7.3 letters Gain in 3 lines (15 letters) at month 6: • 0.3mg ranibizumab: 55.2% • 0.5mg ranibizumab: 61.1% • Sham: 28.8% Mean reduction in foveal thickness at month 6: • 0.3mg ranibizumab: 97.0% • 0.5mg ranibizumab: 97.6% • Sham: 27.9% Safety profile consistent with previous ranibizumab trials	Mean change in baseline BCVA at month 6: • 0.3mg ranibizumab: 12.7 letters • 0.5mg ranibizumab: 14.9 letters • Sham: 0.8 letters Gain in 3 lines (15 letters) at month 6: • 0.3mg ranibizumab: 46.2% • 0.5mg ranibizumab: 47.7% • Sham: 16.9% Mean reduction in foveal thickness at month 6: • 0.3mg ranibizumab: 94.0% • 0.5mg ranibizumab: 97.3% • Sham: 23.9% Safety profile consistent with previous ranibizumab trials
Conclusions	Intraocular injections of 0.3mg or 0.5mg ranibizumab provided rapid, effective and safe treatment for macular edema following BRVO	Intraocular injections of 0.3mg or 0.5mg ranibizumab provided rapid, effective and safe treatment for macular edema following CRVO

"CRVO in a young patient is not common…."
"I would need to evaluate the patient carefully through a detailed history, physical examination and appropriate investigations."

CRVO in Young Patient

1. **Basic evaluation**
   - Medical conditions:
     - HPT, DM, hyperlipidemia, coagulopathy
     - Cardiac disease (mitral valve prolapse), autoimmune disease, AIDS
   - Ocular conditions:
     - Glaucoma
   - Medication (oral contraceptive pills, hormone therapy)

2. **Physical exam**
   - Carotid bruit
   - Heart murmur
   - BP

3. **Laboratory investigation**
   - CBC, ESR
   - Blood sugar levels, lipid levels
   - VDRL, FTA
   - HIV
   - CXR
   - Coagulation (PTT, APTT), homocysteine, antiphospholipid antibody
   - Autoimmune markers

Exam tips:
- Think of SECONDARY causes (page 196).

"The antiphospholipid syndrome refers to a coagulation disorder."
"Characterized by circulating antiphospholipid antibodies…."

Antiphospholipid Syndrome

1. **Classification**
   - Primary:
     - No secondary disease
     - Circulating antiphospholipid antibodies (includes lupus anticoagulant, anticardiolipin antibodies)
     - Affinity for phospholipids (important in conversion of prothrombin to thrombin)
   - Secondary:
     - Systemic lupus, other auto-immune diseases
     - AIDS
     - Phenothiazine and procainamide use

2. **Clinical features**
   - In vitro, antiphospholipid antibodies cause **anticoagulation** (i.e. bleeding)
   - In vivo, they are associated with paradoxically with **coagulation** (i.e. thrombosis):
     - CRVO and BRVO, CRAO and BRAO
     - Retinal vasculitis
     - Choroidal infarction
     - Arteritic anterior ischemic optic neuropathy

CARDIOVASCULAR DISEASE

Overall yield: ✦✦✦   **Clinical exam:**   **Viva:** ✦✦✦   **Essay:** ✦✦   **MCQ:** ✦✦

Q Opening Question: What are Ocular Associations of Cardiac Disease?

"The ocular effects are usually secondary to an embolic phenomenon from cardiac disease."

Cardiac Disease

1. **Embolic (thrombotic, calcific, bacterial material)**
   - Ophthalmic artery:
     - Ophthalmic artery occlusion
   - Retinal artery:
     - Amaurosis fugax
     - CRAO
   - Retinal arterioles:
     - BRAO (cardiac emboli is most common cause of **BRAO** in **younger** persons)
   - Precapillary arterioles:
     - Cotton wool spots, Roth's spot

2. **Generalized decreased perfusion state from heart failure**
   - Fainting spells
   - Ocular ischemic syndrome:
     - "What are the features of ocular ischemic syndrome?" (see page 202)
       - Anterior segment ischemia
       - Hypoperfusion retinopathy

3. **Right heart failure**
   - Superior vena cavae congestion
     - Increase in episcleral venous pressure → glaucoma

> **Notes**
> - "What are the features of ophthalmic artery occlusion?"
>   - Anterior segment ischemia (anterior ciliary artery)
>   - Posterior segment ischemia (posterior ciliary artery)
>   - Ophthalmoplegia (extraocular muscle involvement)
>   - ERG shows decreased "a" and "b" wave amplitude affected)

Q What are the Ocular Associations of Carotid Artery Disease?

"The ocular effects are usually secondary to either a thrombotic or embolic phenomenon."

Carotid Artery Disease

1. **Embolic (cholesterol, fibrinoplatelet, calcific)**
   - Similar spectrum to above (carotid emboli is most common cause of **BRAO** in **older** persons)

2. **Thrombotic**
   - Carotid artery
     - Ocular ischemic syndrome (most common cause of **ocular ischemic syndrome**)

- Ophthalmic artery:
  - Ophthalmic artery occlusion
  - Anterior ischemic optic neuropathy
- Retinal artery:
  - Amaurosis fugax (most common cause of **amaurosis fugax**)
  - CRAO (most common cause of **CRAO**)

3. **Others**
  - Horner's syndrome
  - Stroke (branches of carotid arteries):

- Anterior choroidal artery (homonymous hemianopia)
- Anterior cerebral artery (hemialexia)
- Middle cerebral artery (homonymous hemianopia, Gaze palsies)
- Aneurysm (branches of carotid arteries):
  - Subarachnoid hemorrhage from ruptured aneurysm
  - Compressive III CN palsy

Q What are the Principles of Management of a Patient with Carotid Artery Disease?

Management of Carotid Artery Disease

1. **Modify risk factors**
  - HPT, DM, hyperlipidemia, smoking
2. **Antiplatelet therapy**
  - Aspirin
  - Dipyridamole
  - Clopidogrel
3. **Anticoagulation therapy**
  - Indications:
    - If aspirin fails
    - Recurrent cardiac source of emboli (atrial fibrillation, mitral valve stenosis, etc.)

4. **Carotid endarterectomy**
  - **North American Symptomatic Carotid Endarterectomy Trial (*New Engl J Med* 1998;339:1415–1425)**
    - Indications for carotid endarterectomy:
      - Symptomatic patients with amaurosis, hemispheric TIA, nondisabling strokes
      - Plus 70–99% carotid artery stenosis
    - **Prognosis**
      - 2-year stroke rate is 9% (endarterectomy) vs 26% (no surgery)
  - **European Carotid Endarterectomy Trial (*Lancet* 1998;351:1379–1387)**
    - No benefit with carotid endarterectomy

Q What is Amaurosis Fugax?

"Amaurosis fugax is a transient monocular blindness less than 24 hours by definition."
"The causes can be either systemic or ocular in nature...."

Amaurosis Fugax

1. **Systemic**
  - Carotid artery atherosclerosis (most common cause)
  - Carotid emboli
  - Cardiac emboli
  - Vasculitis:
    - Giant cell arteritis
    - Migraine

- Systemic lupus, polyarteritis nodosa and others
- Coagulation disorders

2. **Ocular**
  - Raised IOP
  - Drusens
  - Papilledema
  - Anterior ischemic optic neuropathy

Exam tips:
- **Causes almost identical to those for retinal artery occlusion (page 233).**

"The ocular ischemic syndrome is a disorder secondary to hypoperfusion of the globe due to either chronic carotid artery obstruction or ophthalmic artery obstruction."

Ocular Ischemic Syndrome

1. **Cause**
   - Carotid atherosclerosis (most common cause):
     - 90% or more carotid artery obstruction before symptoms
     - Bilateral in 20%
   - Generalized decreased perfusion from cardiac failure
   - Others (GCA, arteritis)

2. **Symptoms**
   - Decrease VA (for weeks and months)
   - Aching ocular pain
   - Light-induced visual loss (with prolonged recovery from exposure to bright light)

3. **Signs**
   - **Anterior segment ischemia:**
     - Injected eye
     - Corneal edema
     - Iris neovascularization, iris atrophy, iridoplegia
     - AC flare (more flare than cells)
     - Swollen mature cataract
     - Raised IOP (50%), low IOP (50%)
   - **Posterior segment (hypoperfusion retinopathy):**
     - Vessel tortuosity, venous dilation
     - Microaneurysm, retinal hemorrhage, hard exudate
     - New vessels, VH
     - Choroidopathy (Elschnig's spots, serous RD)
     - Papilledema, macular star

4. **Investigations**
   - FFA:
     - Delayed choroidal filling time (60%)
     - Delayed arteriole-to-venule transit time (95%)
     - Capillary nonperfusion
     - Prominent arteriolar wall staining
   - ERG:
     - Decreased amplitude of both "a" and "b" waves (like ophthalmic artery occlusion, see above)
   - Systemic conditions:
     - ESR, lipids levels

5. **Prognosis**
   - Systemic associations:
     - 50% have ischemic heart disease
     - 25% have previous stroke
     - 20% have severe peripheral vascular disease
   - 5 year mortality is 40% (higher than for CRAO; page 194)

6. **Treatment**
   - Ocular:
     - Laser PRP for new vessels (regression in small percentage)
     - Manage NVG
   - Manage systemic risk factors
   - Carotid endarterectomy

TOPIC 12

RETINOPATHY OF PREMATURITY

Overall yield: ✶✶✶   **Clinical exam:** ✶   **Viva:** ✶✶✶   **Essay:** ✶✶   **MCQ:** ✶✶

Q **Opening Question:** What is Retinopathy of Prematurity?

"Retinopathy of prematurity (ROP) is a proliferative vascular retinal condition."
"It commonly occurs in **premature** and **low birth weight** babies exposed to high ambient **oxygen**."
"There are classically two phases, the active ROP phase and cicatricial ROP phase...."

Retinopathy of Prematurity

1. **Risk factors:**
   - Prematurity <32 weeks
   - Low birth weight <1,500 g
   - Supplemental oxygen
   - Others:
     - Intraventricular hemorrhage
     - Necrotizing enterocolitis
     - Maternal theophylline treatment
     - Abruptio placentae
     - Quality of NICU care
     - Others: Twins, respiratory distress syndrome, history of blood transfusion

2. **Active ROP**
   - Location:
     - Zone I: Circle centered on disc with radius twice the distance from disc to fovea
     - Zone II: Circle from edge of Zone 1 to a point tangential to nasal ora serrata and around to an area near temporal ora
     - Zone III: Remaining crescent from Zone 2 to temporal ora
   - Extent:
     - Number of clock hours

   - Stage:
     - Stage 1: Demarcation line
     - Stage 2: Ridge
     - Stage 3: Extraretinal fibrovascular proliferation
     - Stage 4: Subtotal RD (4a: Extrafoveal; 4b: Foveal involvement)
     - Stage 5: Total RD
   - Plus disease:
     - Dilatation and tortuosity of veins
     - Vitreous haze
     - Engorged iris vessels
     - Poor pupillary reaction

3. **Cicatricial ROP:**
   - 20% of active ROP will progress to cicatricial ROP without treatment
   - Stages:
     - Stage 1: Myopia, pigmentary changes
     - Stage 2: Temporal vitreoretinal fibrosis, dragged disc
     - Stage 3: Peripheral fibrosis and falciform retinal fold
     - Stage 4: Partial RD
     - Stage 5: Total RD, secondary glaucoma

Exam tips:
- **The definition of the various parameters (zones, extent and stage) has to be committed to memory. Many candidates do not define zones well.**

"ROP occurs as a result of failure of vascularization of the immature retina."
"There are two theories...."

Pathogenesis

1. **Normal retinal angiogenesis**
   - Starts at 16 weeks
   - Reaches nasal ora at 36 weeks
   - Complete vascularization at 40 weeks (up to one month post-term)

2. **Biphasic theory of Aston and Patz**
   - High ambient oxygen → vasoconstriction and toxic obliteration of retinal capillaries → on return to room air → relative ischemia develops → angiogenic factors secreted → vascular proliferation

3. **Spindle cell theory of Kretzer and Hittner**
   - Nascent blood vessels form in normally hypoxic uterine condition by canalization and endothelial cell differentiation behind a migrating sheet of spindle cells
   - High ambient oxygen triggers extensive gap junction formation between spindle cells which interferes with migration and canalization of blood vessels
   - Spindle cells secrete angiogenic factors → vascular proliferation

> **Notes**
> - "What is Rush disease?"
>   - Rapidly progressive Stage 3 ROP in Zone 1 or posterior Zone 2
>   - Poor prognosis

Q How do You Screen a Baby for ROP Born at 32 Weeks of Gestation?

"The examination schedule for ROP in our center is...."
"The indications for treatment of ROP are...."

Screening and Management of ROP

1. **Who should be screened?**
   - ≤ 1,500g, born ≤ 32 weeks gestation
   - Selected infants 1,500g–2,000g or born at gestational age >32 weeks, with unstable clinical course

2. **When to start screening?**
   - Median age of ROP = 37 weeks
   - 90% of ROP occur between 34 to 42 weeks
   - Therefore, start screening at 34 weeks (alternatively, can start screening four weeks postnatally)

3. **How often should subsequent screening be?**
   - If first screening examination shows:
     - No ROP → repeat exam in **four weeks** → if no ROP → repeat exam in three months
     - ROP in Zone III → repeat in **two weeks**
     - Prethreshold ROP (Zone I or II) → repeat in **one week** → if threshold ROP → treatment

4. **What are the indications for treatment?**
   - Threshold ROP:
     - Zone I or II
     - Five contiguous clock hours or eight noncontiguous clock hours
     - Stage 3
     - Plus disease
   - Threshold ROP is associated with **50**% risk of having VA 20/200 or worse without treatment
   - More recent evidence support the treatment of prethreshold ROP
     - Early Treatment for Retinopathy of Prematurity Study (ETROP) recommends treatment for:
       - Zone I any stage with plus
       - Zone I Stage 3, no plus
       - Zone II Stage 2 or 3 with plus

5. **What treatments are available?**
    - Prevention: $PaO_2 < 80$ mmHg
    - Cryotherapy:
        - Ablate avascular retina anterior to ridge
        - **Multicenter Cryotherapy for ROP Study** (*Arch Ophthalmol* 1996;114:417–424):
            - 50% reduction in poor VA with cryotherapy
            - 50% reduction in poor fundal status with cryotherapy

    - Indirect laser photocoagulation
    - Vitamin E therapy:
        - Controversial
        - Inhibit gap junction formation in spindle cells
        - Antioxidant
        - Complications (necrotizing enterocolitis, vitreous hemorrhage)
    - Stage 4 ROP might require sclera buckle or vitrectomy

 Clinical approach to dragged disc

"There is dragging of the optic disc by temporal vitreoretinal fibrotic tissues."
"There is also a divergent squint seen."

I'd like to ask patient for a history
- *Prematurity*
- *Contact with dogs*
- *Family history of blindness*

The possible causes are:

1. Proliferative vitreoretinopathy
- *ROP*
- *Familial exudative vitreoretinopathy (AD inheritance)*
- *Incontinentia pigmenti (SLD inheritance)*

2. Uveitis
- *Toxocara*
- *Pars planitis*

3. Tumor
- *Combined hamartoma of RPE and retina*

4. Trauma

Notes
- "Why not earlier?"
    - Limited value in picking up ROP
    - Difficulty in screening (poor pupil dilation, vitreous haze)
    - Complications of mydriatic eyedrops (cardiac, respiratory effects) and ocular examination (oculocardiac reflex, hypotension, apnea)

 Exam tips:
- **Refer to ETROP study (*Arch of Ophthalmol* 2003;121:1684–1696).**

OTHER RETINAL VASCULAR DISORDERS

Overall yield: ✷✷✷ **Clinical exam:** ✷ **Viva:** ✷✷✷ **Essay:** ✷✷ **MCQ:** ✷✷✷✷

Q **Opening Question:** What are the Ocular Effects of Pregnancy?

Ocular Effects of Pregnancy

1. **Physiological**
   - **Lid** — Telangiectasia
   - **Cornea**
     - Decreased corneal sensitivity
     - Corneal edema → increased corneal thickness → change in refractive error
     - Increased incidence of Krukenbergs spindle
   - **IOP** — Increased facility of aqueous outflow and decreased episcleral venous pressure → lower IOP
   - **Lens** — Transient loss of accommodative ability
   - Enlarging pituitary gland → various **VF changes** towards end of term

2. **Pathological (5 "Cs")**
   - **CSR**
     - Secondary to hormonal and hemodynamic changes → change in permeability of blood-retinal barrier
     - Resolve post-partum with residual RPE mottling and pigmentation
   - **CRVO, CRAO, hypertensive retinopathy**
     - Secondary to hypertension
     - CRVO may be sign of impending fit in pre-eclampsia
   - **Cortical blindness**
     - Transient phenomenon, secondary to chronic edema of occipital lobe
   - **Pseudotumor cerebri**
     - Secondary to chronic edema (controversial)

   - **Coagulation disorders**
     - Disseminated intravascular coagulation
     - Thrombotic thrombocytopenic purpura

3. **Preexisting conditions (endocrine and tumors)**
   - **Diabetic retinopathy**
     - Increased incidence of background DR
     - Increased incidence of macular edema
     - Increased progression to PDR
     - Prophylactic photocoagulation important
   - **Grave's disease**
     - Progression during pregnancy
   - **Pituitary adenoma**
     - Normal pituitary gland enlarges with increased prolactin secreting cells
     - May present for the first time during pregnancy
   - **Uveal melanoma**
     - Increased size secondary to increased melanin-stimulating hormone secretion
   - **Meningioma**
     - Secondary to increased estrogen/progesterone
     - May present for the first time during pregnancy
   - **Ocular pharmacology**
     - Avoid FFA → fluorescein can pass through placenta
     - Avoid timolol if breastfeeding
     - Diamox may be teratogenic
     - Topical steroids are not contraindicated

Q **What are the Ocular Effects of Radiation?**

"There are two kinds of radiation: Non-ionizing and Ionizing radiation."

Ocular Effects of Radiation

1. **Non-ionizing radiation**
   - **Microwave (> 12,000 nm):**
     - Cataract
   - **Infrared (12,000–770 nm):**
     - True exfoliation of lens (glassblower's cataract)
   - **Visible light (760–400 nm):**
     - Photic damage:
       - Mechanical (e.g. photodisruption)
       - Thermal (e.g. photocoagulation)
       - Photobiochemical (e.g. solar retinopathy, photic retinopathy)
   - **Ultraviolet (180–390 nm):**
     - Surface epithelial disease and radiation keratitis

2. **Ionizing radiation**
   - Damage depends on tissue sensitivity:
     - Lens > cornea > retina > optic nerve
   - Damage can be:
     - Direct — on actively reproducing cells
     - Indirect — on blood vessels

- **Anterior segment**
  - Lids and conjunctiva:
    - Dermatitis of lids
    - Damage to eyelashes
    - Damage to meibomian glands (dry eyes)
    - Punctal occlusion (wet eyes)
    - Cicatricial conjunctivitis
  - Cornea:
    - Radiation keratitis
    - Limbal stem cell failure
    - Aseptic necrosis and perforation
  - Lens:
    - Cataract
    - Equatorial cells damaged by radiation
- **Posterior segment**
  - Radiation retinopathy (see below)
  - Optic neuropathy

Q **What is Radiation Retinopathy?**

Radiation Retinopathy

1. **Pathology**
   - Damage to retinal vasculature after exposure to ionizing radiation
   - Microangiopathy (like DR)
   - Dose dependent (high risk if > 7,000 rads)

2. **Presentation**
   - Asymptomatic early on
   - Present with decreased VA four months to three years after treatment (external beam or local plaque therapy)
   - Progressive loss of VA

3. **Clinical findings**
   - Retinopathy (hemorrhages, cotton wool spots, hard exudates, microaneurysms)

- Perivascular sheathing, telangiectasia
- Complications
  - New vessels → vitreous hemorrhage, tractional RD, neovascular glaucoma
  - CRAO and CRVO
  - Maculopathy (exudative, edematous, ischemic — like diabetic maculopathy)
  - Papillopathy

4. **Treatment**
   - FFA → look for capillary nonperfusion
   - Focal laser and PRP
   - Papillopathy: Systemic steroids

"Sickle cell disease is a red blood cell disorder."

"Characterized by the presence of abnormal hemoglobin and "sickling" of the red blood cells in conditions of hypoxia."

"The ocular features can be divided into proliferative retinopathy, nonproliferative retinal disease and anterior segment disease...."

Sickle Cell Hemoglobinopathy

1. **Pathogenesis**
   - Mutant S or C hemoglobin allele:
     - Substituted for normal hemoglobin A allele
     - Valine substituted for glutamate at beta-6 chain location of hemoglobin
   - Hypoxia leads to sickling, which causes obstruction of small blood vessels and tissue ischemia (leading to further sickling)

2. **Types (classified on abnormal hemoglobin combinations)**
   - AS (sickle cell trait):
     - 8% of black population
     - Mild systemic disease
   - SS (sickle cell anemia):
     - 0.4% of black population
     - Severe **systemic** disease and anemia
     - Mild ocular disease
   - SC (sickle C disease) and Sthal (sickle cell thalassemia):
     - Mild systemic disease
     - Severe **ocular** disease

3. **Proliferative retinopathy**
   - Stage (note: Stages in ROP are shown in brackets):
     - Stage 1: Peripheral arteriolar occlusion (demarcation line)
     - Stage 2: Peripheral arteriovenous anastomosis (ridge)
     - Stage 3: "Sea-fan" neovascularization (extraretinal fibrovascular proliferation)
     - Stage 4: Vitreous hemorrhage (subtotal RD)
     - Stage 5: RD (total RD)

4. **Non-proliferative retinal disease**
   - "Salmon patch" (fresh intraretinal hemorrhage)
   - "Black sunburst" (old subretinal hemorrhage)
   - "Silver wiring" of peripheral arterioles
   - Angioid streaks
   - Retinal breaks and detachment

5. **Anterior segment**
   - Tortuous "corkscrew" conjunctival vessels
   - Ischemic iris atrophy and rubeosis
   - Hyphema

6. **Management**
   - Management of hyphema:
     - Higher risk of **optic nerve damage** with hyphema (compared to "normal" person)
     - Indication for surgical intervention: > 24 mmHg > 24 hours
   - RD surgery:
     - Risk of **anterior segment ischemia** with scleral buckle

Exam tips:
- **The stages are VERY SIMILAR to ROP stages (page 245).**

Notes
- "How do you prevent anterior segment ischemia during RD surgery?"
  - Intraoperative oxygen, no epinephrine given
  - Minimize manipulation of muscles
  - SRF drainage (lower IOP)
  - Postoperative oxygen
  - Consider vitrectomy instead of scleral buckling
  - Prophylactic laser photocoagulation of all breaks

Q What are the Ocular Effects of Leukemia?

"Ocular effects of leukemia are usually only seen in advanced cases of acute or relapsing disease."
"They are related to both **direct** and **indirect** effects of leukemia (e.g. anemia, immunosuppression).

Leukemia

1. **Direct effects**
   - Anterior segment:
     - Subconjunctival hemorrhage
     - Orbital infiltration
     - Iris:
       - Diffuse white nodular thickening
       - Heterochromia
       - Pseudohypopyon
       - Spontaneous hyphema
     - Secondary glaucoma
   - Posterior segment:
     - "Leopard spot" retina (deposits in choroid)
     - Flame-shaped hemorrhage, hard exudates, cotton wool spots, Roth's spots
   - Venous tortuosity and dilatation, CRVO
   - Neovascularization
   - Exudative RD
   - Optic nerve infiltration

2. **Indirect effects**
   - Anemia (flame-shaped hemorrhage, cotton wool spots, Roth's spots, etc.)
   - Thrombocytopenia
   - Hyperviscosity (ischemic optic neuropathy, proliferative retinopathy)
   - Immunosuppression (opportunistic infections)

Q What are the Causes of Roth's Spots?

"Roth's spots are essentially retinal hemorrhages with a fibrin thrombus occluding the vessel."

Differential Diagnoses of Roth's Spots

1. **Blood disorders**
   - Anemia
   - Leukemia
   - Scurvy
2. **Infective**
   - Infective endocarditis
   - Sepsis
   - AIDs retinopathy
   - Candida retinopathy
3. **Vasculitis**
   - DM
   - Systemic vasculitis (systemic lupus etc.)

Q What are the Ocular Effects of Renal Disease?

Renal Disease

1. **Congenital (concurrent ocular involvement):**
   - **Lowe's syndrome**
     - SLR inheritance
     - Renal problems (aminoaciduria, metabolic acidosis, renal rickets)
     - CNS problems (mental retardation)
     - Ocular effects:
       - Cataract and microphakia
       - Glaucoma
   - **Alport's syndrome**
     - AD inheritance
     - Renal problems (proteinuria, HPT and renal failure)
     - CNS problems (sensorineural deafness)
     - Ocular effects:
       - Anterior polar cataract, anterior lenticonus
       - Posterior polymorphous dystrophy
       - RPE abnormalities (looks like "fundus albipunctatus")
   - **Aniridia**
     - Sporadic form
     - Renal problems (Wilms' Tumor)
     - Ocular effects (page 60)
2. **Acquired (ocular involvement occurs LATER)**
   - **Secondary effects (more common, especially after renal transplant)**
     - HPT retinopathy
     - DM retinopathy
     - Anemia
     - Bleeding diathesis
     - Opportunistic infections (CMV, candida)
     - Steroid induced glaucoma and cataract

- **Primary effects:**
  - Band keratopathy
  - Cataract
- Retinal edema
- Disc edema
- Exudative RD

Q Tell me about Hypertensive Ocular Disease.

"Hypertension can affect the retina, choroid and optic nerve."

Hypertensive Ocular Disease

1. **Hypertensive retinopathy**
   - Pathogenesis
     - Four stages:
       - Vasoconstrictive phase (autoregulatory response)
       - Sclerotic phase
       - Exudative phase
       - Complications phase (macroaneurysms, CRVO)
   - Grading (Keith, Wagener, Barker classification)

Grade	Description
1	Mild narrowing or sclerosis of retinal arterioles ("silver wiring")
2	Generalized and localized narrowing of arterioles, moderate or marked sclerosis of retinal arterioles with exaggeration of arteriolar reflex and arteriovenous compression ("AV nicking")
3	Retinal edema, cotton wool spots, retinal hemorrhages superimposed on sclerotic vessels
4	Diffuse retinal and optic disc edema with narrowing of arterioles ("malignant hypertension")

2. **Hypertensive choroidopathy**
   - "Elschnig's Pearls" (choroidal infarcts)

3. **Hypertensive optic neuropathy**
   - Ischemic optic neuropathy

 Clinical approach to macroaneurysm

"There is an area of flame-shaped hemorrhage and hard exudates at the superotemporal arcade."
"Associated with a localized dilatation of the retinal arteriole at that location."

Look for
- Macular edema/hard exudates at macula
- DR
- HPT changes

I'll like to ask patient for history of
- HPT, DM, hyperlipidemia

In this patient, my management will be
- Conservative (if macular is not involved, macroaneurysm is located at inferotemporal arcade)
- To consider laser photocoagulation (macular edema, hard exudate, superotemporal arcade location)

> **Exam tips:**
> • Hypertensive retinopathy is only ONE of the three manifestations.

Notes

Ocular conditions associated with hypertension
- Retinal vein occlusion
- Retinal artery occlusion
- Retinal artery macroaneurysm
- AION
- Ocular motor nerve palsy
- Uncontrolled hypertension may adversely affect DR

Q **What is Parafoveal Telangiectasia?**

"Parafoveal telangiectasia is an uncommon retinal vascular anomaly that primarily involves the juxtafoveolar capillaries...."

"It can be congenital or acquired, primary (idiopathic) or secondary to underlying systemic disease (e.g. diabetes)...."

Idiopathic Parafoveal Telangiectasia

- Pathogenesis:
  - Poorly understood
  - Characterized by dilatation and tortuosity of retinal blood vessels and multiple aneurysms confined to the parafoveal region. These leak and result in deposition of hard exudates
  - Primarily involves the capillary bed, although arterioles and venules may also be involved
- Gass classification of parafoveal telangiectasia:
  - Group 1: Unilateral
    - Group 1A: Congenital
    - Group 1B: Idiopathic focal
  - Group 2: Bilateral
    - Group 2A: Idiopathic acquired (most common)
    - Group 2B: Juvenile familial occult
  - Group 3: Occlusive

- Group 3A: Associated with systemic disease (e.g. polycythemia, multiple myeloma etc)
- Group 3B: Associated with neurological disease
- Clinical presentation:
  - Patient presents mostly in the 5th to 6th decades with slowly progressive loss of central vision
- FFA:
  - Leakage from telangiectactic vessels confined to the parafoveal region
  - Staining of scars (advanced disease)
- Treatment:
  - There is no definitive treatment, although several modalities have been studied:
    - Laser photocoagulation
    - PDT
    - Intravitreal anti-VEGF
    - Intravitreal steroids

Q **What is Coat's Disease?**

"Coat's disease is an idiopathic, non-hereditary, mostly unilateral retinal vasculopathy characterized by the presence of retinal telangiectasias leading to intraretinal and subretinal exudation, and frequently, exudative RD."

"Coat's disease, Leber's miliary aneurysms and idiopathic parafoveal telangiectasia are thought to represent a spectrum of the same disease, with Coat's disease being the most extensive."

"Before reaching the diagnosis of Coat's disease, it is important to exclude retinoblastoma in a young patient with leukokoria and RD."

Coat's Disease

- Clinical presentation:
  - Mostly in the first decade (average five years) with unilateral visual loss, strabismus or leukokoria
  - Occasionally may present in later childhood, and rarely in adult life
- Examination:
  - Retinal telangiectasia
  - Intraretinal and subretinal yellowish exudation:
    - Often affects areas remote from vascular abnormalities, especially macula
  - Complications:
    - Exudative RD
    - Rubeosis iridis
    - Uveitis
    - Glaucoma
    - Phthisis bulbi
- Investigations:
  - OCT
  - FFA:
    - Leakage from telangiectactic vessels
    - Hypofluorescence: Blockage from hard exudates
  - Ultrasonography ± CT/MRI: Exclude retinoblastoma
- Management:
  - Observation:
    - Mild, non-vision-threatening disease or
    - Total RD with no hope of restoring vision
  - Laser photocoagulation: On telangiectatic vessels
  - Cryotherapy: For telangiectatic vessels
  - Vitreoretinal surgery: Very bullous RD unsuitable for cryotherapy
  - Enucleation: Painful eyes with NVG

RETINITIS PIGMENTOSA

Overall yield: ✪✪✪✪ **Clinical exam:** ✪✪✪✪ **Viva:** ✪✪✪ **Essay:** ✪✪✪ **MCQ:** ✪✪✪✪

Q Opening Question: What is Retinitis Pigmentosa?

"Retinitis pigmentosa refers to a heterogeneous group of photoreceptor dystrophies."
"Characterized by a/the triad of…."

Retinitis Pigmentosa (RP)

1. **Definition**
   - Heterogeneous group of disorders, characterized by a **TRIAD** of:
     - Night blindness
     - Progressive visual field loss from photoreceptor and RPE dysfunction
     - Abnormal ERG findings
   - Prevalence: 1/4,000 to 1/7,000 in population
   - Abnormality of both rods **and** cones, but **rods** are affected more than cones

2. **Clinical features**
   - Symptoms:
     - Bilateral eye involvement, but may be asymmetrical
     - Loss of peripheral vision first
     - Night blindness
   - Signs:
     - Classical **TRIAD** of:
       - Bone-spicule pigmentation
       - Arteriolar attenuation (earliest feature)
       - Waxy optic disc pallor (least reliable feature)
     - Macular involvement, **TRIAD** of:
       - CME
       - ERM
       - Atrophic degeneration
     - Other posterior segment signs, **TRIAD** of:
       - Optic disc drusen
       - Myopic degenerative changes
       - PVD
     - Anterior segment signs, **TRIAD** of:
       - Keratoconus
       - Open angle glaucoma
       - Posterior subcapsular cataract

3. **ERG**
   - Amplitude is markedly subnormal:
     - Both "a" and "b" waves are affected
     - Both rod and cone ERG are affected (although rod abnormality is predominant)
   - Parallel EOG abnormality

4. **"What is atypical RP?"**
   - Variants of RP, characterized by unilateral, asymmetrical and atypical clinical findings
   - Four classical atypical RPs:
     - Retinitis punctata albescens
     - Sector RP
     - Pericentric RP
     - Exudative RP

Exam tips:
- **Remember the different "TRIADS"!**

Clinical approach to retinitis pigmentosa

"On examination of this young patient's fundus...."
"The most obvious lesions are bone spicule-like pigmentations...."
"Distributed along the vascular arcades in the peripheral retina...."
"The retinal vessels are attenuated...."
"The optic disc is pale and waxy in appearance (not common, so be careful here)...."

Look for
- *Macula:*
  - *CME*
  - *ERM*
  - *Atrophic scar*
- *Optic disc:*
  - *Peripapillary atrophy (myopia)*
  - *Optic disc drusen*
- *Other eye:*
  - *Bilateral (if unilateral, think of "pseudo" RP)*

I'd like to
- *Examine anterior segment for evidence of keratoconus, cataract*
- *Check IOP (glaucoma)*
- *Check EOM and presence of ptosis (Kearne-Sayre syndrome)*
- *Examine systemically for diseases associated with RP:*
  - *Hearing (Usher, Refsum's, Kearne-Sayre syndrome)*
  - *Neurologically (Bassen-Kornzweig, Refsum's, Kearne-Sayre syndrome)*
  - *Cardiac (Kearne-Sayre)*
  - *Examine family members for RP*

Q **What are the Differential Diagnoses for RP (Causes of "Pseudo" RP)?**

1. **Drugs**
   - Quinine / hydroxychloroquine
   - Phenothiazine
2. **Infective**
   - Syphilis
   - Rubella
   - Measles
3. **Scarring**
   - Chronic CSR

- Laser PRP scars
- RD
- Trauma
- Uveitis (Vogt-Koyanagi-Harada syndrome)

4. **Vascular**
   - CRAO
   - Ophthalmic artery occlusion
5. **Cancer-related retinopathy**

Exam tips:
- **"Pseudo" RP is usually unilateral, asymmetrical and atypical. Remember "DISC."**
- **Do not confuse "pseudo" RP with atypical RP.**

"Different mutations have been isolated for RP...."

Molecular Genetics of RP

1. **Genes for normal retinal proteins**
   - Rhodopsin (Chromosome **3**)
   - Red and green pigments (Chromosome **X**)
   - Blue pigments (Chromosome **7**)

2. **Rhodopsin mutations**
   - Rhodopsin, Pro23His mutation:
     - **Classic** molecular genetic defect
     - Substitution of histidine with proline at 23 amino acid position

   - 25–30% of AD type of RP
   - Rhodopsin, Pro347LeuHis mutation:
     - Less common
     - Poorer visual prognosis than rhodopsin, Pro23His mutation
   - RDS (retinal degeneration slow) gene mutation:
     - Encodes for peripherin
   - Nonsense mutation in rhodopsin:
     - In AR type of RP

Q How do You Provide Genetic Counseling Advice to Patients with RP?

Genetic Counseling

1. **AD**
   - 20% of all RP
   - Defined as three consecutive generations of parent-to-child transmission
   - Best prognosis
   - Retain VA after 60 years
   - Affected patient has one in two chances of passing defect to child

2. **AR/isolated RP**
   - Worst prognosis
   - Legally blind by 30–40 years

3. **SLR**
   - Same visual prognosis as AR
   - If patient is male, all sons will be normal, all daughters will be carriers

Q What are the Systemic Associations of RP?

"There are numerous systemic diseases associated with RP."
"These disorders have in common several features...."

Systemic Associations

1. **Common features**
   - Systemic:
     - Inherited as AR condition
     - Mental handicap
     - Neurological abnormalities
     - Metabolic abnormalities
     - Skeletal abnormalities
     - Deafness (fairly common)
   - Pigmentary retinopathy:
     - Usually unilateral, asymmetrical and atypical
     - VA may be normal
     - ERG may be normal

2. **Kearns-Sayre syndrome**
   - Key features, **TRIAD** of:
     - Ptosis
     - Chronic progressive external ophthalmoplegia
     - Heart block

3. **Bassen-Kornzweig syndrome**
   - Key features, **TRIAD** of:
     - Ataxia
     - Acanthocytosis (red blood cell abnormality)
     - Abetalipoproteinemia (fat malabsorption)
   - Treatment:
     - Vitamin E may be beneficial (page 413)

4. **Refsum's syndrome**
   - Key features, **TRIAD** of:
     - Phytanic acid metabolic defect
     - Peripheral neuropathy
     - Palpitations (cardiac arrhythmia)

5. **Usher syndrome**
   - Key features, **TRIAD** of:
     - Deafness
     - Ataxia (vestibular dysfunction)
     - Neurological abnormalities

6. **Bardet-Biedl syndrome**
   - Key features, **TRIAD** of:
     - Obesity
     - Hypogenitalism
     - Polydactyly

7. **Laurence-Moon syndrome**
   - Key features, **TRIAD** of:
     - Spastic paraplegia
     - Hypogenitalism
     - Mental handicap

Exam tips:
- This is potentially a difficult question. Discuss first only systemic diseases you are familiar with (e.g. start with Kearns-Sayre syndrome).
- The triad of Bassen-Kornzweig can be remembered by "A."

Q | **What Ocular Conditions are Associated with Deafness?**

Ocular Associations of Deafness

1. **Systemic diseases associated with pigmentary retinopathy**
   - Usher syndrome
   - Kearns-Sayre syndrome
   - Refsum's syndrome
   - Bardet-Biedl syndrome
   - Mucopolysaccharidoses (page 118)

2. **Retinal dystrophies**
   - Leber's congenital amaurosis (page 219)
   - Norrie's disease
   - Alport's syndrome (page 210)

3. **Uveitis**
   - Congenital syphilis
   - Congenital rubella
   - Vogt-Koyanagi-Harada's syndrome

4. **Interstitial keratitis**
   - Cogan's interstitial keratitis

5. **Metabolic diseases**
   - DIDMOAD (diabetes insipidus, diabetes mellitus, optic atrophy and deafness)

FLECK RETINA SYNDROMES AND RELATED DYSTROPHIES

Overall yield: ✸✸　**Clinical exam:** ✸　**Viva:** ✸✸✸　**Essay:** ✸✸✸　**MCQ:** ✸✸✸✸

Q Opening Question: What are Retinal Dystrophies?

"Group of genetically heterogeneous disorders involving the retina…."
"Isolated abnormality in otherwise normal patients or may be associated with systemic abnormalities…."

Retinal Dystrophies Classification

1. **Stationary (congenital stationary night blindness)
   or progressive (most others)**

2. **Anatomical**
   • Diffuse or isolated (photoreceptor, RPE,
     choroidal or vitreous)

   • Widespread (entire retina) or focal (macula)

3. **Age of onset**
   • Congenital, infantile or childhood

Q What are the Fleck Retina Syndromes?

"The classical causes of Fleck retina syndromes are Stargardt's disease, fundus flavimaculatus and familial dominant drusen…."
"Other causes include…."

Fleck Retina Syndromes

1. **RPE dystrophies ("classic" fleck retinas)**
   • Stargardt's disease
   • Fundus flavimaculatus
   • Familial dominant drusen
   • Others:
     • Pattern dystrophy
     • Fleck retina of Kandori
     • Alport syndrome

2. **Photoreceptor dystrophies**
   • Retinitis punctata albescens
     • Atypical RP

   • Fundus albipunctatus
     • Congenital stationary night blindness
       syndrome with abnormal fundus (see below)

3. **Posterior uveitis**
   • Presumed ocular histoplasmosis syndrome
   • Birdshot disease

4. **Others**
   • Crystalline retinopathy
   • Peau d'orange (pseudoxanthoma elasticum)

"Night blindness can be classified as **stationary** or **progressive**."

Night Blindness

1. **Stationary night blindness**
   - Congenital stationary night blindness (CSNB) with normal appearing fundus
   - CSNB with abnormal looking fundus
     - Fundus albipunctata ("What is fundus albipunctata?"):
       · Form of CSNB with abnormality in **visual pigment regeneration**
       · Patients have slow dark adaptation
     - Oguchi's disease ("What is Oguchi's disease?"):
       · Form of CSNB with abnormality in retinal **circuitry**

   - Patients demonstrate **Mizuo's** phenomenon (retina exhibits yellow sheen with light exposure, which disappears with dark adaptation)

2. **Progressive night blindness**
   - Retinal dystrophies:
     - RP and RP variants
   - Choroidal dystrophies:
     - Gyrate atrophy
     - Choroideremia
   - Vitreous dystrophies:
     - Goldmann-Favre disease

"The different causes can be classified into those with gross abnormalities, those with…."

Differential Diagnoses of Poor Vision at Birth

1. **Gross ocular abnormality**
   - Bilateral cataract
   - Bilateral glaucoma
   - Bilateral retinoblastoma

2. **"Normal looking" eyes with nystagmus**
   - Optic nerve hypoplasia (septooptic dysplasia)
   - Macula diseases:
     - Foveal hypoplasia (idiopathic, congenital albinism, aniridia)
     - Juvenile retinoschisis
     - Infectious disease (toxoplasmosis, CMV retinitis)

   - Photoreceptor dystrophies:
     - Leber's congenital amaurosis
     - Achromatopsia (severe photophobia)
     - CSNB

3. **"Normal looking" eyes with no nystagmus**
   - Severe ametropia
   - Cortical blindness
   - Ocular motor apraxia
   - Delayed visual maturation (VA usually normal by six months)

> **Notes**
> - "How do you differentiate Leber's congenital amaurosis, achromatopsia and CSNB?"
>   - ERG:
>   · Leber's: Decreased **rod** and **cone** function
>   · Achromatopsia: Decreased **cone** function
>   · CSNB: Absent **bipolar** cell function (decreased "b" wave)

Leber's Congenital Amaurosis

1. **Definition:**
   - Age-related variant of RP, involving rods and cones

   - Common cause of blindness in children (between 10–18 % of children in blind institutions)
   - Inheritance: AR (some AD cases have been reported)

2. **Presentation:**
   - Poor vision or blindness at birth or first few years of life
   - Nystagmus, roving eye movement, strabismus
   - **Oculodigital syndrome:**
     - Constant rubbing of eyes leading to enophthalmos
   - Children see best under bright light
   - Pupillary reactions to light diminished ("amaurotic pupil")

3. **Clinical features:**
   - Fundus usually "normal" looking
   - Abnormal signs include:
     - Peripheral chorioretinal atrophy with pigmentary changes but classical "bone spicule" pattern is uncommon

- Optic disc pallor and retinal arteriolar attenuation is uncommon
- Disc edema and "**Bull's eye**" **maculopathy**
- Other ocular features:
  - Hypermetropia
  - Keratoconus, keratoglobus
  - Cataract
- Systemic features:
  - Mental handicap, deafness, epilepsy and other neurological abnormalities

4. **ERG**
   - Markedly diminished, even in early cases with normal fundal appearance

---

Notes
- "What are the causes of Bull's eye maculopathy?"
  - Ocular disease:
    - Cone dystrophy
    - Leber's congenital amaurosis
    - Stargardt's disease
  - Systemic disease:
    - Chloroquine toxicity
    - Bardet-Biedl syndrome

Q Tell me about Ocular Albinism.

Ocular Albinism

1. **Pathogenesis**
   - Deficiency of tyrosinase (enzyme converts tyrosine to dopaquinone)
   - Biochemical pathway: Phenylalanine... → L-tyrosine → L-DOPA → dopaquinone → ...melanin

2. **Classification**
   - **Oculocutaneous** (tyrosinase **negative** with no melanin at all)
     - AR
     - Very pale skin and blond hair
     - Ocular features:
       - Translucent, diaphanous iris
       - Axenfeld anomaly
       - Depigmented fundus
       - Fovea hypoplasia
       - Optic disc hypoplasia
       - Refractive errors
     - Neuro-ophthalmic features:
       - Nystagmus

   - Decreased number of uncrossed nerve fibers (abnormal binocular vision)
   - Abnormal visual pathway (from lateral geniculate body to occipital cortex)
   - **Oculocutaneous** (tyrosinase **positive** with variable melanin)
     - Milder version
     - Positive **hair bulb test**:
       - Hair bulb will darker when incubated in a solution with L-dopa or L-tyrosine
     - **Associated systemic diseases:**
       - Chediak-Higashi syndrome (white blood cell defect)
       - Hermansky-Pudlak syndrome (platelet defect)
       - Skin — solar keratosis, basal cell CA, squamous cell CA
   - **Ocular** (decreased melanosomes):
     - **SLR** or AR
     - Ocular features only
     - No systemic features

Gyrate Atrophy

1. **Definition:**
   - Inborn error of metabolism
   - AR
   - Reduced activity of **ornithine ketoacid aminotransferase** (mitochondria enzyme which catalyzes reactions in several amino acid pathways)
   - Gene for enzyme — Chromosome 10

2. **Pathogenesis:**
   - Photoreceptor atrophy with abrupt transition to near normal retina
   - **Not** caused by high levels of ornithine (other metabolic disorders with high ornithine levels do not develop similar changes)

3. **Clinical features:**
   - Symptoms:
     - Onset 10–30 years
     - Night blindness in first decade
     - VF defects
     - Rarely decrease in VA
   - Signs:
     - Characteristic chorioretinal atrophic changes (patchy chorioretinal atrophy with scalloped borders)

   - Differential diagnoses:
     - Choroideremia (SLR, earlier onset, diffuse granular pigmentary changes)
     - High myopia (lacquer cracks, Foster-Fuch's spot, peripapillary atrophy)
     - Generalized choroidal atrophy (AD, widespread choriocapillaris atrophy)
   - Myopia and astigmatism (90%)
   - Posterior subcapsular cataract
   - Abnormal ERG and EOG
   - Abnormal FFA (window defects)

4. **Investigations:**
   - Raised ornithine levels in aqueous, blood, spinal fluid and urine
   - Reduced enzyme activity in different tissues (cultured fibroblasts, lymphoblasts and hair roots)
   - Carriers have 50% of normal enzyme activity

5. **Treatment:**
   - High dose **Vitamin B6** (cofactor in ornithine aminotransferase, stimulates enzyme activity)
   - Protein restriction (reduces arginine levels)
   - Lysine and a-aminoisobutyric acid supplement (augmentation of renal losses of ornithine)

"Juvenile Best disease is also termed vitelliform macular dystrophy…."
"It is a rare autosomal dominant disorder, with macular lesions that evolve through several stages over many years."

Juvenile Best Disease

1. **Pathophysiology**
   - Disorder in the RPE → lipofuscin accumulation in RPE cells and sub-RPE space → secondary photoreceptor loss

2. **Inheritance**
   - AD with variable penetrance
   - Bestrophin (Chr 11q13) implicated

3. **Stages**
   - Stage 0 (pre-vitelliform): Subnormal EOG, asymptomatic, normal fundus
   - Stage 1: Pigment mottling at macula
   - Stage 2 (vitelliform): Well-circumscribed, round egg-yolk ("sunny side up") macular lesion:
     - Infancy or early childhood
     - VA not impaired

   - Stage 3 (pseudo-hypopyon): At puberty:
     - RPE break → accumulation of yellow substance in subretinal space
   - Stage 4 (vitelliruptive): Egg yolk begins to break up ("scrambled egg"), VA drops:
     - Pigment clumping and early atrophic changes may be present
   - Stage 5 (atrophic): Marked decrease in VA

4. **Investigations**
   - EOG: Severely abnormal during all stages
   - ERG: May be normal
   - FFA: Hypofluorescence (blockage by lipofuscin), window defects

5. **Prognosis**
   - Reasonably good till fifth decade

- Causes of poor VA:
  - CNV
  - Macular scarring
- Geographic atrophy
- Macular hole → RD

Q What are Stargardt's Disease and Fundus Flavimaculatus?

"Stargardt's disease and fundus flavimaculatus are genetically inherited retinal dystrophies. They are variants of the same disease, which present at different times and carry different prognoses."
"Fundus flavimaculatus presents in adult life and may not have macular changes, while Stargardt's disease presents in the first and second decades of life, and mainly affects the macula."

Stargardt's Disease and Fundus Flavimaculatus

1. **Inheritance**
   - AR: ABCA4 gene (1p21-22)
2. **Presentation**
   - Stargardt's disease presents in the first and second decades of life with impairment of central vision
   - Fundus flavimaculatus often presents in adult life and may be an incidental finding as vision may not be impaired
3. **Signs**
   - Early findings: Non-specific macular mottling
   - Pisciform flecks at level of deep retina:
     - Stargardt's disease: Flecks located mainly at the macula, "snail-slime" or "beaten-bronze" foveal appearance
     - Fundus flavimaculatus: Flecks at the mid-periphery, may involve posterior pole
   - Geographic atrophy (Bull's eye atrophy) in advanced Stargardt's disease
4. **Investigations**
   - ERG: Photopic ERG may be subnormal
   - EOG: May be subnormal
   - FFA:
     - Dark choroids
     - Flecks may show increased or reduced fluorescence
     - Window defects: May have Bull's eye configuration in Stargardt's disease
5. **Prognosis**
   - Poor for Stargardt's disease
   - Relatively good for fundus flavimaculatus
   - Small minority develop CNV

NEUROOPHTHALMOLOGY

TOPIC 1

OCULAR MOTILITY AND MULTIPLE CRANIAL NERVE PALSIES

Overall yield: ✸✸✸   **Clinical exam:** ✸✸✸✸✸   **Viva:** ✸✸   **Essay:** ✸✸   **MCQ:** ✸✸

Possible Clinical Cases

1. **Neurological lesions**
   - CN III, IV, VI palsies, multiple CN palsies
   - Inter-nuclear ophthalmoplegia (INO), one-and-a-half syndrome
   - Dorsal midbrain syndrome
   - Nystagmus
2. **Pediatrics problems**
   - Esotropia/exotropia
   - Duane's syndrome
   - Brown's syndrome
   - Moebius syndrome
3. **Others**
   - Myasthenia gravis
   - Thyroid eye disease
   - Blow-out fracture
   - Myopathies

 Clinical approach to ocular motility examination

"Examine this patient's ocular motility."

Look at
- *Head posture:*
  - *Head turn — towards side of abduction weakness, e.g. Duane's syndrome, VI CN palsy*
  - *Head tilt — away from side of SO palsy*
  - *Chin down in bilateral SO palsy, chin up in bilateral ptosis*
- *Ptosis — III CN palsy*
- *Primary position — manifest strabismus, e.g. ET, XT, SO palsy*
- *Pupils — anisocoria*

Check versions (both eyes) and ductions (one eye)

(Continued)

(Continued)

Test EOM in all nine positions of gaze

- **Primary**
- **Two horizontal**
  - *VI CN palsy (look at abducting eye)*
  - *INO (look at "ADDUCTING" eye)*
  - *Duane's syndrome (look at palpebral aperture)*
  - *If INO is found on one side, check for one-and-a-half*
- **Two vertical**
  - *III CN palsy*
  - *Supranuclear gaze palsy*
  - *Thyroid (IR restriction)*
  - *Blow-out fracture (IR restriction)*
  - *A and V patterns if ET/XT present*
- **Four vertical in abduction and adduction**
  - *SO palsy (depression in adduction)*
  - *Brown's syndrome (elevation in abduction)*

- **Park Bielchowsky's three-step test**
  - *Primary position*
  - *Head turn*
  - *Head tilt*

Clinical approach to diplopia

"This patient has diplopia. How do you approach the diagnosis?"

I'd like to ask the patient the following questions

- *Blurring of vision or diplopia?*
- *Uniocular or binocular? (Disappear on covering one eye)*
- *Vertical, horizontal or oblique displacement of images?*
- *Is diplopia worse in any position of gaze?*

Test

- *EOM, asking for diplopia*
- *Cover paretic eye in position of maximal separation of images (outermost image will disappear)*

Q **Opening Question:** What are the Possible Causes of Multiple Cranial Nerves Palsies?

Cavernous Sinus Syndrome (III, IV, V, VI CN)

1. **Clinical features**
   - Pure cavernous sinus
     - III, IV, VI plus **V1, V2, V3, Horner's syndrome** (depending on extent of involvement)
   - Superior orbital fissure
     - III, IV, VI plus **V1**
   - Orbital apex
     - III, IV, VI plus **V1 and II**
2. **If VI nerve involved, either**
   - Cavernous sinus syndrome (look for III, IV, V CN palsies and Horner's syndrome)

- Cerebellopontine angle syndrome (look for V, VII, VIII CN palsies and cerebellar signs)
3. **Etiology (note: Classic big four in pathology)**
   - Vascular
     - Aneurysm — intracavernous sinus carotid aneurysm, post-cerebral aneurysm
     - Cavernous sinus thrombosis
     - Migraine
     - Giant cell arteritis
   - Inflammatory
     - Tolosa-Hunt syndrome
     - Meningitis
     - Bacterial — syphilis, TB
     - Viral — herpes zoster
     - Wegener's granulomatosis
     - Sarcoidosis
   - Tumor
     - Primary-pituitary adenoma, meningioma, craniopharyngioma
     - Secondary — nasopharyngeal CA, lymphoma, distant metastasis
   - Trauma
     - Carotid-cavernous sinus fistula

Cerebello-Pontine Angle (V, VI, VII, VIII CN)

1. **Etiology**
   - Tumor
     - Vestibular schwannoma
       - Nasopharyngeal CA
       - Cholesteatoma
       - Clivus meningioma
         - Pontine glioma
         - V CN neuroma
   - Trauma
     - Basal skull fracture
2. **Clinical features of vestibular schwannoma:**
   - V and VIII CN first
     - Corneal reflex lost
     - Nystagmus
   - VI and VII CN next
   - Raised intracranial pressure (papilledema, etc.)

Lateral Medullary Syndrome (V, VIII, IX, X CN)

1. **Etiology**
   - Stroke
   - Multiple sclerosis
2. **Clinical features**
   - V CN and spinothalamic tract (crossed hemihypalgesia)
   - VIII CN (nystagmus)
   - IX and X CN (dysarthria and dysphagia)
   - Sympathetic tract (Horner's syndrome)
   - Cerebellum (nystagmus and other cerebellar signs)

Clinical approach to multiple cranial nerves palsies

"On examination of this patient's ocular motility, there is generalized limitation in all positions of gaze."

Look for
- *Proptosis — carotid cavernous fistula, Tolosa-Hunt syndrome, thyroid eye disease, pseudotumor*
- *Conjunctival injection — carotid cavernous fistula, pseudotumor*
- *Posture of head*
- *Ptosis — III CN palsy, Horner's syndrome*
- *Primary position — manifest strabismus*
- *Pupils — anisocoria*

Check
- *EOM*
  - *Horizontal (VI CN)*
  - *Vertical (III CN)*
  - *Intorsion at abduction (IV CN)*
- *Close eyes (VII CN)*
- *Check pupils (II CN)*
- *Facial sensation (V1, 2, 3 CN), open jaws (V3 CN)*

(Continued)

(Continued)

Exclude

- *Thyroid eye disease*
- *Myasthenia gravis*

I'll like to

- *Check corneal sensation (V1 CN)*
- *Check fundus for papilledema*
- *Examine other cranial nerves*
  - *VIII, cerebellar signs (cerebellopontine angle syndrome)*
- *Refer to ENT to rule out nasopharyngeal CA*

Exam tips:
- **For examinations purposes, there are three syndromes of ophthalmic interest (cavernous sinus, cerebellopontine angle and lateral medullary syndromes).**

The Ophthalmology Examinations Review

THIRD CRANIAL NERVE PALSY

Overall yield: ✸✸✸✸   **Clinical exam:** ✸✸✸✸✸   **Viva:** ✸✸✸   **Essay:** ✸✸   **MCQ:** ✸✸

Q Opening Question: Tell me about III CN Palsy.

"III CN palsy is a common neuroophthalmic diagnostic problem."
"The causes can be divided into…."
"Clinically, III CN palsy can be either medical or surgical III…."

Anatomy	Etiology	Clinical features
Nuclear: • Midbrain • Level of superior colliculus • Ventral to sylvian aqueduct	• Vascular (stroke) • Demyelination (multiple sclerosis) • Tumors	**Nuclear III syndrome:** • Unpaired levator nucleus (bilateral ptosis) • Unpaired Edinger-Westphal nucleus (bilateral mydriasis) • Paired SR nuclei supplying contralateral muscle (contralateral SR palsy) • Paired MR, IR, IO (ipsilateral MR, IR, IO palsies)
Fasciculus: • Through red nucleus • Emerge from midbrain medial to cerebral peduncle	• Weber's syndrome • Benedict's syndrome • Nothnagel's syndrome • Claude's syndrome: Benedict's + Nothnagel's	**Crossed syndromes:** • Pyramidal tract (III CN palsy and contralateral hemiparesis) • Red nucleus (III CN palsy and contralateral hemitremor) • Superior cerebellar peduncle (III CN palsy and contralateral cerebellar ataxia) **Isolated III CN palsy**
Basilar: • Between posterior cerebral and superior cerebellar arteries • Lateral and parallel to posterior communicating artery	• Aneurysm (between posterior communicating and internal carotid) • Raised intracranial pressure (uncal herniation)	

(Continued)

(Continued)

Anatomy	Etiology	Clinical features
Intracavernous: • Pierces dura lateral to posterior clinoid process to enter cavernous sinus • Above IV nerve in lateral wall • Divides into superior and inferior branches	• Causes of Cavernous sinus syndrome (page 224)	**Cavernous sinus syndrome (page 224):** • Multiple CN palsies • Incomplete III • May be pupil sparing (DM) **Isolated III CN palsy**
Intraorbital: • Enters through SOF • Branch to inferior oblique carries parasympathetic fibers	• Vascular (DM) • Trauma	

 Clinical approach to III CN palsy

"This patient has an exotropia in his right eye."
"And fixes with his left eye."

Look for
- *Ptosis not overcome by frontalis action*
- *EOM limitation in all directions except abduction (VI CN)*
- *Watch for aberrant regeneration*
- *Check intorsion in abduction (IV CN)*
- *Check pupils (pupil sparing or not)*

Decide quickly whether you are dealing with medical or surgical III

	Medical III	**Surgical III**
Features	• Age > 60 • Vascular risk factors (DM, HPT, smoking) • Pupil sparing (80%) • Pupil continues to be spared after one week • Complete III CN palsy • Isolated III CN palsy • No aberrant regeneration (see below) • Recovery within 3 months	• Young • No vascular risk factors • Pupil involved (90%) • Progression of pupil involvement • Incomplete III CN palsy • Multiple CN palsies • Aberrant regeneration • No recovery
Common etiology	• **Vascular causes** • DM • Giant cell arteritis (GCA) • Ophthalmic migraine • Inflammatory • Tolosa-Hunt syndrome • Miller Fisher syndrome	• Cerebral aneurysm • Raised intracranial pressure (from uncal herniation) • Tumor

(Continued)

	Medical III	Surgical III
	(Continued)	
Evaluation	• History of DM and HPT • Check BP (HPT) • Headache (GCA, ophthalmic migraine) • Painful III CN palsy (DM, migraine, Tolosa-Hunt syndrome) • Ataxia, areflexia (Miller Fisher)	• Check fundus for papilledema uncal herniation • Examine neurologically • History of head injury • History of headache, nausea and vomiting (raised intracranial pressure) • History of HPT (aneurysm)
Investigations	• CBC, ESR • Fasting blood sugar level • VDRL, FTA • Autoimmune markers	• CT scan (CNS bleed, meningioma, stroke, trauma)

Exam tips:
- **There are two ways to remember etiology:**
  - **Anatomical classification is good for answering essay question.**
  - **Medical/surgical III classification is good for viva/clinical exams.**

Q **How do You Manage III CN Palsy?**

"The management of III CN palsy involves treating the underlying cause, and addressing the diplopia."

1. Underlying cause
- Ligation of aneurysm (endoscopic/surgical)
- Optimize control of diabetes/hypertension/hyperlipidemia if the etiology of III CN palsy is vascular

2. Diplopia
- Non-surgical: Fresnel prisms, uniocular occlusion
- Strabismus surgery (at least 6 months after onset, when all spontaneous improvement has ceased)

"Aberrant regeneration of CN usually follows damage of the nerve by **TRAUMA** or **TUMOR**."
"There are recognized syndromes involving III, VII and IX CN."

Aberrant Regeneration of CN

1. **Aberrant regeneration of III CN palsy:**
   - Lid gaze dyskinesis:
     - Elevation of lid on adduction (inverse Duane's syndrome)
     - Elevation of lid on depression (pseudo Von Graefe's sign)
   - Pupil gaze dyskinesis:
     - Constriction on adduction (pseudo Argyll Robertson pupil)
     - Constriction on depression

2. **Aberrant regeneration of VII CN palsy (crocodile's tears):**
   - Synkinesis between salivation fibers and lacrimation fibers
     - Tearing when eating

3. **Aberrant regeneration of IX CN palsy (Frey's syndrome):**
   - Synkinesis between salivation fibers and sympathetic fibers
     - Flushing and sweating when eating

SIXTH CRANIAL NERVE PALSY

Overall yield: ✸✸✸✸✸ **Clinical exam:** ✸✸✸✸✸ **Viva:** ✸ **Essay:** ✸ **MCQ:** ✸✸

Q **Opening Question:** Tell me About VI CN Palsy.

"VI CN palsy is a common neuroophthalmic diagnostic problem."
"The causes can be divided into…."

Anatomy	Etiology	Clinical features
Nuclear: • Mid-pons, ventral to floor of fourth ventricle • VII CN fasciculus curves around VI CN nucleus	• Vascular (stroke) • Demyelination (multiple sclerosis) • Tumors • Encephalitis	**Nuclear VI syndrome and gaze palsy:** • Abducens nucleus (ipsilateral LR palsy) • PPRF (ipsilateral failure of horizontal gaze) • Facial nucleus (ipsilateral VII CN palsy)
Fasciculus: • Leaves brainstem ventrally at ponto medullary junction	• Raymond's syndrome • Millard Gubler syndrome • Foville's syndrome	**Crossed syndrome:** • Pyramidal tract (VI CN palsies and contralateral hemiparesis) • Pyramidal tract and VII nucleus (VI, VII CN palsy and contralateral hemiparesis) • V, VII nucleus, sympathetic, PPRF (V, VI, VII CN palsy, gaze palsy and Horner's syndrome)
Basilar: • Enters prepontine basilar cistern • Passes upwards close to base of skull, crossed by anterior inferior cerebellar artery • Pierces dura below clinoids • Angles over petrous temporal bone • Passes through Dorello's canal and enters cavernous sinus	Causes of cerebellopontine angle syndrome (page 225): • Vestibular schwannoma • Raised intracranial pressure (false localizing sign) • Nasopharyngeal CA • Basal skull fracture • Clivus meningioma • Gradenigo's syndrome	**Cerebellopontine angle syndrome (page 225)**

(Continued)

Anatomy	Etiology	Clinical features
Intracavernous: • Below III and IV CN • Close to internal carotid artery in the middle of the sinus • Carries sympathetic branches from paricarotid plexus	• Causes of Cavernous sinus syndrome (page 224)	**Cavernous sinus syndrome (page 224)**
Intraorbital: • Enters orbit through SOF within annulus of Zinn to innervate LR	• Vascular (DM) • Trauma	**Isolated VI CN palsy**

Clinical Notes

1. **Isolated medical VI palsy**
   - Same workup as for medical III CN palsy (page 228)
   - Recovery within 4–6 months

2. **Six causes of "pseudo VI CN palsy"**
   - Myasthenia gravis
   - Thyroid eye disease
   - Duane's syndrome
   - Medial wall fracture
   - Esotropia (longstanding)
   - Convergence spasm

3. **Bilateral VI CN palsy**
   - Nuclear:
     - CVA
     - MS
     - Tumor
     - Encephalitis (Wernicke's syndrome)
   - Basilar:
     - False localizing sign
     - Clivus meningioma
   - Intracavernous (big four in pathology):
     - Inflammation (Tolosa-Hunt)
     - Vascular
     - Tumor (nasopharyngeal CA)
     - Trauma (carotid-cavernous sinus fistula)

 Clinical approach to VI CN palsy

"This patient has a right esotropia with abduction weakness."

Look for other CN
- *EOM (III)*
- *Check intorsion in abduction (IV)*
- *Check pupils (II)*

I'll like to
- *Check fundus for papilledema (false localizing, pseudotumor)*
- *Examine neurologically:*
  - *Contralateral hemiparesis (Raymond's syndrome)*
  - *VII CN and contralateral hemiparesis (Millard Gubler syndrome)*
  - *Horizontal gaze palsy, V, VII, Horner's syndrome (Foville's syndrome)*
  - *V, VII, VIII, cerebellar signs (cerebellopontine angle tumor — vestibular schwannoma)*
- *Check ears for otitis media (Gradenigo's syndrome) and battle sign (petrous bone fracture)*
- *Refer to ENT to rule out nasopharyngeal CA*

Exam tips:
- Do not confuse raised intracranial pressure causing uncal herniation (III CN palsy) with false localizing sign (VI CN palsy).

Q   What are Causes of VI CN Palsy in Children?

"VI CN palsy is a common neuroophthalmic diagnostic problem in children."
"First, a squint (ET, Duane's syndrome) must be excluded."
"The causes can be divided into…."

1. **Congenital**
   - Isolated idiopathic
   - Moebius syndrome
2. **Acquired**
   - Trauma
   - Infection:
     - Gradenigo's syndrome (otitis media, V, VI, VII, VIII CN palsies)

- Tumor:
  - Pontine glioma
  - Metastasis form neuroblastoma

Q   What is the Surgical Management of VI CN Palsy?

"Surgical intervention for VI CN palsy is undertaken at least six months after onset, when all spontaneous improvement has ceased."
"The choice of surgery depends on the residual abduction power of LR…."

1. Poor residual LR power
   - Hummelsheim procedure
   - Jensen procedure

2. Some residual LR power
   - Ipsilateral MR recession and LR resection +/− contralateral MR recession

NEUROLOGICAL APPROACH TO PTOSIS

Overall yield: ✸✸✸✸ **Clinical exam:** ✸✸✸✸✸ **Viva:** ✸✸ **Essay:** ✸✸ **MCQ:** ✸✸

Decide Quickly — If

1. Senile aponeurotic ptosis
- Describe:
  - High lid crease
  - Atrophic lid tissues and tarsal plate
  - Deep UL sulcus
- Test:
  - Ptosis in downgaze — more severe
  - EOM full and pupils normal
  - Levator function — usually good

2. Congenital ptosis
- Describe:
  - Absent lid crease
  - Visual axis blocked (if blocked, risk of amblyopia)
- Test:
  - Ptosis in downgaze — lid lag present

- EOM (SR rectus weakness)
- Bell's reflex
- Marcus Gunn Jaw Winking
- Levator function — usually poor
- Check the VA and refraction of patient

3. III CN palsy
- Severe, complete ptosis
- Eye is out and down
- Dilated pupils
- See CN III approach (page 228)

4. Horner's syndrome
- Mild ptosis, overcome by looking up
- Miosis
- Enophthalmos
- See Horner's approach (page 243)

 Clinical approach to ptosis

Describe
- *Unilateral/bilateral*
- *Total/severe/mild*
  - *Shine torchlight to look at visual axis*
  - *Decide whether anisocoria is present now!*
    - *If present, either III CN palsy or Horner's syndrome*
    - *If absent, either myasthenia gravis, congenital ptosis or senile ptosis*
- *Overaction of frontalis*
- *Lid crease, lid sulcus, lid mass*
- *Eye position (squints)*
- *Head tilt*

(Continued)

(Continued)

"This patient has a mild unilateral ptosis in the right lid."
"Associated with smaller pupils in the right eye…."

or

"This patient has severe bilateral ptosis in both lids, covering the visual axis…."
"There is no anisocoria noted…."

Test

- EOM
  - *Upgaze*
    - *Ptosis overcome by frontalis (Horner's syndrome)*
    - *Limitation in upgaze (III CN palsy)*
  - *Downgaze (lid lag in congenital ptosis vs aponeurotic, aberrant III CN regeneration — "pseudo-von Graefes sign")*
  - *Sidegaze (III CN palsy, aberrant III CN regeneration – "reverse Duane's syndrome")*
- *Myasthenia gravis tests — fatigability in upgaze, Cogan's lid twitch, "eyelash" sign, "eyepeek" sign*
- *Lagophthalmos and Bell's (important for management purposes)*
- *Pupils*
- *Marcus Gunn Jaw Winking sign*

I'll like to

- *Measure the degree of ptosis and levator function (important for management purposes)*
- *Perform an SLE and fundal examination*
- *Perform myasthenia gravis tests*

Exam tips:
- **One of the most common clinical examination cases.**
- **See also the ptosis chapter in the oculoplastic section (page 291), III CN palsy (page 228) and Horner's syndrome (page 243).**

MYASTHENIA GRAVIS

Overall yield: ✪✪✪✪ **Clinical exam:** ✪✪✪✪ **Viva:** ✪✪ **Essay:** ✪✪ **MCQ:** ✪✪✪

Q Opening Question: What are the Features of Myasthenia Gravis (MG)?

"Myasthenia gravis is a systemic neurological disorder."
"Caused by a disorder occurring at the **neuromuscular junctions**."
"It has both **systemic** and **ocular** features."

Myasthenia Gravis

1. **Classification:**
   - Ocular:
     - **60%** of MG patients present with ocular features; **90%** will have some ocular involvement in course of disease
     - Prognosis (important):
       - **40%** remain ocular
       - **10%** remission
       - **50%** progress to generalized MG
   - Generalized:
     - Mild
     - Severe acute (respiratory)
     - Severe chronic

2. **Natural history:**
   - Labile phase
   - Slow progressive phase
   - Refractory phase

3. **Ocular features (in 90%):**
   - Ptosis:
     - Fatigable:
       - Enhanced with light and passive elevation of contralateral lid
     - Asymmetrical
     - Variable (different time of day)
     - Shifting (left and right eyes)
     - Cogan's lid twitch
     - Lid hopping/fluttering
   - Ophthalmoplegia:
     - Pupils normal
     - Not consistent with single CN palsy (mimic any of CN palsy)
     - MR first muscle to be involved (therefore need to exclude internuclear ophthalmoplegia)
     - Saccadic abnormalities: Hypermetric and hypometric saccades
     - Accommodative fatigue
   - Orbicularis oculi weakness:
     - "Eyelash" sign (eyelash cannot be "buried" by forcible lid closure)
     - "Eye peek" sign (lids drift open slowly after closure)

4. **Diagnosis:**
   - Tensilon test (**80%** sensitivity)
   - Electromyogram (EMG)
     - Repetitive stimulation at 3 mHz (**50–90%** sensitivity)
       - Look for decremental amplitude with repetitive stimulation
     - Single fiber EMG (**80–95%** sensitivity)
       - Look for variability between individual muscle fibers within a motor unit
   - Anticholinesterase antibody (**70–90%** sensitivity): No correlation with disease severity
   - Anti-skeletal muscle antibody:
     - Increased in females and patients with thymomas
     - Increased risk of bulbar involvement

Exam tips:
- **A differential diagnosis for almost any neuroophthalmic condition.**

Notes
- Osserman's grading
  - I: Ocular
  - II: Generalized
  - III: Fulminant and crisis
  - IV: Late progressive
  - V: Muscle atrophy

Q How do You Perform the Tensilon Test?

"The tensilon test is a diagnostic test for MG with sensitivity of 80%."

Tensilon Test

1. **Preparation:**
   - Edrophonium hydrochloride:
     - Anti-acetylcholinesterase (e.g. increases acetylcholine effects at neuromuscular junction)
     - One vial 10 mg/ml
     - Dilute to 10 ml (concentration: 1 mg/ml)
   - Precaution:
     - Atropine 0.5–1 mg on standby
       - Consider giving IM 0.4mg 15 min before test
     - Resuscitation equipment on standby

2. **Injection (rule of 2s):**
   - IV 2 mg, watch for 2 min
   - If no response, inject another 2 mg, watch for further 2 min
   - If still no response, inject remaining 6 mg, watch for 2 min again

3. **Endpoint:**
   - Most respond within 20–45 seconds
   - Objective endpoints must be determined:
     - Ptosis (measured before and after)
     - Ophthalmoplegia (Hess chart or Lancaster Red-Green Test)

4. **Side effects:**
   - Increased salivation
   - Sweating
   - Perioral fasciculation
   - Nausea
   - Hypotension, bradycardia, arrhythmia
   - Bronchospasm

5. **False positive result:** Eaton-Lambert syndrome, Guillain-Barre syndrome, amyotrophic lateral sclerosis

Exam tips:
- One of few procedures in neuroophthalmology you need to know well.

Q How to Manage a Patient with MG?

"MG is usually co-managed with a neurologist."
"Need to treat both the systemic condition and the ocular complications."

Management of MG

1. **Systemic manifestations:**
   - Anti-acetylcholinesterase (pyridostigmine/mestinon):
     - 30 mg bid dose
   - Thymectomy:
     - Better for generalized MG than ocular MG
   - Immunosuppressive therapy:
     - Prednisolone:
       - Given to reduce dose of pyridostigmine
       - 65% remission, 30% improvement
     - Azathioprine

- Plasmapheresis and IV immunoglobulin — indications:
  - Myasthenic crisis:

2. **Ocular complications:**
   - Lid crutches for ptosis
   - Prisms for ophthalmoplegia

Notes
- Causes of lid retraction in myasthenia gravis:
  - Contralateral lid retraction when there is unilateral ptosis
  - Cogan's lid twitch
  - Thyroid eye disease

Q What are the Drugs to Avoid in MG?

Drugs to Avoid in MG
- **A**minoglycosides (gentamicin)
- Neuromuscular **b**locker (curare, suxamethonium)
- **C**hlorpromazine
- Respiratory **d**epressants (morphine)
- **P**rocainamide
- **P**enicillamine

Exam tips:
- **Remember "ABCD" and "P"!**

NYSTAGMUS

Overall yield: ✪ ✪   **Clinical exam:** ✪   **Viva:** ✪ ✪   **Essay:**   **MCQ:** ✪ ✪

Q **Opening Question:** Tell me about Nystagmus.

"Nystagmus can be defined as...."
"A simple classification is...."

Nystagmus

1. **Definition:**
   - Ocular oscillation which is ....
     - Rhythmic in nature and biphasic with at least one slow phase
     - The slow phase is abnormal and the fast phase is corrective
     - The direction is named after the fast phase

2. **Classification:**
   - Clinical:
     - Primary position or gaze evoked
     - Pendular (two slow phases) or jerk (one quick phase, one slow phase)
     - Horizontal, vertical, rotatory or mixed
     - Conjugate (same in both eyes) or dissociated
   - Etiological:
     - Physiological:
       · End-point nystagmus
       · Optokinetic nystagmus
       · Vestibular nystagmus
   - Motor imbalance
     · Congenital nystagmus
     · Spasmas nutans
     · Latent nystagmus
     · Periodic alternating nystagmus
     · Convergence-retraction nystagmus
     · Downbeat nystagmus
     · Upbeat nystagmus
     · See-saw nystagmus
     · Ataxic nystagmus
   - Sensory deprivation
   - Nystagmoid movements:
     · Ocular flutter and opsoclonus
     · Ocular bobbing
     · Before and after thymectomy
     · Awaiting response to immunosuppression
   - Total body irradiation

Exam tips:
- **Nystagmus is a difficult topic. You need to remember the basic principles and certain types of nystagmus.**

Notes
- Physiological nystagmus:
  - End-point nystagmus
  - Optokinetic nystagmus
  - Vestibular nystagmus

Clinical approach to nystagmus

"This patient has a nystagmus."

Describe

- ***D****irection* — *horizontal/vertical/rotational*
- ***W****aveform* — *pendular/jerk (direction of fast phase)*
- ***A****mplitude* — *large/small (effect of gaze position on amplitude)*
- ***R****est* — *primary position (at rest/gaze evoked)*
- *Frequency* — *fast/slow*

Exam tips:
- **Remember "DWARF."**

Q **What are the Features of Congenital Nystagmus?**

"There are several distinct ocular features of congenital nystagmus."

Congenital Nystagmus

1. **Classification:**
   - Primary/idiopathic
   - Secondary
   - Anterior segment disorders
     - Corneal opacity, cataract, glaucoma
   - Visible posterior segment disorders
     - ROP, optic atrophy, coloboma, macular scar
   - Normal looking eyes:
     - Leber's amaurosis
     - Achromatopsia
     - Cone dystrophy
     - Congenital stationary night blindness

2. **Ocular features:**
   - Starts at birth or 2–3 months after birth (1)
   - No oscillopsia (2)

- Nystagmus is:
  - Binocular (3)
  - Horizontal (4)
  - Conjugate (5)
  - Uniplanar (6)
- Associated with:
  - Head tilt (7)
  - Titubation (8)
  - Null point (9)
  - Dampens on convergence but increases on fixation (10)
  - Diminishes in darkness/during sleep/when eye is covered (11)
  - Latent nystagmus may be present (12)
  - Paradoxical OKN response (13)

Exam tips:
- **A favorite question. Remember all the 13 points but DO NOT say, "There are 13 features…." in case you cannot remember all of them!**

Clinical approach to congenital nystagmus

"On inspection, this young patient has a pendular nystagmus in the primary position."

Describe features
- Binocular (3), horizontal (4), conjugate (5)
- Associated head tilt (7), titubation tremors (8)

Check in different directions of gaze
- Uniplanar in all directions of gaze (6)
- Null point (7)
- Dampens on convergence, but increases on fixation (8)
- Cover one eye, observe for latent jerk nystagmus in contralateral eye (11)

"This patient has congenital nystagmus."

I'd like to
- Ask patient for history of onset of nystagmus (1) and whether patient has symptoms of oscillopsia (2)
- Test for paradoxical response to OKN drum (13)?

Q How would You Manage this Patient?

"My management will be conservative."
"I'll do the following...."

- Refract and prescribe glasses (reading is not impaired)
- Prescribe contact lens if glasses are not suitable
- Give base-out prism to induce convergence

- I will offer surgery only if there is an abnormal head posture (AHP) which is stable:
  - Horizontal AHP: Kestenbaum procedure
  - Vertical AHP: Recess and Resect vertical recti

Q How do You Differentiate a Peripheral from a Central Cause of Vestibular Nystagmus?

"There are several distinct features which will help in differentiating peripheral from central cause of vestibular nystagmus."

Vestibular Nystagmus

	Peripheral	Central
Nystagmus	• Unidirectional, away from site of lesion • May be associated with a rotatory component	• Multidirectional or unidirectional, towards side of lesion
Association	• Dampens on fixation • Rarely lasts more than 3 weeks • Marked vertigo • Tinnitus/deafness	• No dampening • May be permanent • Mild vertigo • No tinnitus/deafness
Location	• Vestibular nerve • Labyrinth	• Cerebellum • Brainstem

"Optokinetic (OKN) nystagmus is induced by looking at the rotation of a striped drum — the OKN drum."
"There is the initial pursuit eye movement following the direction of the rotation...."
"This is followed by the saccade corrective movement in the opposite direction...."

Use of OKN

1. Diagnosis of congenital nystagmus (paradoxical response)
2. Detect internuclear ophthalmoplegia (rotate drum in direction of eye with adduction failure) (see page 253)
3. Detect Parinaud's syndrome (rotate drum downwards to elicit convergence retraction nystagmus) (see page 244)
4. Differentiate organic from nonorganic blindness (see page 285)

5. Differentiate vascular from neoplastic cause in patient with homonymous hemianopia (see page 255):
   - If vascular, lesion is usually confined to occipital lobe (OKN response is symmetrical)
   - If neoplastic, lesion may extend to parietal lobe (OKN response is asymmetrical)

TOPIC 7

PUPILS

Overall yield: ✸✸✸✸ **Clinical exam:** ✸✸✸✸✸ **Viva:** ✸✸✸ **Essay:** ✸✸ **MCQ:** ✸✸

Possible Clinical Cases

1. **Afferent defects**
   - Clinical problem: **RAPD**
   - Optic nerve and tract lesions

2. **Efferent defects**
   - Clinical problem: **Anisocoria**
   - Parasympathetic (III CN palsy) or sympathetic (Horner's syndrome)

3. **Light near dissociation**
   - Clinical problem: **Reaction to accommodation but not to light**

- Causes:
  - Unilateral:
    - Tonic pupil
    - Aberrant III CN regeneration
    - Herpes zoster ophthalmicus
    - Afferent conduction defect
  - Bilateral:
    - Argyll Robertson pupil
    - Dorsal midbrain syndrome
    - Dystrophia myotonica
    - Diabetes
    - Chronic alcoholism

Q Opening Question: What are the Anatomical Pathways of the Pupil Reflexes?

"There are three important pupil reflexes, with different anatomical pathways for each."

Pupil Pathways

1. **Light reflex pathway**
   - 1st order: Retina (ganglion cells) — optic nerve — optic tract — bypasses lateral geniculate body (LGB)
   - 2nd order: Pretectal nucleus
   - 3rd order: Edinger-Westphal nucleus
   - 4th order: Ciliary ganglion — short ciliary nerves — iris constrictor pupillae — **pupil constriction**

2. **Sympathetic pupillary pathway**
   - 1st order: Hypothalamus — brainstem
   - 2nd order: C8 to T2 spinal cord
   - 3rd order: Superior cervical ganglion — pericarotid plexus — ophthalmic division of V

   CN — nasociliary nerve — long ciliary nerve — iris dilator pupillae — **pupil dilation**

3. **Accommodation reflex**
   - Not well defined, the orders are an approximation only (important to emphasize this in the beginning):
   - 1st order: Retina (ganglion cells) — optic nerve — optic tract
   - 2nd order: LGB — optic radiation
   - 3rd order: Visual cortex — visual association areas — internal capsule — brainstem
   - 4th order: Oculomotor nucleus (MR nucleus and Edinger-Westphal nucleus) — **pupil constriction and convergence**

Q What are the Causes of Anisocoria?

"Causes of anisocoria depend on which pupil is the abnormal one…."

Anisocoria

1. **Dilated (mydriatic) pupil abnormal**
   - III CN palsy
   - Tonic pupil:
     - Holmes Adie syndrome
   - Pharmacological mydriasis
   - Iris abnormalities
     - Trauma
2. **Constricted (miosed) pupil abnormal**
   - Horner's syndrome:
     - Brainstem stroke
   - Pancoast syndrome
   - Cluster headache
   - Argyll Robertson pupil
   - Pharmacological
   - Iris abnormalities:
     - Posterior synechiae
   - Pontine hemorrhage

Q What is the Marcus Gunn pupil?

"The Marcus Gunn pupil is also known as the relative afferent papillary defect."
"It is elicited with the **swinging torchlight test**."
"There is **paradoxical dilation** of the pupil when the torchlight is swung from the contralateral eye to the affected eye."

Marcus Gunn Pupil

1. **Etiology:**
   - Optic nerve lesion (most important)
   - Other possible sites:
     - Extensive retinal damage
     - Dense macular lesion
     - Optic chiasma/tract (RAPD in contralateral eye because nasal retina larger than temporal)
     - Dorsal midbrain (RAPD in contralateral eye)
2. **Grading (Bell *et al*. Clinical grading of relative afferent pupillary defects.** *Arch Ophthalmol* 1993;111:938–942):
   - Grade I: Weak constriction then greater dilatation
   - Grade II: No initial constriction, stall, then dilatation
   - Grade III: Immediate dilatation
   - Grade IV: Immediate dilatation following prolonged illumination of the good eye for six seconds
   - Grade V: Immediate dilatation with no secondary constriction

> **Exam tips:**
> - **One of the most important definitions asked in exams.**

Q What is Tonic Pupil? What is the Holmes Adie Pupil? What is the Holmes Adie Syndrome?

Tonic Pupil

1. **Clinical features:**
   - Light-near-dissociation (response to accommodation better than to light)
   - Dilated pupil (pupil small in longstanding Adies)
   - Slow constriction and dilatation
   - Constriction in segments (bag of worms)
   - Asymmetrical accommodation
2. **Investigation:**
   - 0.1% pilocarpine (constriction due to denervation supersensitivity)
3. **Site of lesion:**
   - Ciliary ganglion or short ciliary nerves

4. **Etiology:**
   - Primary = Holmes Adie **pupil:**
     - Monocular (80%)
     - Female (80%)
     - Age 20–40
     - Areflexia (= Holmes Adie **syndrome**)

   - Secondary:
     - Syphilis (bilateral tonic pupil)
     - DM
     - Trauma, surgery
     - Degenerative

Exam tips:
- Tonic pupil ≠ Holmes Adie pupil ≠ Holmes Adie syndrome.

Q **What is Horner's Syndrome?**

"Horner's syndrome is a neurological syndrome caused by lesion in the sympathetic pathway in the head and neck."

Horner's Syndrome

1. **Clinical features:**
   - Miosis
   - Ptosis, inverse ptosis
   - Enophthalmos
   - Heterochromia
   - Ocular hypotony
   - Anhidrosis (if lesion is below superior cervical ganglion)

2. **Investigation:**
   - Cocaine 4–10%
     - Blocks **reuptake** of norepinephrine → pupillary dilatation
     - Confirmation test
     - Affected pupil does not dilate
   - Hydroxyamphetamine 1%
     - Promotes **release** of norepinephrine from terminal axon
     - Differentiates between central/preganglionic from postganglionic
     - Postganglionic lesion (3rd order) pupil fails to dilate
   - Phenylephrine 1%
     - **Denervation supersensitivity**
     - Differentiates central/preganglionic from postganglionic
     - Postganglionic lesion pupil dilates more widely

   - Apraclonidine 0.5%
     - α_1 and α_2 receptor agonist
     - Reverses anisocoria in both central/preganglionic and postganglionic Horner's syndrome

3. **Site and etiology:**
   - Central (first order):
     - Brainstem CVA
     - Trauma
     - Spinal cord tumor
     - MS
     - Syringomyelia
     - Lateral medullary (Wallenburg) syndrome
   - Preganglionic (second order):
     - Pancoast tumor
     - Thyroid CA
     - Vertebral metastasis
     - Subclavian/aortic/common carotid aneurysm
     - Trauma
     - Aortic/common carotid dissection
   - Postganglionic (third order)
     - Internal carotid dissection
     - Cluster headache
     - Cavernous sinus syndrome (Raeder's syndrome)
     - Nasopharyngeal carcinoma

Exam tips:
- **The pharmacological tests for Horner's syndrome are one of the favorite exam questions.**
- **A preganglionic or second order Horner's syndrome is important because of the possibility of Pancoast tumor. Therefore, differentiation of central/preganglionic from postganglionic is important.**

Q **What is the Argyll Robertson Pupil?**

Argyll Robertson Pupil

1. **Clinical features:**
   - Light near dissociation (response to accommodation better than to light)
   - Constricted (miosed) pupil
   - Speed of constriction and dilatation is normal
   - Bilateral pupil involvement common

2. **Investigation:**
   - Cocaine 4–10% (affected pupil does not dilate)

3. **Site of lesion:**
   - Dorsal midbrain (pretectal interneurons to Edinger-Westphal nucleus involved, ventrally located accommodative reflex neurons being spared)

4. **Etiology:**
   - Syphilis
     - Pupil signs:
       - AR pupil **or** tonic pupil
       - Pupillary irregularity (iritis)
       - Poor dilation to atropine
     - Other ocular signs (page 328):
       - Interstitial keratitis
       - Optic atrophy
       - Chorioretinitis
   - DM
   - MS
   - Alchoholism
   - Trauma, surgery
   - Aberrant III CN regeneration

Comparison Between Tonic Pupil and Argyll Robertson Pupil

	Tonic pupil	Argyll Robertson pupil
Demographics	Young	Old
	Female	Male
Pupil	Dilated	Miosed
	Unilateral	Bilateral
	Slow reaction to light and accommodation	Normal reaction to both
Common cause	Holmes Adie pupil or syndrome	Syphilis

Exam tips:
- Argyll Robertson pupil ≠ tonic pupil.
- Argyll Robertson pupil ≠ syphilis.

Dorsal Midbrain Syndrome

1. **Clinical features:**
   - Light-near-dissociation (response to accommodation better than to light)
   - Lid retraction (Collier's sign)
   - Supranuclear gaze palsy (normal vestibular ocular reflex and Bell's reflex)
   - Convergence retraction nystagmus
   - Spasm of convergence
   - Spasm of accommodation
   - Skew deviation

2. **Investigation:**
   - MRI brainstem to exclude lesion on dorsal midbrain

3. **Site of lesion:**
   - Dorsal midbrain (pretectal interneurons to Edinger-Westphal nucleus involved, ventrally located accommodative reflex neurons being spared, similar to AR pupil)

4. **Etiology (by age group):**
   - Hydrocephalus (infant)
   - Pinealoma (10 years)
   - Head injury (20 years)
   - AV malformation (30 years)
   - MS (40 years)
   - Vascular (50 years)
   - Degenerative (Wernicke's) (60 years)

Exam tips:
- Remember the seven classical signs and seven classical causes!

Clinical approach to pupils "Please examine this patient's pupils"

Describe

"On general inspection, there is ptosis/exodeviation."

"Please look at the distant (fixation target)."

"I would like to examine this patient's pupils first in the light and then in the dark."

- *Greater anisocoria in light — dilated pupil abnormalities (III CN, Holmes Adie....)*
- *Greater anisocoria in dark — constricted pupil abnormalities (Horner's....)*

Perform light reflex
- *Direct reflex (consensual reflex)*
- *RAPD*

Decide quickly which scenario

1. RAPD
- *Check EOM (INO, other CN)*

I'll like to check
- *Fundus (optic disc atrophy, retinal lesions)*
- *VA, VF, color vision*

2. Dilated pupil unreactive to light, anisocoria more pronounced in light
- *Ptosis/divergent squint*
  - *Check EOM*
  - *Watch for lid retraction (inverse Duane's syndrome or lid lag (pseudo-von Graefe's sign) from aberrant III CN regeneration)*

(Continued)

"This patient has a complete III nerve palsy."

I'll like to check

- *Fundus (papilledema)*
- *Examine patient neurologically for long tract signs*
- *No ptosis/no divergent squint*
  - *Check EOM*
  - *"I'd like to examine this patient under slit lamp."*
    - *Irregularity of pupils/vermiform movement (Holmes Adie)*
    - *Posterior synechiae (posterior synechiae)*
    - *Rupture sphincter/iris damage (traumatic mydriasis)*

"This patient has tonic pupil."

I'd like to

- *Examine fellow eye (Holmes Adie)*
- *Check tendon reflexes*
- *Perform pharmacological tests (0.1% pilocarpine)*
- *Ask for history of trauma, eyedrop use (can also use 1% pilocarpine to confirm)*

3. Small pupil, both reactive to light, anisocoria more pronounced in the dark

- *Mild ptosis, inverse ptosis*
- *Enophthalmos*
- *Flushing, anhidrosis*
- *Check EOM — ptosis overcome by frontalis*

"This patient has Horner's syndrome."

I'd like to

- *Check IOP (hypotony)*
- *Confirm diagnosis by performing pharmacological tests (cocaine, hydroxyamphetamine)*
- *Examine systematically and neurologically for:*
  - *Neck scars, neck mass (trauma, thyroid CA, lymph nodes)*
  - *Clubbing, hypothenar wasting, finger abduction weakness (Pancoast tumor)*
  - *III, IV, V CN palsies (Cavernous sinus syndrome, Raeder's syndrome)*
  - *VIII, IX, X CN palsies crossed hemiesthesia, cerebellar signs (lateral medullary syndrome)*
  - *Ask for history of pain and headache (cluster headache, carotid artery dissection)*

4. Small pupil, unreactive to light

- *Light-near-dissociation*

"This patient has Argyll Robertson's pupil."

I'll like to

- *Ask for history of DM, HPT, sarcoidosis, syphilis*

TOPIC 8

OPTIC NEUROPATHIES

Overall yield: ✪ ✪ ✪ ✪ ✪ **Clinical exam:** ✪ ✪ ✪ ✪ ✪ **Viva:** ✪ ✪ ✪ **Essay:** ✪ ✪ **MCQ:** ✪ ✪ ✪

Q Opening Question No. 1: What are the Causes of Optic Neuropathy?

"The causes of optic neuropathy can be divided into…."

Optic Neuropathy

1. **Congenital**
   - Hereditary optic neuropathy

2. **Acquired**
   - Optic neuritis (retrobulbar, papillitis, neuroretinitis):
     - Demyelinating
     - Postinfectious
     - Autoimmune diseases (systemic lupus)
     - Idiopathic
   - Ischemic optic neuropathy (anterior ischemic optic neuropathy, posterior ischemic optic neuropathy):
   - Arteritic (giant cell arteritis)
   - Nonarteritic (atherosclerotic)
   - Autoimmune diseases (systemic lupus)
   - Others (hypotension, hypovolemia)
   - Compressive optic neuropathy (tumors)
   - Infiltrative/granulomatous optic neuropathy (sarcoidosis, lymphoma, leukemia)
   - Traumatic optic neuropathy
   - Toxic optic neuropathy
   - Radiation optic neuropathy

> **Exam tips:**
> - Remember the causes of optic neuropathy as **"NIGHT TICS"** (Neuritis, Ischemic, Granulomatous, Hereditary, Traumatic, Toxic, Irradiation and Compressive).
> - But classify it as **"congenital vs acquired."**

Q How do You Differentiate Optic Neuritis From Anterior Ischemic Optic Neuropathy (AION) and Compressive Optic Neuropathy?

	Optic neuritis	Non-arteritic AION	Arteritic AION	Compressive optic neuropathy
Presentation				
1. Age of onset	• 20–40	• 40–65	• 70–80	• Any age
2. Gender	• Female	• Male = Female	• Female	• Male = Female
3. Onset	• Acute and progressive	• Dramatic sudden onset	• Dramatic sudden onset	• Gradual and progressive
4. Pain	• Yes	• No	• Yes	• No

(Continued)

	Optic neuritis	Non-arteritic AION	Arteritic AION	Compressive optic neuropathy
5. Other features	• MS symptoms (e.g. Uhthoff's phenomenon)	• Diabetes, hypertension, atherosclerosis risk factors • Small, crowded disc	• Amaurosis fugax • Giant cell arteritis symptoms (80%) • Jaw claudication • Neck pain • CRP > 2.45 mg/dl • ESR ≥ 47 mm/h • Scalp tenderness • Polymyalgia rheumatica • Malaise/ weight loss	• Headache, nausea and vomiting

Signs

	Optic neuritis	Non-arteritic AION	Arteritic AION	Compressive optic neuropathy
6. VA	• 6/18–6/60	• Severe loss (70%) • Mild loss (30%)	• HM — NPL (50%)	• May be normal
7. Bilateral involvement	• Rare in adults • May occur in children • May alternate between left and right eyes	• Unilateral • Second eye may be involved later on	• Common	• Rare
8. Pupil	• RAPD	• RAPD	• RAPD	• Normal
9. Fundus	• Normal or • Papillitis (pink)	• Disc swelling (sectoral, pale)	• Disc swelling (chalky white disc edema) • Cilioretinal artery occlusion	• Disc swelling (diffuse) • Optociliary shunt (meningioma, optic nerve glioma)
10. Color vision	• Dramatic loss, disproportional to VA loss	• Loss proportional to VA loss		

Investigation

	Optic neuritis	Non-arteritic AION	Arteritic AION	Compressive optic neuropathy
11. VF	• Diffuse (50%) • Central (10%)	• Inferior nasal sectoral defect • Inferior altitudinal defect		• Enlarged blind-spot
12. Blood	• Normal	• ESR raised	• ESR markedly raised • C-reactive protein markedly raised (more sensitive than ESR)	

(*Continued*)

	Optic neuritis	Non-arteritic AION	Arteritic AION	Compressive optic neuropathy
13. FFA	• Mild leakage at disc margins	• Moderate leakage	• Severe leakage • Filling defect seen (decrease capillary and choroidal perfusion)	• Severe leakage
14. VEP	• Latency increase • (Myelination abnormality)	• Amplitude decrease • (axonal abnormality)	• Amplitude decrease • (Axonal abnormality)	• Amplitude decrease • (Axonal abnormality)
15. Other investigations	• MRI		• Temporal artery biopsy	
Prognosis	• 100% recover • 75% to 6/9	• 30% recover • 30% deteriorate • 30% stay the same	• Very poor prognosis • 65% blind in both eyes within a few weeks if left untreated	• Good if compressive lesion removed

Exam tips:
- **The three most important and common causes of optic neuropathy.**
- **Remember that there are five differentiating symptoms, five differentiating signs and five differentiating investigations.**
- **Read treatment of non-arteritic AION from Ischemic Optic Neuropathy Decompression Trial Research Group (*JAMA* 1995;273:625–632).**

Q **How would You Perform a Temporal Artery Biopsy?**

"Temporal artery biopsy is the "gold standard" test for making a diagnosis of temporal arteritis."
"I would commence corticosteroid therapy prior to temporal artery biopsy if the biopsy cannot be performed immediately."
"I would perform temporal artery biopsy ideally within three days of commencing corticosteroid therapy, and preferably not after one week of commencing steroids."

Procedure

1. **Identify branch of superficial temporal artery by palpation or Doppler ultrasound**
2. **Local anesthesia: Lignocaine 1–2% and adrenaline**
3. **Incise skin over the artery with a No. 15 scalpel until subcutaneous fat is seen**
4. **Blunt dissection of space below fat but above superficial temporalis muscle fascia with small curved artery forceps (superficial temporal artery runs within the fascia), avoiding injury to the facial nerve**

5. Carefully dissect superficial temporal artery from fascia with Wescott scissors
6. Tie both ends of segment to be excised with 4/0 silk
7. At least 3cm of artery is excised (because of skip lesions)
8. Cauterize cut ends of artery
9. Close subcutaneous tissue with 5/0 interrupted vicryl suture
10. Close skin with interrupted 6/0 or 7/0 prolene

Complications
- Bleeding
- Damage to branches of the facial nerve
- Failure to identify artery (especially if non-pulsatile)
- Scalp necrosis
- Stroke (rare)

Q Opening Question No. 2: What are the Causes of Optic Atrophy?

"Optic atrophy can be either unilateral or bilateral."

Unilateral optic atrophy	Bilateral optic atrophy	Evaluation
Congenital (not a common cause)	**Congenital**	
1. Hereditary optic neuropathy	1. **Hereditary** optic neuropathy	Family history
• Dominant (Kjer)		
• Recessive (Behr, DIDMOAD)		
• Mitochondrial — Leber's optic neuropathy		
Acquired	**Acquired**	
1. Old **ischemic** optic neuropathy	1. **Pituitary** tumor	CT scan
2. **Compressive** optic neuropathy/pituitary tumor	2. Chronic **papilledema** (secondary OA)	Drug history, anemia Serum vitamin levels
3. **Infiltrative** optic neuropathy:	3. Toxic optic neuropathy	ESR
• Sarcoidosis	4. Consecutive ischemic optic neuropathy	History of MS, VDRL
• Malignancies (lymphomas, optic nerve tumors)	5. Consecutive optic neuritis	FTA
4. Old optic neuritis	6. Radiation optic neuropathy	History of nasopharyngeal CA
5. Traumatic optic neuropathy	7. Chronic glaucoma	IOP, VF
6. Radiation optic neuropathy		
7. Chronic glaucoma		
8. Toxic optic neuropathy:		
• TB drugs (ethambutol, isoniazid, streptomycin),		
• Chloramphenicol, digitalis, chloroquine		
• Toxins (lead, arsenic, methanol)		
• Thiamine, vitamin B2, B6, B12, niacin, folate deficiency		
• Tobacco-alcohol toxicity		
9. Others — PRP, retinitis pigmentosa		

Clinical approach to optic atrophy

"The most obvious abnormality is a pale optic disc."

Comment on
- *Sectoral pallor, altitudinal pallor, bow tie, cupping*

I'll like to
- *Test for RAPD*
- *Check EOM for other CN involvement*
- *Examine the fellow eye*

If unilateral, think of
- *Old optic neuritis (internuclear ophthalmoplegia, other CN palsies)*
- *AION (vascular risk factors)*
- *Compressive optic neuropathy (headache, nausea, vomiting, optociliary shunt, Foster Kennedy syndrome)*
- *Traumatic optic neuropathy (history of trauma)*
- *Radiation (history of DXT)*

If bilateral, think of
- *Pituitary tumors (bitemporal VF defect)*
- *Consecutive optic neuritis*
- *Toxic optic neuropathy (ethambutol and other drugs)*
- *Hereditary optic neuropathy (Leber's optic neuropathy)*

Exam tips:
- **Very similar answer to causes of optic neuropathy but this question requires a more "clinical" approach.**
- **Causes are listed slightly differently for unilateral vs bilateral optic atrophy. The common ones are in bold.**

Q **Opening Question No. 3:** What are the Causes of Optic Disc Swelling?

"Optic disc swelling can be either unilateral or bilateral."
"The causes are either congenital or acquired."

Unilateral disc swelling	Bilateral disc swelling
Acquired	**Acquired**
1. **Optic neuritis**	1. **Papilledema**
2. **Ischemic optic neuropathy**	• Space occupying lesion
3. **Compressive optic neuropathy**	• Idiopathic intracranial hypertension
4. Infiltrative optic neuropathy	• Malignant HPT
5. Traumatic optic neuropathy	2. **Pseudopapilledema**
6. Toxic optic neuropathy	• Drusen
7. Radiation optic neuropathy	• Congenital optic disc anomaly
	3. Consecutive ischemic optic neuropathy

(Continued)

(*Continued*)

Unilateral disc swelling	Bilateral disc swelling
PLUS	4. Consecutive optic neuritis
8. Ocular disease — central retinal vein occlusion, posterior uveitis, posterior scleritis	5. Compressive optic neuropathy
	6. Toxic optic neuropathy
9. Orbital disease — pseudotumor, thyroid eye disease	7. Diabetic papillopathy (may be unilateral)
Congenital (not as common as acquired)	**PLUS**
1. Hereditary optic neuropathy	7. Ocular disease — posterior uveitis, posterior scleritis
	8. Orbital disease — pseudotumor, thyroid eye disease
	Congenital (not as common as acquired)
	1. Hereditary optic neuropathy

Exam tips:
- Unilateral disc swelling — cause of optic neuropathy plus ocular and orbital diseases.

OPTIC NEURITIS AND MULTIPLE SCLEROSIS

Overall yield: ✵✵✵✵✵ **Clinical exam:** ✵✵✵✵ **Viva:** ✵✵✵ **Essay:** ✵✵ **MCQ:** ✵✵✵

Q Opening Question No. 1: What is the Anatomy of the Optic Nerve?

"Optic neuritis is the second cranial nerve."
"It is divided into four segments."

Segment	Length	Diameter	Blood supply
Intraocular • Optic disc • Prelaminar • Laminar • Postlaminar	1 mm	1.5 × 1.75 mm	• Retinal arterioles from CRA • Peripapillary choroidal vessels* • Circle of Zinn Haller* • Pial branches*
Intraorbital	25 mm	3 mm	Pial branches of CRA
Intracanicular	4–10 mm	3 mm	Ophthalmic artery branches
Intracranial	10 mm	7 mm	Internal carotid artery and ophthalmic artery branches

*From posterior ciliary arteries

Exam tips:
• A "gift" question and one of the favorite anatomy questions. Answer it well.

Q Opening Question No. 2: Tell me About Optic Neuritis.

"Optic neuritis is an acute inflammatory optic nerve disease."

Optic Neuritis

1. **Classification**
   • Etiological:
     • Idiopathic/demyelination
     • Secondary to:
       · Autoimmune diseases
       · Infectious diseases (e.g. syphilis, viral infection)
   • Anatomical
     • Sarcoidosis
     • Retrobulbar neuritis:
       · Common variant in adults
       · Frequently associated with multiple sclerosis

- Papillitis:
  - Common variant and usually bilateral in children
- Neuroretinitis:
  - Associated with viral infection, cat scratch disease, Lyme's disease, syphilis
  - Not associated with multiple sclerosis

- Usually self-limiting and resolves within 6–12 months

2. **Clinical features and investigations (see page 248)**
3. **Prognosis (see below)**
4. **Treatment (see below)**

Notes
- Signs of optic nerve dysfunction:
  - Decrease in VA
  - RAPD
  - Dyschromatopsia (usually red-green)
  - Diminished light-brightness and contrast sensitivity
  - Visual field defects

Q **What is the Prognosis of a Patient with Optic Neuritis Diagnosed Two Days Ago?**

Prognosis

1. **Recovery**
   - Onset within a few days, maximal impairment within 1–2 weeks
   - Recovery begins within 2–3 weeks, maximal at 6 months
   - Almost 100% have some recovery
   - Full recovery in **75%**

2. **Recurrence**
   - No recurrence in **75%**

3. **Risk of MS**
   - MS develops in **75%** of women (35% in men)
   - Risk factors:
     - Patient:
       - Age 20–40
       - Female sex

- White race
- Family history of MS
- Winter onset
- Ocular:
  - History of Uhthoff's phenomenon
  - FFA leakage around disc margin
  - Recurrence of optic neuritis
  - Optic neuritis in fellow eye
- Systemic:
  - History of nonspecific neurological symptoms
  - HLA DR2
  - CSF oligoclonal bands
  - MRI periventricular lesions ($\geq$ 3, each $\geq$ 3 mm in size)
- If MRI normal, risk of developing MS only 16% in 5 years

Exam tips:
- "3R" for "recovery, recurrence and risk of MS."
- 3/4 rule for the chance of each outcome.
- Risk factors for MS: 4 patient factors, 4 ocular factors, 4 systemic factors.

Q **What are the Main Findings of the Optic Neuritis Treatment Trial (ONTT)?**

"The ONTT is a multicenter trial to evaluate treatment of optic neuritis with steroids."
"There were 457 patients enrolled."
"The patients were randomized to three treatment regimes."

Treatment Regimes

1. **IV steroids**
   - 3 days IV methylprednisolone (1g/day) plus 11 days of oral prednisolone (1mg/kg/day)
2. **Oral steroids**
   - 14 days of oral prednisolone
3. **Placebo**
   - 14 days of oral placebo

Results

1. **Recovery**
   - IV steroids vs placebo: **Faster** recovery, but final VA same, although color vision, contrast sensitivity and VF better
   - Oral steroids vs placebo: no difference
2. **Recurrence**
   - IV steroids vs placebo: **No** difference
   - Oral steroids vs placebo: **Higher** recurrence
3. **Risk of MS**
   - IV steroids vs placebo: **Lower** risk in first two years but same after that
   - Oral steroids vs placebo: No difference
   - **MRI** important predictor of MS (≥ 3, each ≥ 3 mm or more in size increases risk by 12 times)

Exam tips:
- **An easy way to commit to memory the effects of each type of treatment on the "3Rs" of prognosis.**
- **One of the few big trials you are expected to know well.** *N Engl J Med* **1992; 581–88,** *Surv Ophthalmol* **1998;43:291,** *Arch Ophthalmol* **1997;115:1545–1552.**

Q **What are the Main Findings of the Controlled High Risk Subjects Avonex Multiple Sclerosis Prevention Study (CHAMPS)?**

"The CHAMPS is a prospective randomized study designed to determine whether the effect of early treatment with interferon beta-1a (Avonex) delayed the risk of developing clinically definite multiple sclerosis."
"There were 383 patients enrolled, who had their first demyelineating event (including optic neuritis, myelitis, brainstem-cerebellar syndromes) and had at least two MRI white matter abnormalities characteristic of MS."
"The patients were randomized to two treatment regimes."

Treatment Regimes

Group 1: ONTT protocol of IV and oral steroids followed by weekly intramuscular 30µg interferon beta-1a
Group 2: ONTT protocol of IV and oral steroids followed by weekly intramuscular injection of placebo

Results

1. **Interferon beta-1a reduces the three-year likelihood of conversion to clinically definite MS**
2. **MRI findings:**
   - Reduction in volume of brain lesions in interferon beta-1a group
   - Fewer new/enlarging lesions and fewer gadolinium enhancing lesions in interferon beta-1a group

Trial terminated because of clear benefit of treatment over placebo.
Benefit of interferon beta-1a also shown in other trials (including Rebif), and continues over a 10-year period of observation (CHAMPIONS study)

- **Side effects of interferon beta-1a:**
  Depression, fluid-like symptoms, liver toxicity, anaphylaxis

"Multiple sclerosis is an idiopathic demyelination disorder of the CNS."
"MS does not involve the peripheral nervous system."
"The CNS lesions are separated in **TIME** and **SPACE**."
"Diagnosis is therefore made when there are two or more different neurological events occurring at different times."

Multiple Sclerosis

1. **Systemic features**
   - Hemisphere:
     - Dementia
     - Hemiparesis, dysphasia, hemianopia
   - Brain stem:
     - Dysarthria, dysphagia
     - Nystagmus, ataxia, diplopia
   - Spinal cord:
     - Motor
     - Sensory
     - Bladder, bowel and sexual disturbances
   - Transient disturbances:
     - Lhermitte's sign
     - Uhthoff's phenomenon
     - Trigeminal neuralgia

2. **Ocular features**
   - Sensory (hemisphere lesions)
     - **Optic neuritis:**
       - One-third of MS will present with optic neuritis
       - Two-thirds will have optic neuritis in course of disease
       - Risk of MS with optic neuritis (see above)
     - Posterior visual system lesions (VF defects)
   - Motor (brainstem lesions)
     - Gaze abnormalities:
       - **Internuclear ophthalmoplegia:**
         - One-third of MS will present with INO

- Two-thirds will have INO in course of disease
- Clinical features (see below)
   - Horizontal gaze palsy
   - One-and-a-half syndrome
   - Ocular dysmetria
   - Dorsal midbrain syndrome
   - Skew deviation
   - Nystagmus
   - Isolated CN involvement
   - Paroxysmal eye movement disorders
- Rare:
   - Intermediate uveitis
   - Retinal periphlebitis

3. **Investigations**
   - Lumbar puncture:
     - Oligoclonal bands
     - Leukocytosis
     - IgG > 15% total protein
   - VEP:
     - Increase in latency typically exceeds decrease in amplitude
   - MRI:
     - Periventricular and corpus callosum plaques
     - Acute lesions may enhance with gadolinium

"INO is motor abnormality caused by lesions in the medial longitudinal fasciculus (MLF)."

1. **Classical feature (triad)**
   - Failure of adduction of ipsilateral eye (e.g. side of MLF lesion)
   - Ataxic nystagmus of contralateral eye on abduction
   - Normal convergence (posterior INO)

2. **Other clinical features**
   - Horizontal:
     - Slowing of saccades in adducting eye
     - Horizontal nystagmus of adducting eye

- Vestibuloocular reflex (VOR) impaired (note: VOR is not intact because lesion is not supranuclear)
- Abnormal convergence (note: Cogan's anterior INO, implies lesion extents to midbrain convergence center)
- Manifest exotropia (wall-eyed bilateral INO or WEBINO)
- Vertical:
   - Vertical nystagmus
   - Vertical pursuit impaired

- Vertical VOR impaired
- Upgaze maintenance impaired

3. **Investigations**
   - OKN drum:
     - Slowing of saccades in adducting eye (to elicit, rotate drum in direction of ipsilateral MLF lesion)

- ENG (electronystagmogram):
  - Reduction of peak velocity of adduction

4. **Etiology**
   - MS (40%)
   - CVA (40%)
   - Others (tumor, trauma, infection)

Exam tips:
- There are 10 clinical features of INO (not three).

Clinical approach to INO

"The most obvious abnormality is a failure of adduction of the right eye."
"With a horizontal nystagmus seen in the left eye."

Examine
- *Exclude one-and-a-half syndrome (failure of abduction of ipsilateral eye and adduction of contralateral eye)*
- *Vestibulo-ocular reflex/Doll's eye reflex (should be impaired)*
- *Convergence (if impaired, implies Cogan's anterior INO)*
- *Vertical movements*

I'd like to
- *Examine pupils for RAPD (old optic neuritis inflamed optic nerve)*
- *Examine fundus (optic atrophy)*
- *Examine neurological system (signs of MS or stroke)*
- *Ask for history of trauma*

Exam tips:
- An extremely common clinical exam case. Usually asked to examine the ocular movements.
- Remember to look at the adducting eye when testing for horizontal movements!

Q **What are the Supranuclear Disorders of Ocular Motility?**

"Supranuclear disorders of ocular motility are characterized by the absence of diplopia, and the presence of normal vestibulo-ocular reflexes."

1. **Horizontal gaze palsies:**
   - Parapontine reticular formation (PPRF) lesions: Ipsilateral horizontal gaze palsy
   - Medial longitudinal (MLF) lesions: Internuclear ophthalmoplegia
   - PPRF and MLF lesions: "One-and-a-half syndrome"

2. **Vertical gaze palsies:**
   - Parinaud dorsal midbrain syndrome
   - Progressive supranuclear palsy (Steele-Richardson-Olszewski syndrome)

VISUAL FIELD DEFECTS IN NEUROOPHTHALMOLOGY

Overall yield: ✪✪✪   **Clinical exam:** ✪✪✪✪   **Viva:** ✪✪   **Essay:** ✪   **MCQ:** ✪✪

Q Opening Question: What are the Ocular Manifestations of a Meningioma Compressing the Left Optic Tract?

Lesion in Left Side of the Visual Pathway

1. **Left optic nerve**
   - Decrease in VA in **left** eye
   - Decrease in color vision in **left** eye
   - RAPD in **left** eye
   - Optic disc swelling or atrophy in **left** eye
   - Dense central/diffuse scotoma in **left** eye

2. **Optic chiasm**
   - Bitemporal hemianopia (classic)
   - Dense central/diffuse scotoma (optic nerve)
   - Incongruous homonymous hemianopia (optic tract)
   - Bitemporal central scotoma (macular fibers)
   - Junctional scotoma (junction of optic nerve and chiasma)
   - Other features of chiasmal syndrome (see pituitary disorders, page 260)

3. **Left optic tract**
   - Incongruous **right** homonymous quadrantanopia
   - RAPD in **right** eye

4. **Left parietal lobe**
   - Incongruous **right** lower homonymous quadrantanopia
   - Pursuit defect to **left**
   - Hemiparesis or hemianesthesia in **right** side of body

   - OKN asymmetry (defect when drum rotates towards left)
   - Dominant parietal lobe (Gerstmann syndrome)
     - Aphasia/agraphia/acalculia
     - Left-right disorientation
   - Non-dominant parietal lobe
     - Neglect/inattention
     - Impaired constructional ability
     - Dyscalculia

5. **Left temporal lobe**
   - Incongruous **right** upper homonymous hemianopia
   - Formed visual hallucination
   - Auditory hallucinations
   - May be complicated by motor seizures

6. **Left visual cortex**
   - Congruous **right** homonymous hemianopia
   - OKN symmetry
   - Unformed visual hallucination
   - Other features of visual cortex involvement (see stroke, migraine and other vascular disorders, page 266)

Clinical approach to visual field examination

"Please examine this patient's visual field."

Common clinical syndromes

- *Bitemporal hemianopia*
- *Homonymous hemianopia*
- *Bitemporal or homonymous quadrantanopia*
- *Altitudinal hemianopia*

Preliminary instructions

"I am going to test the area that you can see."
"Please cover your left eye and look at my nose."
"Is there any part of my face that is not clear?"
"How many fingers are there?"
"Now look at my face and do not move your eyes…."

Quadrant testing

"How many fingers are there?"

Neglect testing

"How many fingers are there altogether?"

Central scotoma testing
Test fellow eye

*"This patient has **bitemporal hemianopia**, my clinical diagnosis is a **pituitary lesion**."*

I'd like to

- *Check EOM (see-saw nystagmus, CN palsies)*
- *Check fundus (bow-tie atrophy, papilledema)*
- *Ask history of diplopia (nonparetic), metamorphopsia, visual hallucination*
- *Look for features of **hypersecretion** from an adenoma*
  - *Growth hormone (acromegaly)*
  - *Prolactin (history of amenorrhea, galactorrhea, infertility in females or impotence in males)*
  - *ACTH (Cushing's syndrome)*
- *Assess for **etiology** of pituitary lesion — ask for history of*
  - *Trauma*
  - *Radiation*
  - *Shock, blood loss during pregnancy (pituitary apoplexy)*
  - *Adrenalectomy for Cushing's (Nelson's syndrome)*
  - *Secondaries to pituitary, infiltrative lesions (TB, sarcoidosis)*

Or

*"This patient has **right homonymous hemianopia**, my clinical diagnosis is a **left postchiasmal lesion**."*

I'd like to

- *Check fundus (optic atrophy, papilledema)*
- *Perform full Humphrey VF to assess congruity of lesion*
- ***Left optic tract***
  - *Incongruous **right** homonymous quadrantanopia*
  - *RAPD in **right** eye*

(Continued)

(Continued)

- **Left parietal lobe**
  - Incongruous **right** lower homonymous quadrantanopia
  - Check EOM (failure of pursuit to **left**)
  - Check for **right** hemiparesis or hemianesthesia
  - Assess reading (alexia) and writing (agraphia)
  - OKN asymmetry (move drum towards **left**)

- **Left temporal lobe**
  - Incongruous **right** upper homonymous hemianopia
  - Formed visual hallucination

- **Left occipital lobe**
  - Congruous **right** homonymous hemianopia
  - Assess visual attention (inattention) and visual recognition (agnosia)
  - OKN symmetry
  - Unformed visual hallucination

Exam tips:
- Alternate question can be "What are the ocular manifestations of stroke involving the right optic radiation?"
- Few important principles to remember
  1. VF defect becomes more congruous as you move further back along the visual pathway.
  2. Visual hallucination is formed in temporal lobe lesions vs unformed for cortex lesions.
  3. OKN asymmetry indicates that a lesion has involved the parietal lobe (usually a tumor) as compared with OKN symmetry in a pure cortex lesion (usually a stroke) (page 240).

PITUITARY AND CHIASMAL DISORDERS

Overall yield: ✮✮✮✮ **Clinical exam:** ✮✮✮✮ **Viva:** ✮✮✮ **Essay:** ✮✮ **MCQ:** ✮✮✮✮

Q **Opening Question:** Tell me about the Pituitary Gland.

1. **Anatomy**
   - Situated in sella turcica of sphenoid bone
   - Anterior lobe:
     - Secretes ACTH, GH, Prolactin, FSH, LH and TSH
   - Posterior lobe:
     - "Secretes" ADH and oxytocin (actual hormones produced from hypothalamus)
   - Relationship with chiasma:
     - **Central:**
       - 80%
       - Classic "chiasmal syndrome" features (see below)
       - Optic chiasmal VF defect: Bitemporal hemianopia, involving the superior fields first
     - **Prefixed** (chiasma is **anterior** to pituitary gland):
       - 10%
       - Optic tract features
       - Optic tract VF defect: Incongruous homonymous hemianopia
       - Macular involvement: Bitemporal central scotoma
     - **Postfixed** (chiasma is **posterior** to pituitary gland):
       - 10%

   - Optic nerve features (RAPD, color vision, etc)
   - Optic nerve VF defect: Dense central/ diffuse scotoma
   - Optic nerve and chiasmal junction: Junctional scotoma (von Willebrand's knee)

2. **Spectrum of pituitary disorders**
   - Tumors:
     - Pituitary adenoma
     - Craniopharyngioma
     - Meningioma
     - Others:
       - Chordoma
       - Nasopharyngeal CA
       - Rathke's pouch cyst
       - Secondaries
   - Vascular (aneurysm)
   - Inflammation (Tolosa-Hunt syndrome, meningitis)
   - Demyelination (MS)
   - Trauma, surgery and DXT
   - Non-neoplastic masses: Fibrous dysplasia, sphenoidal sinus mucoceles, arachnoid cysts

"Pituitary adenomas are benign tumors of the pituitary gland."
"They can be classified as either secreting or nonsecreting, which can be subdivided into chromophobes, acidophils…."
"Or classified as either microadenoma or macroadenoma, defined as…."
"The clinical presentation is that a combination of local mass effects and systemic endocrine effects."

Classification		Hormones	Clinical features
Secreting (75%)	Chromophobes (50%)	Prolactin	• Infertility-amenorrhea-galactorrhea in women (like a lactation state, except you cannot get pregnant!) • Hypogonadism, impotence, sterility, decreased libido, gynecomastia and galactorrhea in men
	Acidophils (20%)	GH	• Acromegaly in adults (see below) • Gigantism in children
	Basophils (5%)	ACTH FSH and TSH	• Cushing's disease (causing Cushing's syndrome) • FSH and TSH tumors are extremely rare
Nonsecreting (25%)			
Microadenoma		Less than 10 mm in diameter	• Usually that of secreting adenomas • Nonsecreting microadenomas are not discovered!
Macroadenoma		More than 10 mm in diameter	• Mass effects • Usually nonsecreting in nature

1. **Localized mass effects**
   - Chiasmal syndrome (see below)
   - Compression of other adjacent structure:
     - Cavernous sinus (CN palsies)
     - Pituitary gland (hypopituitarism)
     - Raised intracranial pressure (papilledema)
2. **Endocrine effects**
   - Hypersecretion
3. **Management**
   - Investigation:
     - Skull XR (note: In practice, skull XR is not very useful):
       - Expansion or ballooning of fossa
       - Erosion of clinoid
       - "Double floor" sign (asymmetrical fossa expansion)
     - CT scan/MRI
   - Endocrine evaluation: Prolactin, FSH, TSH, GH
   - Treatment:
     - Factors to consider:
       - Age
       - Presenting problem (vision, mass effect, endocrine effect)
       - Size and stage of tumor
     - Surgery (transphenoidal, transethmoidal, craniotomy)
     - Bromocriptine for prolactinomas (increases prolactin inhibition factor)/somatostatin for GH tumors
     - Radiotherapy (complications include radiation optic neuropathy and panhypopituitarism):
       - Gamma-knife stereotactic radiotherapy

Exam tips:
- The clinical presentation is often a combination of either: Endocrine effects (from secreting tumors) or mass effects (from macroadenomas).
- Most ophthalmologists end up seeing macroadenomas with mass effects on the chiasma.
- To aid memory (not exactly accurate!), microadenomas = secreting adenomas = endocrine effects; macroadenomas = nonsecreting adenomas = mass effects.

Q What are the Ocular Manifestations of a Pituitary Adenoma Pressing on the Chiasma?

Clinical Features of the Chiasmal Syndrome
- VF defects (depending on location of chiasma):
  - Bitemporal hemianopia involving superior fields first (classic VF defect)
  - Incongruous homonymous hemianopia (optic tract)
  - Bitemporal central scotoma (macular fibers)
  - Dense central/diffuse scotoma (optic nerve)
  - Junctional scotoma (junction of optic nerve and chiasma)
- Optic atrophy (spectrum of changes):
  - Normal looking disc
- Temporal pallor (papillomacular bundle)
- Bow tie atrophy
- Dense optic atrophy
- Hemifield slip (nonparetic diplopia)
- Postfixation blindness
- Visual hallucination
- See-saw nystagmus

Exam tips:
- The "chiasmal syndrome" is an important syndrome and bitemporal hemianopia is but one of five different VF defects.

Q What are the Ocular Features of Acromegaly?

Acromegaly
- **A**ngioid streaks
- **C**hiasma syndrome
- **R**etinopathy (DM and HPT retinopathy)
- **O**ptic atrophy, papilledema
- **M**uscle enlargement

Exam tips:
- Remember the clinical features as "ACROM."

Q What is Pituitary Apoplexy?

Pituitary Apoplexy
- Infarction of pituitary gland
- Tumor outgrows blood supply or tumor compresses hypophyseal portal vessels
- Presents with **hyperacute** chiasmal syndrome
- Treatment: High dose steroids/surgery

Q Tell me about Craniopharyngioma.

"Craniopharyngioma is an intracranial tumor arising from remnants of Rathke's pouch."

Craniopharyngioma

1. **Histological features**
   - Solid component with squamous epithelium and calcification
   - Cystic component with greenish fluid
2. **Clinical presentation — depends on growth of tumor**
   - Superiorly into ventricles (most common, hydrocephalus and raised intracranial pressure)
   - Anteriorly to frontal lobe (dementia)
   - Anteroinferiorly to optic nerve and chiasma (chiasmal syndrome)
   - Posteroinferiorly to hypothalamus and pituitary gland (diabetes insipidus and hypopituitarism)
   - Children often present with panhypopituitarism secondary to hypothalamic dysfunction (dwarfism, delayed sexual development, obesity), while adults often present with visual impairment and visual field defects
3. **Diagnosis**
   - CT scan/MRI (suprasellar **calcification** in 70%)
4. **Treatment: Surgical excision +/− postoperative radiotherapy**
   - Recurrence common and requires lifelong follow-up

Notes
- Differential diagnoses of bitemporal visual field defects:
  - Chiasmal lesions
  - Dermatochalasis of upper lids
  - Tilted discs
  - Optic nerve colobomas
  - Nasal retinitis pigmentosa
  - Nasal retinoschisis
  - Functional visual loss

Q What is the Empty Sellar Syndrome?

"The empty sellar syndrome is a neurological condition in which the subarachnoid space extends into the sella, remodeling the bone and enlarging the sella."

Empty Sellar Syndrome

1. **Classification**
   - Primary:
     - Common, 25% of autopsies
     - Transfer of CSF pressure through a congenitally large opening in diaphragm sella
     - Risk factors: Multiparous women, elderly atherosclerotic patients, idiopathic intracranial hypertension
   - Secondary:
     - Pituitary surgery
     - DXT
     - Pituitary apoplexy (need to exclude concomitant pituitary adenoma)
2. **Clinical features**
   - VA usually normal
   - Decrease VA rare
     - Due to herniation of suprasellar contents (e.g. optic nerve) into sella or vascular compromise
   - VF defects:
     - Binasal (classically)
     - Bitemporal, altitudinal and generalized constriction of VF possible
   - Headache
   - Elevated prolactin levels
3. **Diagnosis**
   - CT scan/MRI

PAPILLEDEMA AND INTRACRANIAL TUMORS

Overall yield: ✪✪✪✪ **Clinical exam:** ✪✪✪✪ **Viva:** ✪✪✪ **Essay:** ✪✪ **MCQ:** ✪✪

Q Opening Question: What are the Clinical Features of Papilledema?

"Papilledema is bilateral optic nerve head swelling secondary to raised intracranial pressure. It can be divided into four stages...."

"Clinical features are related to either vascular or mechanical changes of the optic disc...."

Papilledema

Stage	Vision	Optic disc vascular changes	Optic disc mechanical changes
Early	• VA normal	• Hyperemia of margins • Loss of spontaneous venous pulsation (absent in 20% of normal individuals) • Indistinct disc margins	• Blurring of margins (superior and inferior margin first) • Edema of peripapillary nerve fiber layer
Established	• Transient visual disturbances • VA normal or impaired • Enlarged blind spot	• Venous tortuosity and dilation • Peripapillary flame-shaped hemorrhage • Cotton wool spots • Hard exudates • Obscuration of small vessels traversing disc	• Elevated disc • Obliteration of cup • Retinal/choroidal folds
Longstanding	• VA impaired • Constricted VF	• Vascular changes resolves	• "Champagne cork" appearance • Optociliary shunts • Drusen-like crystalline deposits
Atrophic	• VA severely impaired		• Secondary optic atrophy

"Idiopathic Intracranial Hypertension (IIH) is a neurological syndrome of raised intracranial pressure in the absence of...."

Idiopathic Intracranial Hypertension

1. **Definition (important)**
   - Raised intracranial pressure
     - > 250 mm water (need lumbar puncture) — lateral decubitus position
   - In **absence** of (triad):
     - Space occupying lesion (need CT scan)
     - Hydrocephalus (need CT scan)
     - Abnormal CSF (need lumbar puncture)

2. **Etiology**
   - Associated with obesity
   - Exclude:
     - Sagittal sinus thrombosis (most important to exclude. Need MRV to diagnose)
     - Metabolic disorders (Cushing's disease, Addison's, hypoparathyroidism)
     - Vitamin A toxicity (see page 413) and lead poisoning
     - Drugs (steroids, nalidixic acid, amiodarone, tetracycline)

3. **Clinical features**
   - Headache (90%)
   - Visual loss:
     - Transient (70%) or persistent (30%)
     - Variable (different time of day)
     - Shifting (left and right eyes)
     - Loss of contrast sensitivity
     - VF loss (essentially like VF defects in **papilledema):**
       - Enlargement of blind spot and constriction of VF
       - Other VF defects (nasal defects, central defects)
   - Tinnitis (60%)
     - IIH has been called "otitic hydrocephalus" precisely because of this symptom
   - Others (photopsia, retrobulbar pain, diplopia)

4. **Investigations**
   - CT scan/MRI:
     - Normal looking ventricles
     - Small ventricles
   - Empty sella (see page 261)
   - Venous sinus thrombosis
   - Lumbar puncture
   - Metabolic/endocrine evaluation
   - Perimetry

5. **Prognosis**
   - Spontaneous remission (3–12 months)
   - May be remitting and relapsing or develop into chronic condition
   - Recurrence (10%)
   - Visual loss risk factors:
     - Vascular disease (HPT, DM, anemia)
     - Raised IOP
     - Recent weight gain

6. **Treatment**
   - Conservative: Lose weight, discontinue inciting drug, treat systemic disorders
   - Indications for treatment:
     - Severe symptoms (headache)
     - Visual loss
     - High CSF pressure
   - Repeat lumbar puncture:
     - 25% remit after first lumbar puncture
     - However, CSF usually replenishes within 1–2 hours
   - Diuretics (acetazolamide):
     - Oral diamox 500 mg bid for 4–6 weeks
     - Topiramate (anticonvulsant that also inhibits carbonic anhydrase)
     - If there is no response, consider
   - Steroids:
     - Dexamethasone 4 mg 6 hourly for 1–2 weeks
     - If no response, consider
   - Optic nerve sheath decompression or ventriculo/lumbo — peritoneal shunt
   - Stenting of transverse sinus

"The ocular features of a meningioma include general signs due to raised intracranial pressure."
"And focal signs depending on where the meningioma is...."

Ocular Signs of Intracranial Tumors

1. **General (raised intracranial pressure)**
   - Symptoms:
     - Visual blurring (transient or persistent)
     - Diplopia
   - Signs:
     - Papilledema and optic atrophy
     - Foster Kennedy syndrome
       - **Triad** of optic atrophy in one eye, papilledema in other eye and anosmia

   - VI CN palsy (false localizing sign)
   - III CN palsy (uncal herniation)

2. **Focal**
   - Supratentorial (mainly sensory)
   - Suprasellar/sphenoidal ridge/midbrain (both sensory and motor)
   - Infratentorial (mainly motor)

Exam tips:
- The ocular features of ANY brain tumor can be divided into general signs due to raised intracranial pressure (see papilledema above) and focal signs, depending on location of tumor.
- For neuroophthalmology and strokes (see page 255), for migraines and other vascular disorders (see page 265).

Principles of Management

1. **Histological diagnosis**
   - Access via burr hole or craniotomy
   - Guidance via free hand or stereotactic technique

2. **Curative excision for benign tumors (e.g. meningioma)**

3. **Palliative excision for malignant tumors (e.g. glioblastoma)**

4. **Adjunctive therapy (e.g. DXT, chemotherapy)**

STROKES, MIGRAINES & OTHER VASCULAR DISORDERS

Overall yield: ✪✪✪✪ **Clinical exam:** ✪✪ **Viva:** ✪✪✪ **Essay:** ✪✪✪ **MCQ:** ✪✪

Q Opening Question: What are the Ocular Manifestations of Strokes?

"Strokes cause a variety of different ocular syndromes."
"Depending on the **arterial system** and **location** of the stroke...."
"The ocular features can be either **sensory** or **motor**...."

Vertebrobasilar System Stroke

1. **Vertebral or basilar artery**
   - Complete brainstem infarct:
     - CN involvement:
       - III, IV, VI CN palsies (ophthalmoplegia)
       - V CN palsy (loss of corneal reflex)
       - VII CN palsy (lagophthalmos)
       - VIII CN palsy (nystagmus)
     - PPRF, convergence center, MLF involvement:
       - Conjugate gaze palsies
       - INO, WEBINO (see page 253)
       - One-and-a-half syndrome (see page 254)
       - Parinaud's syndrome (see page 244)
     - Sympathetic involvement:
       - Horner's syndrome
   - Midbrain:
     - Crossed syndromes (Weber's syndrome, Benedikt's syndrome and others)
   - Pons:
     - Crossed syndromes (Millard Gubler and others)
   - Medulla:
     - Lateral medullary syndrome (posterior inferior cerebellar artery):
       - V CN palsy and spinothalamic tract involvement (crossed hemianesthesia)
       - VIII CN palsy (vertigo and nystagmus)
       - IX and X CN palsy (dysarthria and dysphagia)
       - Sympathetic involvement (Horner's syndrome)
       - Cerebellar involvement (ataxia and other cerebellar signs)

2. **Posterior cerebral artery**
   - Lateral geniculate body (posterior choroidal artery):
     - Incongruous homonymous hemianopia
     - Homonymous sectoranopia (wedge-shaped)
   - Anterior visual cortex (see below):
     - Congruous homonymous hemianopia with macular sparing
     - Others

3. **Cerebellar arteries**
   - Cerebellar involvement (see nystagmus, page 238)

Carotid System Stroke

1. **Internal carotid artery**
   - Amaurosis fugax (see below and page 201)
   - Venous stasis retinopathy (page 202)
   - Ischemic optic neuropathy (page 247)
   - Central retinal artery occlusion (page 193)
   - Anterior segment ischemia (page 202)

2. **Anterior cerebral artery**
   - Hemialexia (page 283)
3. **Anterior choroidal artery**
   - Important branch of internal carotid artery
   - Causes **full blown CVA** (hemiplegia, hemianesthesia)
   - Involves different parts of the visual pathway:
     - Optic tract:
       - Incongruous homonymous hemianopia
     - Lateral geniculate body (compare with posterior choroidal artery involvement above):
       - Homonymous superior and inferior sectoranopia
     - Optic radiation:
       - Incongruous homonymous hemianopia
4. **Middle cerebral artery**
   - Involves different parts of cortex and visual pathway (anterior to posterior):

- Frontal eye fields:
  - Conjugate gaze palsy (saccade defect)
- Parietal eye fields:
  - Conjugate gaze palsy (pursuit defect)
- Posterior parietal regions:
  - Alexia and agraphia (see page 283)
- Lateral geniculate body:
  - Homonymous sectoranopia
- Optic radiation:
  - Incongruous homonymous hemianopia
- Posterior visual cortex:
  - Congruous homonymous central field defect ("macular VF defect")
  - Balint's syndrome:
    - Ocular apraxia (cannot move eyes on command but can move spontaneously!)
    - Visual inattention (eyes wander around)

Exam tips:
- **Knowledge of the anatomy of the blood supply to the brain is important.**
- **Alternate questions can be, "What happens when the basilar artery is blocked?" or "What are the ocular manifestations of middle cerebral artery stroke?"**

Q **What are the Ocular Signs in Visual Cortex Lesions?**

"The ocular manifestations of visual cortex lesions depend on the area and extent of the involvement."
"The signs are either predominantly anterior cortex or posterior cortex."
"And the ocular features can be either VF defects or various psychosomatic syndromes...."

Visual Cortex

1. **Visual field defects**
   - Congruous homonymous hemianopia with macular sparing (**anterior** cortex, posterior cerebral artery)
   - Congruous homonymous central field defect/"macular VF defect" (**posterior** cortex, middle cerebral artery)
   - Temporal crescent unilateral VF defect (most **anterior** portion of visual cortex)
     - This is the only **monocular** VF defect in the visual pathway posterior to the chiasma!
   - Others:
     - Bilateral homonymous hemianopia with macular sparing (bilateral anterior cortex)
     - Bilateral homonymous altitudinal defect:
       - Inferior (bilateral involvement of superior cortex)

- Superior (bilateral involvement of inferior cortex)
- Checkerboard defect (homonymous anopia, superior defect in one eye, inferior defect in other)

2. **Psychosomatic syndromes**
   - Cortical blindness (page 283)
   - **Anton's** syndrome (cortical blindness plus denial of blinding)
   - **Riddoch's** phenomenon (can see moving targets but not stationary targets)
   - **Balint's** syndrome (ocular apraxia, visual inattention)
   - OKN asymmetry (see OKN, page 240)
   - Unformed visual hallucinations (see visual hallucinations, page 282)

Exam tips:
- An alternate question can be, "What are the ocular features of a meningioma impinging on the visual cortex?"
- Differentiate signs of the anterior visual cortex (supplied by posterior cerebral artery) from those of the posterior visual cortex, where the macular representation is localized (supplied by middle cerebral artery).
- Note that macular area is supplied by the middle cerebral artery!

Q **What is Amaurosis Fugax?**

"Amaurosis fugax is an ocular transient ischemic attack (TIA)."
"The etiology is usually…."

Amaurosis Fugax

1. **Most common ocular TIA (transient ischemic attack)**
2. **Due to cholesterol/platelet emboli from carotid atheroma**
3. **Clinical notes**
   - Visual loss:
     - Transient, lasting less than 10 minutes to 2 hours (never more than 24 hours by TIA definition)
     - Starts in the central VF, expanding outwards or altitudinal (curtain like effect)
   - Contralateral hemiplegia (12.5%)
   - Carotid bruit (20%)
4. **Treatment and prognosis**
   - Carotid ultrasound
   - Carotid endarterectomy (NASCET results):
     - Carotid stenosis < 50% (no benefit)
     - Carotid stenosis > 70% (eight-year benefit)
     - Carotid stenosis 51 to 69% (consider this only if other risk factors are present)
   - Carotid artery stenting:
     - Carotid Revascularization Endarterectomy vs Stenting Trial (CREST) (*N Engl J Med*;2010: Epub):
       - Risk of stroke, MI or death similar between stenting and endarterectomy groups
       - During periprocedural period, higher risk of stroke with stenting, and higher risk of MI with endarterectomy
     - European International Carotid Stenting Study (*Lancet* 2010;375:985–997):
       - Stents had a higher rate of complications compared to endarterectomy (stroke, myocardial infarction, death)
   - Commonest cause of death: Cardiac causes (not stroke!)

Exam tips:
- This is an important differential diagnosis of sudden visual loss and an extremely common problem referred to by ophthalmologists in emergency room settings "requiring decisions made on the spot (see page 201)."
- Read results of the North American Symptomatic Carotid Endarterectomy Trial (NASCET) *N Engl J Med* 1998;339:1415–25.

Q **Tell me about Migraines.**

"Migraine is a **neurovascular** disorder."
"It can be classified into…."
"The ocular features can be either sensory or motor….."

Migraine

1. **Classification**
   - Without aura:
     - Common migraine (= classic migraine without the aura)
   - With aura:
     - Classic migraine
     - Migraine equivalent
       - Aura without headache

- Ophthalmoplegic migraine
  - Painful III, IV and V CN palsies
- Retinal migraine
  - Photopsia
- Basilar migraine
  - III, IV and V CN palsies
  - Fortification spectra
- Cluster headache (variant of migraine)

2. **Ocular features of classic migraine**
   - Sensory
     - Excitatory:
       - Fortification spectra:
         - Zig-zag patterns

- Gradual build up
- Starts in central VF, expanding outwards to peripheral VF
- Photopsia
- Metamorphopsia
- Inhibitory:
  - Blurring of vision
  - Amaurosis fugax
  - Scotoma
- Others:
  - Photophobia
- Motor:
  - III, IV and V CN palsies

Exam tips:
- **This is important because the migraine is one of the most common neurological conditions and often presents with ocular symptoms first.**

Q **Tell me about Carotid Cavernous Fistula.**

"Carotid cavernous fistula (CCF) is an **arteriovenous fistula** which connects the carotid artery and the cavernous sinus."
"It can be divided into…."

	Direct CCF	Indirect CCF
Classification	• Barrow's Type I (internal carotid artery to cavernous sinus)	• Type II (meningeal branches of internal carotid artery to cavernous sinus) • Type III (meningeal branches of external carotid artery to cavernous sinus) • Type IV (meningeal branches of both internal and external carotid artery to cavernous sinus)
Etiology	• Head trauma with base of skull fracture (young men) • Spontaneous rupture from atherosclerosis (postmenopausal hypertensive women)	• Congenital malformation (associated with Ehlers-Danlos or pseudoexanthoma) • Spontaneous rupture from atherosclerosis (postmenopausal hypertensive women)

Clinical features	• Acute pulsatile proptosis (with thrill and bruit)
	• Severe EOM impairment (abolished by carotid compression)
	• Anterior segment:
	  • Engorged corkscrew episcleral vessels
	  • Glaucoma (from increased episcleral venous pressure, orbital congestion, secondary angle closure, neovascular glaucoma from CRVO)
	  • Anterior segment ischemia
		• Slowly progressive proptosis (with thrill and bruit)
		• Mild EOM impairment (VI CN palsy)
		• Subtle anterior segment signs
		  • Dilated cockscrew episcleral vessels
		  • Raised IOP
		  • Increased ocular pulsation

(Continued)

	Direct CCF	Indirect CCF

	• Posterior segment:
	  • CRVO
	  • Optic nerve head swelling (ON compression)
		• Posterior segment:
		  • Features of venous congestion

Blinding complications	• Glaucoma • Exposure keratopathy • Optic nerve compression • Ocular ischemia	

Investigation	• CT scan ("What are CT scan features?"):
	  • Proptosis
	  • Distended superior ophthalmic vein
	  • Enlarged EOM
	  • Bowing of cavernous sinus
	• Orbital Doppler
	  • Dilated superior ophthalmic vein
	  • Reversal of flow
	• Carotid angiogram
	  • Indicated if surgery considered
		• Similar

Indications for treatment	• Blinding complications • Severe diplopia • Severe bruit	

Treatment	• Most fistula close spontaneously
	• Interventional radiology (embolization):
	  • Balloon, glue, sphere
	  • Complications (stroke in 5%, failure of procedure common)
	• Surgery (progressive carotid artery ligation)
		• Most fistula close spontaneously

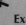

Exam tips:
- **Common differential diagnosis of unilateral proptosis (page 307).**

Notes
- Glaucoma in CCF:
  - Increased episcleral venous pressure ishemia → secondary open angle glaucoma
  - Anterior segment ischemia → neovascular glaucoma
  - Congestion of uveal tissues → angle closure glaucoma

NEUROOPHTHALMIC MANIFESTATIONS OF CEREBRAL ANEURYSMS

Overall yield: ✹✹ **Clinical exam:** **Viva:** ✹✹ **Essay:** ✹ **MCQ:** ✹✹

Q Opening Question: Tell me about Cerebral Aneurysms.

"Cerebral aneurysms are saccular or fusiform dilatations of intracranial arteries."

Cerebral Aneurysm

1. **Prevalence and presentation**
   - 1–6% of population in autopsies, of which 20–30% have multiple aneurysms
   - Presentation:
     - **90%** present acutely with subarachnoid hemorrhage from ruptured aneurysm
     - **10%** present with chronic mass effects:
       - Headache is most common symptom
       - The median time of signs due to mass effect to aneurysm rupture is **14 days** (therefore important to diagnose aneurysm early to prevent devastating subarachnoid hemorrhage)

2. **Etiology**
   - Primary/idiopathic
   - Hypertension
   - Others (rare):
     - Connective tissue disorders (Ehlers-Danlos syndrome, polycystic kidneys)
     - Bacterial/fungal aneurysm
     - Traumatic

3. **Location**
   - Anterior to the Circle of Willis **(70%)**:
     - Anterior cerebral artery, anterior communicating artery, internal carotid artery at bifurcation and posterior communicating artery
     - Supraclinoid:
       - Sensory: Optic nerve, chiasma and tract involved

   - Infraclinoid:
     - Motor: III, IV and VI CN involved:
       - Anterior (V1 CN involved)
       - Middle (V1 and V2 CN involved)
       - Posterior (V1, V2 and V3 CN involved)
   - Middle cerebral artery **(20%)**
   - Posterior to Circle of Willis **(10%)**

4. **Ocular features**
   - Acute with subarachnoid hemorrhage:
     - Increased intracranial pressure (see page 262)
     - Terson syndrome
   - Chronic with mass effects:
     - Motor **(70%)**:
       - Infraclinoid aneurysms
       - Painful, incomplete, pupil-involved III CN palsy (60% of aneurysms will have III CN involvement)
       - Multiple CN involvement (IV, VI and V, depending on location)
     - Sensory **(20%)**:
       - Supraclinoid aneurysms
       - Chiasmal syndrome (see page 260)
     - Mixed motor and sensory **(10%)**:
       - Cavernous sinus carotid artery aneurysms
       - Triad of pulsatile proptosis (with bruit), conjunctival injection and VI CN palsy (see carotid cavernous fistula, page 268)

Q How would You Manage a Patient Suspected of Having a Cerebral Aneurysm?

Management of Cerebral Aneurysm

1. **Investigations**
   - CT scan:
     - Sensitivity = 60%
     - If subarachnoid hemorrhage has occurred, sensitivity increases to 90%
   - MRI:
     - Sensitivity = 80%
     - MR angiogram, sensitivity = 90%
   - Carotid angiogram:
     - Gold standard, sensitivity = 95%
     - Need four vessel angiograms to see both anterior **and** posterior circulations

2. **Treatment**
   - Medical:
     - Control of BP
     - Antivasospasm
     - Anticonvulsant
     - Antiedema (dexamethasone)
   - Surgical:
     - Clipping of aneurysm
     - Proximal ligation of parent artery
   - Interventional radiology: Embolization of aneurysm with coils

NEUROCUTANEOUS SYNDROMES

Overall yield: ✪✪✪✪   **Clinical exam:** ✪✪✪✪   **Viva:** ✪✪   **Essay:** ✪   **MCQ:** ✪✪✪✪

Q Opening Question: What is Neurofibromatosis?

"Neurofibromatosis (NFM) is one of the neurocutaneous syndromes." "With systemic and ocular features."

Classical Neurofibromatosis

1. **Hereditary pattern**
   - AD (with incomplete penetrance and expressitivity)
   - Chromosome 17 mutation

2. **Skin features**
   - Café au lait spots
   - Neurofibroma
   - Plexiform neurofibroma
   - Axillary freckles

3. **CNS features**
   - Neural tumors in brain, spinal cord, CN and peripheral nerves (neurofibroma, glioma, schwannoma)

4. **Ocular features**
   - Orbital features:
     - Lid plexiform neurofibroma and ptosis
     - **Nonaxial pulsatile** proptosis (congenital defect of sphenoid bone with spheno-orbital-encephalocele)
     - **Axial nonpulsatile** proptosis (optic nerve glioma)
     - **Nonaxial nonpulsatile** proptosis (other orbital nerve tumors, e.g. neurilemmoma)

   - Ocular features:
     - Prominent corneal nerves
     - Lisch nodules
     - Ectropion uvea
     - Glaucoma — 50% have unilateral UL neurofibroma/facial hemiatrophy
     - Choroidal hamartomas

5. **Others**
   - Skeletal abnormalities:
     - Short stature
     - Scoliosis
     - Macrocephaly
     - Facial hemiatrophy
   - Childhood malignancies
   - Hypertension from pheochromocytoma

6. **Diagnostic criteria for neurofibromatosis type I (NF-1) (≥ 2 of the following)**
   - ≥ 6 cafe au lait spots
   - ≥ 2 neurofibroma or ≥ 1 plexiform neurofibroma
   - Axillary/inguinal freckles
   - Optic nerve/chiasmal glioma
   - ≥ 2 lisch nodules
   - Osseous lesions e.g. sphenoid dysplasia
   - First degree relative with NF-1

Exam tips:
- **Remember that ALL the syndromes have the three cardinal sites of involvement: Skin, CNS and eye(s).**

Q | **What is the Difference between Neurofibromatosis Type I and II?**

Type II or Central NFM

- Rarer
- Chromosomal 22 mutation
- Less café au lait spots
- Ocular features include:
  - Bilateral vestibular schwannomas (V, VI, VII, VIII palsies)
  - Posterior subcapsular cataracts
  - Combined hamartomas of retina and RPE
  - No risk of glaucoma, no Lisch nodules

- Diagnostic criteria for neurofibromatosis type II (NF-2):
  - Bilateral vestibular schwannomas or
  - First degree relative with NF-2 and either unilateral vestibular schwannoma or any two of the following:
    - Meningioma
    - Glioma
    - Schwannoma
    - Juvenile posterior subcapsular lenticular opacities/juvenile cortical cataract

---

Clinical approach to neurofibromatosis

"This patient has multiple nodules on his face and neck."

Look for

- *Lid neurofibroma and ptosis (plexiform neurofibroma)*
- *Anterior segment:*
  - *Prominent corneal nerves*
  - *Lisch nodules*
  - *Ectropion uvea*
- *Proptosis:*
  - *Pulsatile, no bruit (spheno-orbital encephalocele)*
  - *Nonpulsatile (optic nerve glioma)*

"This patient has neurofibromatosis."

I'd like to

- *Check IOP and gonioscopy (glaucoma)*
- *Check pupils for RAPD (optic nerve glioma, meningioma) and then dilate the pupils to….*
- *Examine fundus (optic atrophy, papilledema, optociliary shunts, choroidal hamartomas)*
- *Examine systemically for other features of NFM:*
  - *Skin (café au lait, axillary freckles, plexiform neurofibromas, neurofibromas on other parts of body)*
  - *Skeletal (short stature, scoliosis, macrocephaly, hemiatrophy of face)*
  - *Neurologically (CNS tumors)*
  - *BP (HPT from pheochromocytoma)*
- *Examine family members*

What is Tuberous Sclerosis?

"Tuberous sclerosis is one of the neurocutaneous syndromes."
"With systemic and ocular features."
"The **classical triad** consists of: Mental handicap, epilepsy and adenoma sebaceum."

Tuberous Sclerosis

1. **Hereditary pattern**
   - AD
   - Chromosome 9 mutation
2. **Skin features**
   - **Adenoma sebaceum**
   - Ash leaf spots
   - Shagreen patches
   - Café au lait
   - Skin tags
3. **CNS features**
   - Astrocytic hamartoma:
     - **Epilepsy**
   - Hydrocephalus
   - **Mental handicap**
4. **Ocular features**
   - Retinal astrocytoma
   - Hypopigmented iris and fundal lesions
5. **Others**
   - Visceral hamartoma:
     - Kidneys
     - Heart
     - Subungal areas

Q **What is the Sturge-Weber Syndrome?**

"Sturge-Weber syndrome is one of the neurocutaneous syndromes."
"With systemic and ocular features."

Sturge-Weber Syndrome

1. **Hereditary pattern**
   - None (like Wyburn Mason syndrome)
2. **Skin features**
   - Nevus flammeus/cavernous hemangioma/port wine stain:
     - First and second divisions of V CN
     - Hypertrophy of face
3. **CNS features**
   - Angioma of meninges ("Which layer is involved?" Answer: Pial) and brain:
     - Ipsilateral to side of facial angioma
     - Parietal and occipital lobe
     - May calcify and show up in Skull XR as "**tram track** sign"
   - Epilepsy, hemiparesis and hemianopia
4. **Ocular features**
   - Glaucoma:
     - **30%** of patients
     - Ipsilateral to side of facial angioma
     - Higher risk if upper lid involved
   - Choroidal hemangioma:
     - **40%** of patients
     - Ipsilateral to side of facial angioma
     - Diffuse type of choroidal hemangioma (**not** circumscribed type of choroidal hemangioma)
   - Episcleral, iris and ciliary body hemangiomas

 Clinical approach to Sturge Weber syndrome

"This patient has a port wine stain…."
"In the distribution of the 1st and 2nd divisions of the Trigeminal nerve."

Look for
- *Hypertrophy of face on side of hemangioma*
- *UL involvement — ptosis*
- *Episcleral hemangioma*

(Continued)

(Continued)

- *Iris, ciliary body hemangioma (lens subluxation)*
- *Trabeculectomy*

I'll like to

- *Exclude glaucoma (30%), check IOP and look at optic disc*
- *Perform gonioscopy (hemangioma, angle anomaly, increased episcleral venous pressure)*
- *Check fundus for diffuse choroidal hemangioma (40%)*
- *Examine patient neurologically (hemangiomas of brain)*

Exam tips:
- Note that cavernous hemangioma (Sturg Weber syndrome) is not the same as the benign capillary hemangioma (page 310).

Notes
- "What are the mechanisms of glaucoma?"
  - Raised episcleral venous pressure
  - Angle abnormally
  - Ciliary body angioma

Q What is Ataxia Telangiectasia?

"Ataxia telangiectasia is one of the neurocutaneous syndromes."
"With systemic and ocular features."

Ataxia Telangiectasia

1. **Hereditary pattern**
   - AR
   - Chromosome 11 mutation
2. **Skin features**
   - Cutaneous **telangiectasia**
3. **CNS features**
   - **Cerebellar ataxia**
   - Mental handicap

4. **Ocular features**
   - Conjunctival telangiectasia
   - Oculomotor defects:
     - Nystagmus
     - Oculomotor apraxia
     - Strabismus

Q **What is the Von Hippel-Lindau Syndrome?**

"Von Hippel-Lindau syndrome is one of the neurocutaneous syndromes."
"With systemic and ocular features."

Von Hippel-Lindau Syndrome

1. **Hereditary pattern**
   - AD
   - Chromosome 3 mutation
2. **Skin features (not prominent)**
   - Café au lait
   - Melanocytic nevi
3. **CNS features**
   - **Hemangioblastoma**
     - Cerebellum
     - Brainstem
     - Spinal cord
     - May cause polycythemia

4. **Ocular features**
   - Capillary hemangioma of retina
     - Treatment: Laser photocoagulation (small lesions), cryotherapy (peripheral lesions), PDT, IVTA, intravitreal anti-VEGF
   - Hypertensive retinopathy (pheochromocytoma)
   - Papilledema (CNS hemangioblastoma)
5. **Others**
   - Visceral tumors:
     - Cysts of kidney, pancreas, liver, epididymis, ovary and lungs
     - Hypernephroma
     - Pheochromocytoma

Q **What is Incontinentia Pigmenti?**

"Incontinentia pigmenti is one of the neurocutaneous syndromes."
"With systemic and ocular features."

Incontinentia Pigmenti

1. **Hereditary pattern**
   - Sex linked dominant (one of only few disease)
2. **Skin features**
   - Stage 1: Erythema and bullae at extremities
   - Stage 2: Wart-like changes
   - Stage 3: Hyperpigmented macules in "**christmas tree**" pattern on trunk

3. **CNS features**
   - Epilepsy
   - Mental retardation
   - Hydrocephalus
4. **Ocular features**
   - **Proliferative retinopathy** (like retinopathy of prematurity)

Notes
- Ocular conditions with X-linked inheritance
- X-linked dominant:
  - Incontinentia pigmenti
  - Alport's syndrome
  - Aicardi syndrome

- X-linked recessive:
  - Norrie's disease
  - Juvenile retinoschisis
  - Choroideremia
  - Ocular albinism
  - Lowe syndrome

"Wyburn Mason syndrome is one of the neurocutaneous syndromes."
"With systemic and ocular features."

Wyburn Mason Syndrome

1. **Hereditary pattern**
   - None (like Sturg Weber syndrome)
2. **Skin features (not prominent)**
3. **CNS features**
   - Arteriovenous malformation in CNS:
     - Epilepsy

   - Hemiparesis
   - Mental retardation
4. **Ocular features**
   - **Racemose angioma**

HEAD INJURY

Overall yield: ✸✸   **Clinical exam:**   **Viva:** ✸✸   **Essay:** ✸   **MCQ:** ✸✸

Q Opening Question: What are the Ocular Signs in Head Injury?

"Ocular signs are important in head injuries because they have immediate localizing and prognostic values."

"They can be divided into…."

Ocular Signs of Head Injury

1. **Visual pathway signs:**
   - Retina and optic disc:
     - Papilledema
     - Purtscher's retinopathy
   - Optic nerve:
     - Traumatic optic neuropathy (see below)
   - Optic chiasma:
     - Infrequent, usually from frontal contusion
   - Retrochiasmal:
     - Homonymous hemianopia (secondary to occipital ischemia)

2. **Motor signs:**
   - III, IV and VI CN palsies, conjugate gaze palsies, INO:
     - Difficult to diagnose
     - Observe spontaneous eye movements
     - Oculocephalic reflex may help

3. **Pupillary signs:**
   - Fixed dilated pupil:
     - Transtentorial/uncal herniation (III CN palsy)
   - Traumatic III CN palsy
   - Traumatic mydriasis
   - Orbital blow out fracture
   - Small pupil:
     - Horner's syndrome
     - Traumatic miosis
     - Pontine hemorrhage
     - Hutchinson's pupil (early stages of transtentorial herniation)

4. **Late signs:**
   - Subdural hematoma:
     - Late III CN palsy (transtentorial herniation)
     - Late VI CN palsy (raised intracranial pressure)
   - Aberrant III CN regeneration
   - Carotid cavernous fistula
   - Late Horner's syndrome

Q How do You Manage a Patient with Severe Head Injury?

"The aim of management is to limit the extent of the **primary damage** and to prevent **secondary brain damage**."

Management of Head Injury

1. **Primary brain damage:**
   - Open laceration
   - Contusion
   - Diffuse axonal injury
   - Brainstem injury

2. **Secondary brain damage:**
   - Hemorrhage

- Extradural:
  - Lucid interval
  - Trauma to temporal bone area/pterion area with rupture of middle meningeal artery
  - III CN palsy on ipsilateral side (herniation of uncus on same side)

- Treatment:
  - Immediate clot evacuation, with good prognosis
- Subdural:
  - Usually associated with diffuse cerebral damage
  - Bilateral III CN palsy
  - Treatment:
    - Immediate clot evacuation, with poorer prognosis
- Subarachnoid/intraventricular:
  - Treatment:
    - Conservative management
- Intracerebral:
  - Treatment:
    - Dependent on size, if large, may need to evacuate

- Cerebral edema:
  - IV mannitol
  - Hyperventilate to vasoconstrict cerebral vessels
  - Intraventricular drain to monitor intracranial pressure and drain cerebrospinal fluid simultaneously
- Cerebral hypoxia:
  - Give oxygen
  - IV fluids (improve BP)
- Infection:
  - IV antibiotics
- Epilepsy:
  - Antiepileptics

Q **What are the Features of Traumatic Optic Neuropathy?**

"Traumatic optic neuropathy is an important complication of head injury."
"It occurs in about **2%** of all head injuries."

Traumatic Optic Neuropathy

1. **Classification**
   - **Mechanical** compression from fracture fragment
   - Indirect damage from **edema/ischemia**

2. **Clinical features**
   - Ipsilateral frontotemporal contusion
   - Severe enough to have some loss of consciousness
   - Instantaneous decrease in VA
   - Need to differentiate from ON avulsion, CRAO and ophthalmic artery occlusion
   - Improve in one-third to half of cases

3. **Management**
   - Mechanical compression from fracture fragment:
     - CT scan good for diagnosis (bony fragments)
     - Surgical decompression
   - Indirect damage from edema/ischemia:
     - MRI better for diagnosis
     - Medical decompression is controversial:
       - High dose steroids:
         - No contraindication for steroids (e.g. sepsis)

- Follows regime from NASCIS (National Acute Spinal Cord Injury Study) (*JAMA* 1997;277:1597–1604)
  - IV 30 mg/kg bolus dose, followed by:
    - 5.4 mg/kg for next 24 hours (injury < 3 hours)
    - 5.4 mg/kg for next 48 hours (injury 3–8 hours)
  - Oral steroids tapering dose for 15 days
- Optic Nerve Trauma Study (*Ophthalmology* 1999;106:1268–1277):
  - Failed to find benefit of either corticosteroids or optic canal surgery
  - But was a non-randomized study and there was no uniformity of adminis-tered corticosteroid treatments
- Surgical decompression:
  - If no improvement with steroids
  - Optic nerve **canal** decompression via transethmoidal approach (not the same as optic nerve **sheath** decompression!)
  - No contraindication to surgery

Exam tips:
- **A controversial area. Read latest results from National Acute Spinal Cord Injury Study (NASCIS), *JAMA* 1997;277:1597–604.**

COMA, DISORDERS OF HIGHER FUNCTIONS & PSYCHIATRIC DISEASES

Overall yield: ✺ ✺   **Clinical exam:**   **Viva:** ✺ ✺   **Essay:** ✺ ✺ ✺   **MCQ:** ✺ ✺

Q **Opening Question:** What are the Ocular Features Seen in Patients in Coma?

"The neuroophthalmic signs include the eyelids, pupil, fundus and ocular motility."

Neuroophthalmic Signs in Coma

1. **Eyelid signs**
   - Eye opening:
     - Glasgow Coma Scale
     - Spontaneous, to speech, to pain
   - Eye closure:
     - Closure (intact lower pons)
     - Tone of closure proportional to depth of coma
     - Asymmetrical closure (VII CN palsy on one side)
   - Blinking:
     - Spontaneous blinking (intact reticular system)
     - Reflex blinking:
       - To light or threat (intact anterior visual pathway, brainstem and VII CN)
       - To sound (intact VIII and VII CN)
       - To corneal reflex (intact V and VII CN)

2. **Pupillary signs**
   - Fixed, dilated pupil:
     - Unilateral (III CN palsy with transtentorial herniation)
     - Bilateral (atropine poisoning, barbiturate poisoning, severe hypoxia-ischemia)
   - Marcus Gunn pupil (optic nerve or chiasm damage, pituitary apoplexy)
   - Small pupil:
     - Unilateral (Horner's syndrome)
     - Bilateral (pontine hemorrhage, opiates poisoning, severe metabolic damage, thalamic and basal ganglia damage)

3. **Fundus**
   - Papilledema (space-occupying lesion)
   - Retinal hemorrhage (subarachnoid hemorrhage)

4. **Eye motility**
   - Spontaneous eye movement:
     - Roving, bobbing, ping-pong movements (brainstem damage)
   - Sustained conjugate eye deviation:
     - Horizontal deviation ("What are the possible causes?")
       - **Ipsilateral hemispheric lesion:**
         - Oculocephalic reflex/caloric stimulation positive
         - Associated contralateral hemiparesis
       - **Contralateral pontine lesion:**
         - Oculocephalic reflex/caloric stimulation negative
         - Associated ipsilateral hemiparesis
       - **Contralateral thalamic lesion** (also known as the "wrong way deviation")
     - Downward deviation:
       - Dorsal midbrain lesion
     - Upward deviation:
       - Hypoxia-ischemia
   - Sustained disconjugate eye deviation:
     - III, IV, VI CN palsies, internuclear ophthalmoplegia
     - Skew deviation (brainstem lesion)

Q What are the Doll's Eye Reflex and Caloric Tests?

"The Doll's eye reflex is a head rotation test for the oculocephalic reflex."
"Caloric stimulation is a similar test of the oculocephalic reflex."

Oculocephalic Reflex

1. **Anatomical pathway**
   - Afferent: Labyrinth — VIII CN — gaze centers in brainstem
   - Efferent: Medial longitudinal fasciculus – III, IV, VI CN

2. **Normal response**
   - Rotation of head to one side (Doll's eye test):
     - Conjugate movement of eye to **other** side

- Cold water in ear to one side (caloric test):
  - Conjugate movement of eye to **same** side
  - Nystagmus to opposite side (**COWS**)

3. **Patient with coma and normal response**
   - Metabolic coma
   - Barbiturate poisoning

4. **Patient with coma and abnormal response**
   - Indicates brainstem damage

> **Exam tips:**
> - **This is an uncommon question, but is still an important neurological test.**
> - **Remember the mnemonic "COWS" for cold water stimulation and nystagmus response: Cold Opposite, Warm Same.**

Q Tell me about the Psychiatric Conditions with Ocular Manifestations.

"Psychiatric diseases are associated with a variety of different ocular manifestations."

Psychiatric Conditions with Ocular Manifestations

1. **Visual symptoms in patients with psychiatric disorders**
   - Visual hallucinations from **traditional psychiatric diseases** (e.g. schizophrenia)
   - Palinopsia:
     - Persistence of image after its removal
     - Causes:
       - Lesion in non-dominant parieto-occipital lobe
       - Drugs (cocaine abuse)
       - Metabolic (hyperglycemia)
   - Release hallucinations following visual loss:
     - Crossed modality hallucinations (e.g. "hear" a vision)
     - Perceive various images in blind field
     - Associated with various VF defects

2. **Charles Bonnet syndrome**
   - Visual hallucination in patients with **visual impairment**
   - First described in cataract-induced blindness
   - Variable onset
   - Duration episodic or continuous

- Images of humans, animals, flowers
- Usually colorful, well-defined, bright and rich in theme
- Individual's emotional response: Surprise, indifference, curiosity, but **NOT** fear

3. **Psychiatric consequences of visual loss**
   - In children, can lead to:
     - Developmental delay
     - Associated hearing loss
     - Grieving process
   - In adults, can lead to:
     - Grieving process
     - Depression
     - Personality change
     - Communication problems

4. **Drug complication**
   - **Ophthalmic** complications of psychiatric drugs:
     - Chlorpromazine (cataract and retinal toxicity)
     - Thioridazine (retinal toxicity)
     - Anticholinergics (acute angle closure glaucoma)
     - Lithium (nystagmus)

- **Psychiatric** complications of ophthalmic drugs:
  - Beta-blockers (depression, fatigue, hallucinations)
  - Topical anti-cholinergics (tachycardia, transient delirium)
- Diamox (depression, decreased libido)
- Drug **interactions**:
  - Beta-blockers and phenothiazines (increased levels of both)
  - Effect of epinephrine prolonged in patients with tricyclic-antidepressants

Q What is Visual Hallucination?

"Visual hallucination is visual perception **without** retinal stimulus."
"It can be divided into **physiological** and **pathological**, and **unformed** or **formed**...."

Visual Hallucination

1. **Physiological**
   - Unformed hallucination:
     - Entoptic phenomenon (phosphenes, lightning streaks of Moore's)
   - Formed hallucination:
     - Hypnagogic (occurs when person is falling asleep)
     - Hypnopompic (occurs when person is waking up)
2. **Pathological**
   - Unformed hallucination:
     - Migraine
     - Epilepsy (occipital lobe)
     - Optic neuritis
     - Retinal detachment
   - Formed hallucination:
     - Epilepsy (temporal lobe)
     - Drugs (barbiturate, LSD, levodopa)
     - Alcohol
   - Release hallucination:
     - Charles Bonnet syndrome

Q Tell me about Alexia.

"Alexia is the inability to read."
"It can be divided into...."

Alexia

1. **Classification**
   - With agraphia:
     - Inability to read or write
     - Site of lesion: Left angular gyrus
     - Associated with Gerstmann syndrome
   - Without agraphia:
     - Able to write but unable to read what he/she has written!
     - Site of lesion: Left occipital lobe (i.e. pure visual sensory lesion)
     - Associated with right homonymous hemianopia
   - Hemialexia:
     - Site of lesion: Splenium of corpus callosum
2. **Etiology**
   - Stroke, tumor, trauma

Q Tell me about Metamorphopsia.

"Metamorphosia is the distortion of shape or size of objects."
"It can be divided into...."

Metamorphopsia

1. **Peripheral causes**
   - Macular edema and central serous retinopathy
   - Epiretinal membrane
   - Chiasmal syndrome (hemifield slip) (page 260)
2. **Central causes (occipital and temporal lobe)**
   - Migraine
   - Epilepsy
   - Drug intoxication

"Cortical blindness is decreased vision secondary to **bilateral** retrogeniculate lesions."

Cortical Blindness

1. **Clinical features**
   - Decreased VA may be mild to NPL
   - Decreased VA symmetrical in both eyes
   - Normal fundi, normal pupils
   - Anton's syndrome — denial of blindness (page 267)
   - Various degrees of dementia, memory loss

2. **Location**
   - Bilateral retrogeniculate lesions
   - Unilateral retrogeniculate lesions **do not** lead to cortical blindness

   - 25% of patients with unilateral occipital CVA develop contralateral CVA resulting in cortical blindness within four years

3. **Etiology**
   - Vascular (stroke, severe hypotension, post angiography)
   - Infection (meningitis, encephalitis)
   - Demyelination (multiple sclerosis)
   - Tumors
   - Trauma

OTHER NEUROOPHTHALMIC PROBLEMS

Overall yield: ✱   **Clinical exam:** ✱   **Viva:** ✱   **Essay:** ✱   **MCQ:** ✱✱

Q **Opening Question:** How do You Tell if a Blind Patient is Malingering/Has a Nonorganic Cause?

"There are several clues to differentiate organic vs nonorganic blindness...."

Nonorganic Blindness

1. **Clues:**
   - Walks with normal gait
   - Wears sunglasses in darkened room
   - Avoids "looking" at doctor when talking
   - Normal pupils and normal anterior and posterior segment examination

2. **Differentiating from total blindness:**
   - Evoke lid/eye movements with visual stimuli (a blind person should have no movements):
     - Visual threat
     - OKN drum
     - Mirror test of Troost's (movement of eye with rotation of mirror)
   - Test proprioception (should be normal in a blind person):
     - "Index finger" test ("point your index fingers at each other")
     - "Sign your name" test
   - Visual evoked potential

3. **Differentiating from partial blindness:**
   - Look for discrepancies in vision tests:
     - Failing to improve linearly with increasing target size or decreasing target distance
     - Improvement with lens of minimal optical power
     - Normal or incongruous results on testing stereopsis, color vision, contrast sensitivity
   - OKN response at maximum distance
   - Four prism diopter lens (conjugate movement in direction of apex of prism)
   - Refraction with fogging (for unilateral poor vision)
   - Visual field: Tunnel vision (failure for the visual field to become wider with increasing distance from the patient)

Clinical approach to optic disc coloboma

"On examination of the optic disc, there is an inferonasal defect seen."
"Otherwise the retina looks normal, there is no retinal detachment seen."

Look for
- *Obvious dysmorphic features (trisomy 13, 18)*
- *Choanal atresia (CHARGE syndrome)*

"This patient has optic disc coloboma."

I'd like to
- *Examine anterior segment for:*
  - *Post embryotoxon*
  - *Posterior lenticonus*
  - *Lens and iris coloboma*
- *EOM for squint and nystagmus*
- *Systemically for other features:*
  - *Cardiac*
  - *Neurologically*

 Clinical approach to optic disc drusen

"On examination of the fundus, the most obvious abnormality is an optic disc swelling."
"However, the disc has a waxy, yellowish, lumpy appearance."
"There is no optic cup."
"The blood vessels are normal looking, not tortuous or dilated and elevated from the disc."
"There is no associated rim hemorrhages seen."
"This appearance is consistent with a diagnosis of optic disc drusen."

Look for
- *Retinitis pigmentosa*
- *Angioid streaks*
- *Fellow eye (bilateral)*
- *Obvious systemic features (neurofibromatosis, tuberous sclerosis, pseudoxanthoma elasticum, Paget's disease)*

I'll like to confirm my diagnosis with
- *B-scan under low gain (acoustically solid optic disc)*
- *FFA (**autofluorescence**, no vessel leakage)*

Clinical approach to optic disc pit

"On examination of the fundus, the most obvious abnormality is a round defect at the temporal edge of the optic disc."
"The disc margin is otherwise distinct and has a normal optic cup."
"The blood vessels are normal looking."
"This appearance is consistent with a diagnosis of optic disc pit."

Look for
• *Central serous retinopathy*

I'd like to perform a
• *VF to look for enlarged blind spot*

OCULOPLASTIC AND ORBITAL DISEASES

THE EYELIDS AND ORBIT

Overall yield: ✱✱✱   **Clinical exam:**   **Viva:** ✱✱   **Essay:** ✱   **MCQ:** ✱✱✱✱

Q **Opening Question No. 1:** What is the Anatomy of the Eyelid?

"The eyelid is divided into the **upper lid** and **lower lid**."
"They each have **anterior** and **posterior** lamellas separated by the **orbital septum**."

Eyelid Anatomy

1. **Anterior lamella**
   - Skin
     - Thinnest skin in body
     - No subcutaneous fat
   - Orbicularis oculi:
     - Three portions:
       - Orbital
       - Palpebral:
         - Preseptal
         - Pretarsal
       - Lacrimal (Horner's muscle)
     - Nerve supply: VII CN (temporal and zygomatic branches)

2. **Orbital septum**
   - Extension of periosteum from orbital rim to tarsus

   - Separates preaponeurotic fat pad from levator and lower lid retractors

3. **Posterior lamella**
   - Tarsal plate:
     - Fibrous skeleton of lids
     - Meibomian glands are embedded within structure
     - 25 mm × 10 mm in upper lid but only 25 mm × 4 mm in lower lid (therefore upper lid tarsus can be used for lid grafts)
   - Tarsal conjunctiva:
     - Tightly adherent to tarsus

> **Exam tips:**
> - **One of the more common basic science questions in examinations.**

Q **Opening Question No. 2:** Tell me about the Levator Palpebrae Superioris.

"The levator muscle is an important extraocular muscle in the superior orbit."
"The main function is in raising the upper lid."

Levator Palpebrae Superioris

1. **Anatomy**
   - 4 cm long, ending 10 mm behind orbital septum to extend as an aponeurosis
   - Aponeurosis fuses with septum 4 mm above tarsus
   - Identified by pre-aponeurotic fat pad

   - Muller's muscle arises from posterior layer of levator inferior to Whitnall's ligament and inserts on superior tarsal border

2. **Origin**
   - Lesser wing of sphenoid

3. **Insertion (four classical sites)**
   - Skin crease
   - Medial and lateral palpebral ligaments (including Whitnall's ligament)
   - Anterior surface of tarsal plate (lower 1/3, **NOT** upper 1/3!)

   - Pretarsal orbicularis

4. **Nerve supply**
   - III CN (upper division)

> **Exam tips:**
> - **Probably the most important oculoplastic muscle.**
> - **Note the importance of the number 4.**

Q **What is the Physiology of the Blinking Reflex?**

"There are three types of blinking."

Blinking

1. **Voluntary blinking**
   - **Palpebral and orbital** portion of orbicularis oculi

2. **Reflex**
   - Stimuli:
     - Sensory stimuli
     - Optical stimuli
   - **Palpebral** portion of orbicularis oculi

3. **Spontaneous/involuntary**
   - Absent until about 3 months of life
   - No stimuli needed
   - Rate: 12/min
   - Amplitude: 9.5 mm (slightly less than palpebral aperture)
   - Duration: 0.3 s (less than a second)
   - **Palpebral** portion of orbicularis oculi

Q **Opening Question No. 3:** Tell me about the Anatomy of the Orbit.

Anatomy of Orbit

1. **Gross anatomy**
   - Pyramidal-shaped, with base anteriorly and apex posteriorly
   - 30 ml volume
   - Medial and lateral wall of orbit are 45° to each other
   - Medial walls of the two orbits are parallel to each other, while lateral walls are perpendicular to each other
   - Orbital axis 22.5° to sagittal plane

2. **Bony orbit**
   - Medial wall (lacrimal, maxilla, ethmoid, body of sphenoid)
   - Floor (maxilla, zygomatic, palatine)
   - Lateral (zygomatic, greater wing of sphenoid)
   - Roof (frontal, lesser wing of sphenoid)

PTOSIS

Overall yield: ✪✪✪✪✪   **Clinical exam:** ✪✪✪✪   **Viva:** ✪✪✪   **Essay:** ✪✪   **MCQ:** ✪✪✪✪

Q Opening Question No. 1: What are the Types of Ptosis?

"Ptosis is defined as an abnormally **low position** of the upper lid in respect to the globe."
"It can be divided into **congenital** or **acquired** forms…."

Classification of Ptosis

1. **Congenital**
   - Levator maldevelopment (see below)

2. **Acquired**
   - Neurogenic:
     - III CN palsy
     - Horner's syndrome
     - Marcus Gunn Jaw Winking syndrome
     - Myasthenia gravis
   - Myogenic:
     - Chronic progressive external ophthalmoplegia (CPEO)

   - Muscular dystrophies
   - Aponeurotic:
     - Senile ptosis
     - Post-surgery
     - Post-trauma
   - Mechanical:
     - Lid mass
     - Scarring

> **Exam tips:**
> - See also ptosis in the neuro-ophthalmology section (page 233).
> - The causes of acquired ptosis are listed from proximal (nerves, neuromuscular junction) to distal (muscles, lids).

Q Opening Question No. 2: Tell me about Congenital Ptosis.

"Congenital ptosis is defined as an abnormally low position of the upper lid with respect to the globe."
"Occurring at birth or soon after birth…."

Classification of Congenital Ptosis

1. **Primary**
   - Levator maldevelopment (see below)

2. **Secondary**
   - Neurogenic:
     - Marcus Gunn Jaw Winking
     - III CN misdirection
     - Congenital Horner's syndrome
     - Myasthenia gravis
   - Myogenic:
     - Blepharophimosis

   - Congenital fibrosis
   - Chronic progressive external ophthalmoplegia (CPEO)
   - Aponeurotic:
     - Post-trauma (birth trauma from forceps delivery)
   - Mechanical:
     - Lid mass
     - Scarring

Exam tips:
• The causes are classified exactly like that of acquired ptosis.

Q What are the Differences Between Congenital and Senile Ptosis?

Primary Congenital Ptosis vs Aponeurotic Senile Ptosis

	Congenital ptosis	Senile ptosis
Age	Young	Old
Laterality	Usually unilateral (75%)	Usually bilateral but may be asymmetrical
Severity	Severe	Milder
Upper lid crease	Absent	High*
On downgaze	Lid lag	Ptosis is worse*
Levator function	Poor	Good*
Other signs	Superior rectus weakness (10%)	Thinning of eyelids* Deep upper lid sulcus*
Treatment	Brow suspension usually needed	Aponeurosis repair

*Five cardinal features of aponeurotic ptosis

Q Tell me about Marcus Gunn Jaw Winking Syndrome.

"The MG Jaw Winking syndrome is an uncommon cause of congenital ptosis."

Marcus Gunn Jaw Winking Syndrome

1. Synketic innervation of levator and pterygoid muscle by V CN
2. Movement of jaw (to opposite side) leads to retraction or wink
3. Frequently associated with monocular elevation deficit (double levator palsy), anisometropia, amblyopia and superior rectus weakness
4. Treatment depends on severity of ptosis vs degree of winking:
   • For severe winking (synkinetic excursion >2 mm), consider complete extirpation of levator (including transaction of medial and lateral horns) plus brow suspension
   • For mild winking (synkinetic excursion <2 mm), mullerectomy and levator resection may be sufficient

Q Tell me about the Blepharophimosis Syndrome.

"Blepharophimosis is a rare cause of congenital ptosis."

Blepharophimosis Syndrome

1. AD inheritance
2. Defined as a narrowing of horizontal palpebral aperture (note: NOT vertical!)
3. Five classical features:
   • Ptosis with poor levator function and absent lid crease (note: Just like other congenital ptosis)
   • Telecanthus (note: Defined as medial canthal distance > half of interpupillary distance, due to laxity of medical canthal tendons)
   • Epicanthus inversus
   • Lateral ectropion of lower eyelid (note: One of only a few causes of lower lid ectropion)
   • Hypoplasia of nasal bridge and orbital rim

- Other features:
  - High arched palate
  - Protruding ears
  - Cardiac defects
  - Infertility (mainly in females, therefore transmitted by males only)

4. **Treatment depends on severity of ptosis, other lid problems and presence of amblyopia**
   - Treat amblyopia

- Correct lid defects first (telecanthus and epicanthus inversus) at age 3–4 years
- Correct ptosis later (bilateral brow suspension) 6 months later
- Correct lateral ectropian in teens

Clinical approach to congenital ptosis

"This young boy has a right ptosis...."

Look for
- *Visual axis blockage (potential for amblyopia)*
- *Check levator function (determine type of operation)*
- *Check EOM (aberrant III CN, SR weakness)*
- *Jaw movement (Marcus Gunn Jaw Wink)*
- *Bell's Reflex (determine extent of correction)*
- *Refraction (astigmatism?)*
- *Iris color (congenital Horner's syndrome)*

Exam tips:
- **Do not forget to test for Jaw Winking!**

Q **How do You Manage a Patient with Ptosis?**

"The management of a patient with ptosis depends on...."
*"They can be **conservative** (eyelid crutches) or **surgical**...."*

Management of Ptosis

1. **Factors to consider:**
   - Cause of ptosis
   - Severity of ptosis
   - Levator function

2. **Type of surgery:**
   - Levator function good (> 10 mm):
     - Ptosis severe (> 2 mm) — aponeurotic repair

- Ptosis mild (< 2 mm) — Fasanella servat (tarsomullerectomy)
- Levator function moderate (4 to 10 mm):
  - Levator resection
- Levator function poor (< 4 mm):
  - Brow suspension

"The common postoperative complications are corneal exposure and either over or undercorrection...."
"Other complications include...."

Complications of Ptosis Surgery

1. **Corneal exposure**
2. **Over and undercorrection**
3. **Contour defects: Lateral droop and medial flare**
4. **Less common complications:**
   - Lash ptosis and entropion

- Lash eversion and ectropion
- Conjunctival prolapse
- Contralateral ptosis
- Orbital hemorrhage (rare)

ENTROPIAN AND ECTROPIAN

Overall yield: ✪✪✪   **Clinical exam:** ✪✪   **Viva:** ✪✪✪   **Essay:** ✪✪   **MCQ:** ✪✪✪✪

Q Opening Question No. 1: Tell me about Entropian.

"Entropian is an **inversion** of the eyelid."
"It can be divided into…."

Classification of Entropian

1. **Congenital**
   - Rare, associated with congenital epiblepharon

2. **Acquired**
   - Involutional
   - Cicatricial, e.g. trachoma:
     - Infectious, e.g. trachoma

- Noninfectious, e.g. ocular cicatricial pemphigoid
- Stevens-Johnson syndrome, chemical injury, chronic blepharitis
- Acute spastic:
  - Spasm of orbicularis oculi (ocular irritation or essential blepharospasm)

> **Notes**
> - "What are the pathogenic mechanisms? How do you test for them?"
> - **Five classic mechanisms:**
>   - Overriding of preseptal to pretarsal orbicularis oculi (test by closure of eyelids)
>   - Horizontal lid laxity (test by pulling lid away from globe and watching lids "snap" back)
>   - Weakness of lower lid retractors (test by downgaze to see position of lower lid)
>   - Tarsal plate atrophy (test by palpation of tarsal plate)
>   - Atrophy of retrobulbar fat leading to relative enophthalmos

Q How do You Manage a Patient with Entropian?

"The management of a patient with entropian depends on
- Cause of entropian
- Severity of entropian
- Length of cure required and
- Specific pathogenic mechanisms…."

"They can be conservative or surgical…."

Management of Entropian

1. **Involutional entropian**
   - Temporary cure required — transverse lid everting sutures
   - Long term cure required:
     - No excess horizontal laxity — Weis procedure (transverse lid split and everting sutures)
     - Excess horizontal laxity — Quickert's procedure (Weis procedure **plus** horizontal lid shortening)
     - Recurrence of entropian after Weis or Quickert's procedure — Jones procedure (plication of lower lid retractors)

2. **Cicatricial entropian**
   - Management of trichiasis/distichiasis:
     - Epilation

   - Electrolysis
   - Cryotherapy
   - Lash excision
   - Mild — anterior lamellar repositioning with lid split at gray line
   - Moderate — anterior
   - Severe — rotation of terminal tarso-conjunctiva and posterior lamellar graft or advancement

3. **Congenital entropian**
   - Hotz procedure (tarsal fixation of pretarsal skin and orbicularis)

4. **Acute spastic**
   - Conservative (taping of lids, eyelid everting sutures, Botox injection)

> **Exam tips:**
> - **Need to know basic surgical steps for each entropian operation. Prepare your own surgical notes!**

Q **Opening Question No. 2:** Tell me about Ectropian.

"Ectropian is an **eversion** of the eyelid."
"It can be divided into…."

Classification of Ectropian

1. **Congenital**
   - Rare condition, associated with blepharophimosis or congenital ichthyosis

2. **Acquired**
   - Involutional

   - Cicatricial
     - Infectious
     - Noninfectious (e.g. SJS)
   - Paralytic (see facial nerve palsy — page 302)

> **Exam tips:**
> - **Very similar classification to entropian. Substitute "acute spastic" in entropion for "paralytic" in ectropian.**

> **Notes**
> - "What are the mechanisms?"
>   - Weakness of pretarsal orbicularis oculi (test by closure of eyelids)
>   - Horizontal lid laxity (test by pulling lid away from globe and watching lid "snap" back)
>   - Tarsal plate atrophy (test by palpation)
>   - Laxity of medical and lateral canthal ligaments

Q How do You Manage a Patient with Ectropian?

"The management of a patient with ectropian depends on
- Cause of the ectropian
- Extent of ectropian (medial or entire lid) and
- Whether horizontal lid laxity is present or not...."

"They can be conservative or surgical...."

Management of Ectropian

1. **Involutional ectropian**
   - Medial lid involvement only:
     - No horizontal lid laxity — medial conjunctivoplasty (excision of a diamond of tarso-conjunctiva)
     - Mild horizontal lid laxity — Lazy-T procedure (medial conjunctivoplasty **plus** full thickness lid excision)
     - Severe horizontal lid laxity — medial canthal tendon plication
   - Entire lid:
     - Mild:
       - No excess skin — Bick's procedure (horizontal lid shortening)
       - Excess skin — Kuhnt-Szymanowski procedure (Bick's procedure **plus** blepharoplasty)
     - Moderate — lateral tarsal strip procedure
     - Severe — wedge resection with lateral tarsal strip

2. **Cicatricial ectropian**
   - Mild — Z-plasty
   - Severe — Skin grafts or flaps

3. **Congenital ectropian**
   - Skin grafts

4. **Paralytic**
   - See facial nerve palsy (page 302)

LID TUMORS

Q Opening Question: Tell me about Eyelid Tumors.

"Eyelid tumors can be classified into **benign** and **malignant** tumors…."
"Malignant eyelid tumors can be further classified into…."

Classification of Malignant Tumors

1. **Primary**
   - Basal cell CA (BCC)
   - Squamous cell CA (SCC)
   - Sebaceous gland CA
   - Malignant melanoma
   - Kaposi's sarcoma

2. **Secondary**
   - Lymphoma
   - Maxillary CA
   - Others

Clinical Approach to Classification

1. **Pigmented eyelid mass**
   - BCC
   - Nevus
   - Malignant melanoma
   - Nevus of Ota

2. **Non-pigmented eyelid mass**
   - Epithelial:
     - Papilloma — sessile, pedunculated
     - Keratoacanthoma — central crater with keratin plug
     - Actinic keratosis — rough, dry scales
     - Seborrheic keratosis — greasy, brown, friable
     - BCC — shiny
     - SCC — crusting, erosions, fissures
   - Subepithelial:
     - Solid:
       · Sebaceous gland CA
       · Meibomian cyst
     - Cystic:
       · Cyst of Moll
       · Cyst of Zeiss
       · Sebaceous cyst

Q How do You Manage a Patient Who Presents with a 6-Month History of Slowly Growing Eyelid Lump?

Clinical Approach

1. **History**
   - Demographics:
     - Older age, white race
   - Risk factors:
     - Prior skin CA
     - Excessive sun exposure
     - Previous radiation, burns, arsenic treatment
   - Tumor characteristics:
     - Growth, change in size
   - Pain
   - Discharge, bleeding
   - Change in color

2. **Examination of tumor**
   - Size and shape
   - Destruction of eyelid margin architecture
   - Loss of cilia
   - Ulceration
   - Telangiectasia

- Loss of fine cutaneous wrinkles
- Palpable induration well beyond margin

3. Other examinations
- Punctal involvement
- Fixation to deep tissue and bone

- Proptosis
- EOM
- CN
- Regional lymph nodes
- Systemic features

 Clinical approach to lid mass

"On inspection, there is a nodular, shiny mass at the lower lid."

Describe
- *Size "Measuring about 1 cm in diameter"*
- *Color "Pearly-white color"*
- *Margin "With distinct margins"*
- *Ulceration "There is a central ulcer with rolled borders"*
- *Areas of pigmentation "There are patches of pigmentation"*
- *Telangiectasia, bleeding, crusting "However, no telangiectasia, bleeding or crusting can be seen"*
- *Eyelid margin architecture, loss of cilia, punctal involvement*

"This patient has a basal cell CA."

I'd like to
- *Examine tumor under slit lamp*
- *Check lymph nodes*
- *Ask for duration and change in size of lid mass, history of occupational sun exposure, prior DXT*

Q **Tell me about Basal Cell Carcinoma.**

"BCC is the most common human malignancy...."
"Classically, there are three types...."

Basal Cell Carcinoma

1. Epidemiology
- 90% of BCC located in head and neck region
- 90% of malignant eyelid tumors
- Most common site: Lower eyelid, followed by medial canthus, upper eyelid and lateral canthus (note: Sequence is like extraocular muscle involvement sequence in **thyroid eye disease**!)
- Worst prognosis: **Medial canthus** (due to infiltration into lacrimal system)

2. Classification
- Nodular:
  - Shiny translucent nodule
  - **Pearly white** appearance
- Ulcerative:
  - Rolled border

- **Rodent ulcer**
- Sclerosing:
  - Multicentric involvement
  - Chronic **blepharitis**

3. Histology
- Nodular and ulcerative:
  - **Nests and cords** of proliferating epidermal basal cells
  - Palisade of nuclei at edge of tumor
  - Cracking artifact (artifactious separation between tumor and stroma)
  - Collagen deposition in dermis
- Sclerosing
  - Branching cords penetrate into dermis, like tentacles ("**indian file**" arrangement)
  - Striking **dermal fibrosis**
  - Difficult to see edge of tumor

Q Tell me about Squamous Cell Carcinoma (SCC).

"SCC is the second most common eyelid malignancy...."
"It can arise de novo or from a precancerous lesion...."

Squamous Cell Carcinoma

1. **Epidemiology**
   - **5–10%** of eyelid malignancy
   - Worse prognosis as compared with BCC

2. **Classification**
   - Arise **de novo**
   - **Precancerous** lesion:
     - Actinic keratosis
     - Bowen's disease

3. **Histology**
   - Arise from **prickle** cell layer
   - Dysplastic cells
   - Multinucleated giant cells
   - Well to moderate to poorly differentiated
   - **Intradermal keratin pearls** (keyword)

Q Tell me about Sebaceous Cell CA.

"Sebaceous cell CA is a rare malignancy of the eyelid...."
"There are two types...."

Sebaceous Cell Carcinoma

1. **Epidemiology**
   - 1–5% malignant eyelid tumors
     Most common site: **Upper eyelid**
     ("Why?" More meibomian glands in upper lid!)
   - Arise from:
     - Meibomian glands
     - Glands of Zeiss
     - Sebaceous glands of eyebrow and caruncle
   - Worst prognosis of three classical eyelid tumors.
     Mortality in 30%

2. **Classification**
   - Nodular:
     - Looks like chalazion
   - Superficial spreading:
     - Pagetoid spread within epithelium of palpebral, forniceal and bulbar conjunctiva
     (therefore looks like chronic blepharitis, chronic conjunctivitis or superior limbic keratitis!)

3. **Histology**
   - Cords and lobules of poorly differentiated infiltrative sebaceous cells
   - Cells have a **foamy** appearance (contain fat — fresh histological specimen must be sent for special fat stains)
   - Types of growth:
     - Lobular pattern
     - Papillary pattern
     - Comedo-acinar pattern
     - Combined

Notes
- "What are the bad prognostic features?"
  - Site: Upper lid involvement
  - Site: 10 mm or more
  - Duration: 6 months or more
  - Origin: Meibomian as compared with Zeiss
  - Type: Superficial spreading type (pagetoid spread)
  - Grade: Undifferentiated

Q Tell me about Malignant Melanoma.

"Malignant melanomas are rare eyelid malignancies…."
"There are three types…."

Malignant Melanoma

1. **Classification**
   - Nodular
   - Superficial spreading
   - Arising from lentigo maligna
2. **Staging**
   - Clark (five levels of invasion: Level 1: Epidermis, Level 5: Subcutaneous)
   - Breslow (thickness)
3. **Suspicious nevus (ABCDE)**
   - **A**symmetry
   - **B**orders irregular
   - **C**olor mottled
   - **D**iameter large
   - **E**nlargement over time

Q What are the Principles in the Treatment of Malignant Eyelid Tumors?

"The management of malignant eyelid tumors involves multiple modalities…."
"We can use surgery, radiotherapy, chemotherapy and cryotherapy…."

Principles of Surgery

No. 1: Remove as much tumor as possible, preserving as much normal tissue as possible

No. 2: Keep 3 mm margin of normal tissue

No. 3: Use either frozen section or Moh's technique (serial frozen section during surgery)

No. 4: If tumor is > 4 mm from margin and not fixed to tarsal plate, can consider **partial thickness excision of tumor** with direct closure of margins

No. 5: If tumor is < 4mm from margin or fixed to tarsal plate, need **full thickness lid excision**

No. 6: Reconstruct both anterior and posterior lamella **separately (posterior lamella may not be needed if less than half of lid involved)**

No. 7: Reconstruct either anterior or posterior lamella with a **graft** and the other layer with a flap (keep blood supply)

No. 8: Aim to provide stable eyelid margin and smooth internal surface

Size of defect	Upper lid	Lower lid
Less than a third of eyelid margin	• Direct closure • Consider lateral cantholysis	• Direct closure • Consider lateral cantholysis
A third to half of eyelid margin	• Tenzel semicircular flap	• Tenzel semicircular flap
More than half of eyelid margin	• Bridging grafts: Cutler-Beard procedure (full thickness lower lid advancement)	• Hughes procedure (posterior lamellar tarsoconjunctival flap form upper lid and anterior lamellar skin graft) • Hewes procedure (lateral tarsal transposition of tarso-conjunctiva) combined with anterior lamellar skin graft • If vertical extent of defect > 5 mm, then use Mustarde cheek rotation procedure (anterior lamellar skin flap with posterior lamellar mucosal graft)

Exam tips:
- Keep basic principles in mind and remember one surgery approach.
- Remember to give your own scenario, "For example, if a patient has a small lower lid tumor...."

Q What are the Types of Lid Grafts Available?

Lid Grafts

1. **Anterior lamellar skin graft**
   - Skin upper lid or lower lid of either the same or fellow eye
   - Retroauricular skin (full thickness)
   - Supraclavicular skin
   - Inner arm skin

2. **Posterior lamellar mucosal graft**
   - Tarsal plate + conjunctiva of upper lid or lower lid of either the same or fellow eye

   - Hard palate (keratinized epithelium — bandage contact lens needed in early postoperative period and better suited to lower lid use)
   - Buccal mucosa
   - Ear cartilage
   - Perichondrium

TOPIC 5

FACIAL NERVE PALSY

Overall yield: ✦✦✦✦ **Clinical exam:** ✦✦✦ **Viva:** ✦✦✦ **Essay:** ✦✦✦ **MCQ:** ✦✦✦✦

Q **Opening Question:** Tell me about Facial Nerve Palsy.

"Facial nerve palsy is a common neurological condition."
"The causes can be divided into…."

Classification of Facial Nerve Palsy

1. **Upper motor neuron (supranuclear causes)**
   - CVA (different CVA syndromes)
   - Tumors

2. **Lower motor neuron (nuclear and infranuclear causes)**
   - Idiopathic:
     - Bell's palsy
   - Infectious:
     - Herpes zoster (Ramsay Hunt syndrome)
     - Acute or chronic otitis media
     - Others: Syphilis, mumps, meningitis
   - Tumors:
     - Parotid gland tumors

   - Cerebellopontine angle tumors (acoustic neuroma, nasopharyngeal CA)
   - Others: Sarcoma, leukemia
   - Trauma:
     - Temporal bone fracture
     - Facial trauma
   - Vascular:
     - Pontine stroke
   - Metabolic:
     - DM, uremia

Exam tips:
- A common examination topic. Alternate questions may be, "What is the anatomy of the facial nerve?" and "Why are the upper facial muscles spared in supranuclear facial nerve palsies?"

Notes
- "What is Bell's palsy?"
  - Sir Charles Bell was the founder of Royal College of Surgeons of Edinburgh and described the anatomy of the VII CN pathway
  - Most common cause of lower motor neuron VII CN palsy
  - Etiology: Controversial, either ischemia, viral infection or demyelination
  - Prognosis:
    - 75% spontaneous full recovery
    - 25% recovery incomplete with **aberrant regeneration:**
      - Crocodile tears: Tearing at mealtimes, due to synkinetic innervation of submandibular and lacrimal gland

(Continued)

- Reverse jaw winking: "Twitching mouth with attempted blinking, due to synkinetic innervation of orbicularis and mouth muscles"
- Treatment:
  - Oral steroids initiated within the first week associated with a better outcome
  - May be combined with oral antivirals

Q How do You Manage a Patient with Facial Nerve Palsy?

"The management of a patient with facial nerve palsy depends on…."
- Age of patient (younger patients tolerate exposure better)
- Prognosis for recovery:
  - Cause of the palsy
  - Duration of treatment needed (e.g. Bell's palsy will recover)
- Risk of exposure:
  - Lagophthalmos
  - Bell's phenomenon
  - Corneal sensation
  - Dry eye

"They can be conservative or surgical…."

Management of Facial Nerve Palsy

1. **Temporary treatment required for acute corneal symptoms**
   - Conservative:
     - Artificial tears and ointments
     - Taping of lids at night
     - External gold weights
     - Botox
     - Moist chamber goggles
   - Surgical:
     - Tarsorrhaphy

2. **Permanent treatment required:**
   - Surgery aims to manage:
     - Exposure
     - Lower lid paralytic ectropian
     - Brow ptosis
   - Exposure:
     - Punctal occlusion
     - Medial canthoplasty
     - Lateral tarsorrhaphy
     - Gold weights (implanted)
     - Mullerectomy/levator recession
   - Ectropian present:
     - No MCT laxity: Medial canthoplasty
     - MCT laxity: Medial wedge resection
       - May be combined with lateral tarsal strip
     - Fascia lata sling for extreme cases

Clinical approach to facial nerve palsy

"This patient has a right facial asymmetry."

Look for
- *Facial nerve paralysis:*
  - *Brow ptosis*
  - *Loss of forehead wrinkle*
  - *Ectropian*
  - *Loss of nasolabial fold*
  - *Drooping of outer angle of mouth*
  - *Asymmetry of blink reflex*

(*Continued*)

(Continued)

- *Corneal exposure and tearing*
- *Esodeviation (VI CN palsy)*

Examine

- *Eye closure (lagophthalmos, Bell's palsy)*
- *EOM (VI CN)*
- *Hearing (VIII CN)*
- *Corneal sensation (V CN)*
- *Check of cause of palsy (neck scars, parotid mass, vesicles on ears)*

I'll like to

- *Check for hyperacusis, taste on anterior 2/3 of tongue*
- *Check fundus for papilledema*
- *Examine neurologically:*
  - *VII and contralat hemiparesis (Millard Gubler syndrome)*
  - *VII and gaze palsy, V, VIII, Horner's syndrome (Foville's syndrome)*
  - *VII, V, VIII, cerebellar signs (cerebellopontine angle tumor — nasopharyngeal CA)*
- *Examine slit lamp for evidence of corneal exposure*
- *Refer to ENT to rule out nasopharyngeal CA*

THYROID EYE DISEASE

Overall yield: ✪✪✪✪✪ **Clinical exam:** ✪✪✪✪✪ **Viva:** ✪✪✪✪ **Essay:** ✪✪✪✪ **MCQ:** ✪✪✪✪

Q Opening Question No. 1: What is Dysthyroid or Thyroid Eye Disease (TED)?

"TED is a chronic **inflammatory** disease of the eye which usually occurs...."
"In patients with **systemic thyroid disease**...."
"Commonly in **middle aged women**...."
"It is believed to be **autoimmune** in nature...."
"The systemic features include...."
"The ocular features include...."

Q Opening Question No. 2: What are the Ocular Signs in Thyroid Eye Disease?

"The eye signs of thyroid eye disease can be classified into...."

Ocular Features of Thyroid Eye Disease

1. **Extraocular**
   - Proptosis
   - Lid signs:
     - Lid retraction, lid lag, lid swelling, lid pigmentation
   - Restrictive myopathy

2. **Intraocular**
   - Anterior segment:
     - Conjunctival injection and chemosis
     - Superior limbic keratitis
     - Dry eyes
     - Exposure keratopathy
     - Episcleritis/scleritis
     - Glaucoma
   - Posterior segment:
     - Choroidal folds
   - Macular edema
   - Optic nerve swelling

3. **Signs of disease activity (modified Mourits score)**
   - Lid edema (0–1)
   - Lid injection (0–1)
   - Conjunctival chemosis (0–2)
   - Conjunctival injection (0–2)
   - Pain on eye movements (0–1)
   - Retro-orbital pain at rest (0–1):
     - Total score of four or more is indication of active disease
     - Active disease needs treatment for control of inflammatory process first

Exam tips:
- **This is a very common question, but always poorly answered! Many candidates get stuck with describing in detail the different eyelid signs. You should quickly cover the entire spectrum of manifestations before concentrating on one aspect.**

Blinding Complications of TED

1. ON compression
2. Severe exposure keratopathy

3. Glaucoma (rare)

1. Age of patient (older patients — poorer prognosis)
2. Race (Asian patients have higher incidence of optic neuropathy)
3. Nature of disease onset (acute onset worse)
4. Thyroid function:

   • Thyroid dysfunction (hyper or hypothyroid) associated with poorer prognosis

   • Pretibial myxedema
   • High autoantibody levels
5. Smoking (important!)

Pathology of TED

1. Acute phase
   • Hypertrophy of extraocular muscles (accumulation of **glycosaminoglycan**s — keyword in TED pathology)
   • Increase in inflammatory cells

   • Proliferation of other tissues (fat, connective tissue, lacrimal gland)
2. Chronic phase
   • Fibrosis of muscles
   • Increase in chronic inflammatory cells

"The management of TED involves a team approach, with the general **systemic** condition managed by the physician."
"The specific **ocular** management will depend on several factors."

• **Activity** of disease
• Nature and **severity** of ocular involvement
• **Stability** of disease
• Thyroid status and general health of patient

"When surgery is indicated, the **sequence** of surgery is: 1) Orbital decompression, 2) strabismus surgery, and finally 3) lid surgery."
"In patients with...."

Management of TED

Active disease:
   • Immunosuppression is the key
   • NSAIDs rarely effective
   • High-dose pulsed intravenous steroids are the treatment of choice:
     • Oral steroids less effective
   • Methotrexate may be used for long-term maintenance/avoidance of side effects of steroids
   • Orbital radiation may be used if steroids contraindicated

1. Mild TED with lid and soft tissue involvement only (80%)
   • Conservative treatment:
     • Tear replacement and lubricants for dry eyes and mild exposure keratopathy
     • Sunglasses for photophobia
     • Sleep with head elevated and diuretics for lid swelling
     • Chemical sympathectomy (adrenergic blocking agents, e.g. reserpine, propranol)
     • Topical steroids for superior limbic keratitis

- Antiglaucoma medication for raised IOP
- Monitor patient at regular intervals:
  - VA and clinical examination
  - Visual fields
  - Hess chart, binocular fields
- **Lid surgery** is performed only when restrictive myopathy and proptosis are corrected (**key principle in the management of TED**):
  - Mild lid retraction (< 2mm): Mullerectomy
  - Moderate retraction (2–4 mm): Levator recession with LCT lengthening
  - Severe retraction (> 4mm): Lid spacer (hard palate, dermis-fat graft, auricular cartilage)
  - Other lid pathology that may require surgery: Epiblepharon, fat prolapsed and dermatochalasis

2. **Moderate TED where restrictive myopathy predominates (15%)**
- Conservative:
  - Correct with prisms
  - Botox injections
- What are the indications for surgery?
  - Diplopia in primary gaze or downgaze
  - Stable myopathy for six months
  - No evidence of acute congestive TED
- Type of surgery:
  - IR recession
  - Adjustable squint surgery

3. **Severe TED with severe proptosis and ON compression (5%)**
- What are the indications for orbital decompression?
  - ON compression
  - Severe exposure keratopathy
  - Severe proptosis with choroidal folds and macular edema
  - Cosmesis (less common)
- Involves medical decompression, surgical decompression or radiotherapy
- Types of surgical decompression:
  - Two wall:
    - Floor and posterior portion of medial wall
  - Three wall:
    - Two wall **plus** lateral wall
  - Four wall:
    - Three wall **plus** sphenoidal bone at apex
- Complications:
  - Retrobulbar hemorrhage/soft tissue edema — potential for ON compression
  - Strabismus, hypoglobus
  - Lid position changes

Exam tips:
- **Again, this is a very common question. You need to quickly cover all aspects of the management before going into specific details.**

Notes
- "What is chemical sympathectomy?"
- Indicated in several situations in the management of TED:
  - Temporary relief while waiting for spontaneous correction or surgical intervention
  - Subacute lid retraction of less than six months' duration
  - Diagnostic test to assess role of Muller's muscle in lid disease

"TED is the most common cause of lid retraction, but other causes include...."

Causes of Lid Retraction

1. **"M" causes**
   - Myasthenia Gravis (contralateral ptosis, Cogan's lid twitch)
   - Myotonic (hyperkalemia, hypokalemia, dystrophia myotonica)
   - Marcus Gunn Jaw Winking syndrome
   - Metabolic diseases (uremia, cirrhosis)

2. **"P" causes**
   - Parinaud's syndrome (Collier's sign)
   - Parkinson's disease (progressive supranuclear palsy)
   - Ptosis of opposite eye
   - Palsy (aberrant III CN regeneration)

Exam tips:
- Causes are "M" and "P."

Q What are the Mechanisms of Lid Retraction in TED? What are the Types of Surgery Available to Correct Lid Retraction?

Pathophysiology of lid retraction in TED	Surgery to correct lid retraction
Contraction/fibrosis of levator palpebrae superioris (LPS)	LPS recession Blepharoplasty Lateral tarsorrhaphy
Contraction/fibrosis of inferior rectus (IR) with secondary overaction of LPS	IR recession
Sympathetic overaction with overstimulation of Muller's muscle	Mullerectomy
Proptosis	Orbital decompression

Q Why does Ptosis Sometimes Occur in TED?

Ptosis in TED
- LPS aponeurosis dehiscence (aponeurotic ptosis)
- Associated myasthenia gravis
- CN III palsy (orbital apex compression)
- Pseudoptosis (proptosis in fellow eye)

Clinical approach to proptosis

Thyroid eye disease (TED)

Inspection (eight features to describe)

"On inspection, this middle aged lady has...."

- *Unilateral or bilateral proptosis*
- *Axial in nature (use torchlight to look at light reflex, then look at proptosis from behind patient)*

(Continued)

- *Attentive gaze (Kocher's sign) and infrequent blinking (Stellwag's sign)*
- *Squint*
- *Fullness of eyelids (Enoth's sign)*
- *Lid retraction (Dalrymple's sign)*
- *Chemosis or conjunctival injection*
- *Goitre (ask patient to swallow)*

Test lid and EOM

"Please follow this target, move your eyes, do not move your head."

- *Test downgaze first to look for lid lag (Von Graefe's sign)*
- *Then test for upgaze to look for restriction in upgaze*
- *Test all other EOM*
- *Do not forget to test convergence (Mobius sign)*
- *May also see lower lid lag on testing upgaze (Griffith's sign)*
- *Close lids to look for lagophthalmos and Bell's reflex*
- *Test pupils*

Palpation

"I'm going to gently touch your eyes, let me know if you feel any pain."

- *Orbital rim*
- *Pulsation/thrill*

Look for systemic features

- *Hands: Pulse, sweat, tremor, acropachy*
- *Thyroid goitre*
- *Pretibial myxedema*

I'd like to

- *Objectively measure the proptosis*
- *Examine the anterior segment under slit lamp for: Chemosis, superior limbic keratitis, exposure keratopathy, keratoconjunctivitis sicca*
- *Check IOP in primary and upgaze position*
- *Check fundus for: Disc pallor or swelling, choroidal folds*
- *Test VA, color vision, VF, Hess test*
- *Investigate systemic complications: Thyroid function test, etc.*

Nonthyroid eye disease

Inspection

- *Unilateral or bilateral*
- *Axial or nonaxial proptosis (use torchlight, then look from behind)*
- *Fullness of eyelids laterally (lacrimal gland)*
- *Conjunctival injection (pseudotumor, CCF), cockscrew vessels (CCF)*

Test lid and EOM

- *EOM*
- *Lagophthalmos*
- *Pupils*

Palpation

- *Lacrimal mass*

(Continued)

- *Orbital rim*
- *Globe retropulsion*
- *Pulsation/thrill*

Others (ABC)
- *Auscultate for bruit (CCF)*
- *Bend down (varix, lymphangioma)*
- *Check lymph nodes*

I'd like to check
- *Fundus for: Disc pallor, optociliary shunts, choroidal folds*

Exam tips:
- **One of the most common clinical ocular examinations [the others being: Ptosis (page 233, pupils (page 245) and extraocular movements (page 223)].**
- **The KEY is to make a quick decision as to whether the proptosis is related to TED or nonthyroid eye disease.**

Exam tips:
- **Common exam causes include: Carotid cavernous fistula (CCF), cavernous hemangioma and lacrimal gland tumors.**

Q What is Grave's Disease?

Grave's Disease

1. **Definition**
   - Grave's disease is an autoimmune systemic disease and is the most common cause of hyperthyroidism

2. **Pathophysiology of Grave's disease**
   - Lymphocytes → TSH receptor antibody (TRAB) → bind to TSH receptor in thyroid gland → goitre and hyperthyroidism

3. **Clinical features**
   - Three cardinal features:
     - Hyperthyroidism
     - Pretibial myxedema
     - TED

4. **Sequence of presentation**
   - 20% TED → hyperthyroidism
   - 40% TED and hyperthyroidism present simultaneously
   - 40% hyperthyroidism → TED

5. **Prevalence**
   - 30% of patients with hyperthyroidism have TED

6. **Investigation**
   - Thyroxine levels
   - TRAB
   - TSI (thyroid stimulating immunoglobulin):
     - Correlates well with bioactivity of eye disease

Q How do You Manage a Patient with Grave's Disease?

Management of Grave's Disease

1. **Medical**
   - Carbimazole:
     - Blocks all T4 production
     - 30–40 mg everyday or twice a day
   - 3–12 weeks until patient is euthyroidic:
     - Decremental regimen — 15 mg everyday → 10 mg every day maintenance

- Block and replace — maintain at 30–40 mg everyday **plus** supplemental thyroxine
  - Advantages: Tasteless, cheap, small risk of teratogenicity
  - Side effects: Skin rashes, loss of hair, neutropenia
- Propylthiouracil — indications:
  - Allergy to carbimazole
  - Pregnancy
  - T3 thyrotoxicosis
  - But bitter, expensive and not as efficacious
- Prognosis:
  - Treat for one year:
    - 50% relapse after one year
    - 70% still have abnormal TRAB
- On treatment:
  - 90% of lid retraction improvement
  - 30% of restrictive myopathy improvement
  - Only rarely does proptosis improve

2. **Surgical treatment**
  - Indications:
    - Failed medical treatment or relapse
    - Allergic to medicine
    - Large goitre
  - Prognosis:
    - 60% become euthyroidic
    - 30% become hypothyroidic
    - 10% will relapse

3. **Radioiodine (I^{131})**
  - Indications:
    - Failed medical treatment or relapse
    - Allergic to medicine
    - Contraindication to surgery (elderly, cardiac disease)
  - Prognosis:
    - Euthyroidic within three months
    - 50% become hyperthyroidic after one year
    - Incidence of hypothyroidism: 4% per year (therefore patient needs T4 replacement for life)
  - Disadvantages:
    - Worsens TED (need prednisolone to control inflammation)
    - Acute bout of thyroiditis with release of T4 (in elderly, need to make sure patient is euthyroidic first)
    - Risk of gastric cancer

PROPTOSIS & ORBITAL TUMORS

Overall yield: ✪✪✪✪ **Clinical exam:** ✪✪✪ **Viva:** ✪✪✪ **Essay:** ✪✪✪ **MCQ:** ✪✪✪✪

Q Opening Question: How do You Differentiate a Capillary from Cavernous Hemangioma?

	Capillary hemangioma	Cavernous hemangioma
Pathology	• Vascular **hamartoma**. Abnormal growth of blood vessels, with varying degrees of endothelial proliferation	• Benign, encapsulated **tumor** consisting of large, endothelial-lined channels, vascular walls with smooth muscles and stroma
Demographics	• Infant • Females > males • Most common benign orbital tumor in **childhood** • Progressive slow growth in first year of life • Spontaneous involution by age 5–7	• Adult 20–30 years • Usually woman • Most common benign orbital tumor in **adults** • Progressive slow growth throughout life
Others	• Associated with dermal hemangioma and deep visceral capillary tumors (Kasabach-Merritt syndrome — hemangioma, anemia and thrombocytopenia, Maffucci syndrome)	• May be associated with Sturge-Weber syndrome (page 274)
Presentation	• **Superficial hemangioma** — hemangioma confined to dermis, single or multiple • **Deep hemangioma** — posterior to orbital septum, present with **nonaxial proptosis** that increases in size with valsalva maneuver or crying • **Combined** superficial and deep • **Poor vision: Amblyopia from ptosis (superficial) or astigmatism (deep)**	• **Deep hemangioma** — presents with **axial proptosis** from intraconal tumor • **Usually presents with hyperopia**
CT scan	• **Either** intra- or extraconal mass • Moderate to poorly defined margins	• Well-encapsulated **intraconal** tumor • No bony erosion • Enhances with IV contrast
Angiography	• Multiple feeder arteries and draining veins (therefore hemodynamically rapid)	• No feeding arteries or veins. Staining in late arterial phase (low flow lesion)

(Continued)

	Capillary hemangioma	**Cavernous hemangioma**
Management	• Indications for removal: 　• Systemic complications: 　　• High output cardiac failure 　　• Kasabach-Merritt syndrome 　• Ocular complications: 　　• Amblyopia (from astigmatism, anisometropia, strabismus and ptosis) 　　• Proptosis (ON compression and exposure keratopathy) 　　• Tissue necrosis • Treatment options: 　• Systemic steroids 　• Intralesional steroids 　• Antifibrinolytic agents (aminocaproate, tranexamic acid) in Kasabach-Merritt syndrome (2 Rs, 2 Ts) 　• Angiographic embolization 　• Radiotherapy Surgical excision — difficult	• Mainly observation in absence of symptoms

---

Q **How do You Differentiate a Lymphangioma from an Orbital Varix?**

	Orbital lymphangioma	**Orbital varix**
Pathology	• Isolated vascular **choristoma** • Various types of tortuous vessels containing blood or clear fluid	• Dilated venous outflow channels, with well-defined endothelial lined channels containing blood • Non-encapsulated • Similar to cavernous hemangioma but with more smooth muscle in vessel walls
Demographics	• Early **childhood**	• Late **middle age**
Presentation	• **Superficial lymphangioma** — transilluminable cystic lesion beneath skin of eye lid • **Deep lymphangioma** — nonaxial proptosis that does not increase in size with valsalva maneuver. Acute episodes of spontaneous hemorrhage in tumor • Combined superficial and deep	• Deep varix — **intermittent proptosis** and pain with exertion. Increases in size with valsalva maneuver • Superficial varix — swelling of lids and conjunctiva • Combined superficial and deep
CT scan	• Low-density cyst-like mass • Enhancement of • Enlargement of bony orbit	• Abnormally dilated irregular veins • Mulitlobular lesions (hemorrhage)

	Orbital lymphangioma	Orbital varix
Venography	• No arterial or venous connection	• Venous connection may be present
Management	• Surgical removal • Prognosis is guarded because lesion is large, friable, infiltrate normal orbital tissue, not encapsulated and bleeds easily	• Surgical removal • Prognosis is also guarded because lesion is friable and bleeds easily and excision may be incomplete

Exam tips:
• An easy way to remember is to compare the features of lymphangioma with those of capillary hemangioma (both occur in childhood and have similar clinical). Then compare the features of varix with those of cavernous hemangioma.

Q **Tell me about Lacrimal Gland Tumors.**

"Lacrimal gland tumors are common causes of nonaxial proptosis."
"Classified according to epithelial or nonepithelial origin."
"Benign or malignant."
"The clinical presentation is…."
"The pathological features include…."

Classification, Clinical Features and Management

Type	Frequency	Tumor	Clinical features	Management
50% epithelial	50% benign	• Pleomorphic adenoma	• **Older** patients • Chronic presentation • **Painless** • Nonaxial proptosis • CT scan — affect usually orbital lobe with pressure changes in bony orbit	• **Excision** biopsy (keyword) • Lateral orbitotomy • Malignant transformation — 10%
	50% malignant	• 50% adenoid cystic carcinoma, of which 50% is basaloid variant (worst prognosis) • Other malignant tumors (50%) include: Pleomorphic adenocarcinoma, mucoepidermoid CA, monomorphic adenocarcinoma	• **Younger** • More acute history • **Pain** (perineural spread — keyword) • CT scan — usually affect orbital lobe with destructive changes in bony orbit	• **Incisional** biopsy (keyword) • Orbital exenteration • Mid facial resection • Radiotherapy

(Continued)

Type	Frequency	Tumor	Clinical features	Management
50% nonepithelial	50% benign	• Inflammation (dacryoadenitis)	• Signs of orbital inflammatory disease	• Antibiotics • Steroids
	50% malignant	• Lymphoma	• **Older** • Acute history • **Pain** • **Bilateral** tumor common • CT scan — affect **both** orbital and palpebral lobe and molds to the shape of globe	• Radiotherapy • Chemotherapy

Exam tips:
• Famous "Rule of 50" (refers to new cases in tertiary oncology referral center). In the general ophthalmology setting, closer to 80:20 nonepithelial:epithelial ratio.

Q What is the Pathology of Pleomorphic Adenoma? Adenoid Cystic Carcinoma?

Pathology of Lacrimal Gland Tumors

1. **Pleomorphic adenoma**
   • Involves orbital lobe
   • Mixture of **epithelial** tissues (nests/tubules in two layers) and **stromal** tissues (connective tissues, cartilage, bone, myxoid tissues) (hence the term "pleomorphic"!)
   • Pseudocapsule from compression of normal tissue by slow growing tumor

2. **Adenoid cystic carcinoma**
   • Involves orbital lobe
   • Classic type: **Swiss cheese** appearance (keyword)
   • Other varieties: Basaloid variant (worst prognosis), comedo acinar, sclerosing, tubular
   • No capsule (invades surrounding tissue, including nerves hence "perineural spread")

Q Tell me about Lymphoma Involving the Eye.

"Lymphoma is a malignant lymphoproliferative disease which can affect the ocular structures in a number of ways…."
"Orbital lymphoma is a spectrum of disease which can range from…."

Lymphoma and the Eye

1. **Orbital lymphoma**

2. **Anterior segment**
   • Conjunctival lymphoma
   • Cornea (crystalline keratopathy)
   • Uveitis (masquerade syndrome)

3. **Posterior segment**
   • Vitritis (masquerade syndrome)
   • Subretinal infiltrate
   • Primary intraocular lymphoma

Orbital Lymphoma

Types	Histology	Prognosis
Orbital **inflammatory** disease (pseudotumor)	• **Hypocellular** lymphoid lesion • Mature lymphocytes • Mixture of different cells (polyclonal proliferation) • Fibrous stroma	Benign
Benign reactive lymphoid hyperplasia	• **Hypercellular** lesion • Mature (T cell) lymphocytes • Reactive stroma • Patternless or follicular	20% become malignant
Atypical lymphoid hyperplasia	• **Hypercellular** lesion • Borderline maturity • Diffuse or follicular pattern	30% become malignant
Malignant lymphoma	• **Hypercellular** lesion • Immature malignant (**B cell**) cells • Monomorphous (monoclonal proliferation) • Follicular (10%) or diffuse (90%) pattern • Commonest type is MALT lymphoma	Malignant 50% associated with systemic lymphoma (20% with preceding history of lymphoma)

Q **Tell me about Rhabdomyosarcoma.**

"Rhabdomyosarcoma is the most common **primary malignant** tumor of the orbit in children."
"It is a tumor of connective tissues that has the capacity to differentiate towards muscle...."
(Note: Does not *arise* from extraocular muscles!)

Rhabdomyosarcoma

1. **Histology**
   - Embryonal:
     - Most **common**
     - Undifferentiated connective tissues
   - Alveolar:
     - Most **aggressive**
     - Fibrovascular strands floating freely in alveolar spaces
   - Pleomorphic:
     - **Best** prognosis but rarest
     - Most differentiated and pathologically looks like muscles
     - Usually in **older** individuals
     - (**Note:** Very much like pleomorphic adenoma of lacrimal gland!)
   - Botyroid:
     - Rare variant of embryonal
     - Not primarily found in orbit, usually invades orbit from paranasal sinus
     - Grape-like form

2. **Clinical presentation**
   - First decade (7–8 years)
   - Rapid progressive proptosis
   - Severe inflammatory reaction:
     - Main differential diagnoses in children: Chloroma, Ewing's sarcoma, neuroblastoma, orbital cellulitis
   - Nonaxial proptosis (mass in upper orbit)

3. **Management**
   - Radiotherapy
   - Chemotherapy (vincristine, dactinomycin, cyclophosphamide)
   - Exenteration

Q **How do You Differentiate an Optic Nerve Glioma from Meningioma?**

	ON glioma	ON meningioma
Gross pathology	• **Fusiform** enlargement of ON • Expansile intraneural or invasive perineural form (usually seen associated with neurofibromatosis)	• **Tubular** enlargement of ON
Histopathology	• Growth pattern: Intrinsic or extrinsic • Arises from **glial tissue** (astrocytes, oligodendrocytes, ependymal cells) • Spindle-shaped cells • **Rosenthal** fibers (keyword) • Microcystic degeneration • Meninges show reactive hyperplasia, dura is normal	• Arises from **meninges** (arachnoid layer — meningo epithelial cells) • Plump cells arranged in whorl-like pattern • **Psammoma** bodies (keyword) • **Intranuclear cytoplasmic inclusions** • **Dural invasion**
Demographics	• **Young girls** (2–6 years)	• **Late middle age women**
Presentation	• Axial proptosis occurs early • VA decrease occurs early • EOM normal • Optociliary shunt uncommon • **Associated with Type I neurofibromatosis** in 20–49% (keyword)	• Axial proptosis occurs late • VA decrease occurs late, may have gaze evoked amaurosis • EOM impaired • **Optociliary shunt** (keyword) common • Associated with neurofibromatosis uncommon
CT scan/MRI	• **Fusiform enlargement** (keyword) • Isodense to bone • Enlarged ON canal • Chiasmal involvement may be present • Mucinous degeneration • No central lucency (optic nerve)	• **Tubular enlargement** (keyword) • Hyperdense to bone (calcification) • Normal ON canal • Sphenoidal bone **hyperostosis** (keyword) • ON sheath **enhancement** on MRI (keyword)
Management	• Conservative treatment if VA good • Surgical removal if VA poor and life threatening • Radiotherapy	• Conservative treatment if VA good • Surgical removal if VA poor and life threatening • Radiotherapy

EPIPHORA

Q Opening Question: What are the Causes of Epiphora in Adults?

"Epiphora can be divided into...."

Functional classification	Etiology
Hypersecretion (1)	1. Entropian, ectropian 2. Trichiasis 3. Keratoconjunctivitis sicca 4. Corneal/conjunctival diseases

Obstruction
• Canalicular
  • Complete (2)
  • Partial (3)
• Nasolacrimal duct (NLD)
  • Complete (4)
  • Partial (5)
	1. Congenital — atresia
	2. Acquired
	  • Involutional
	  • Infection — canaliculitis, dacryocystitis
	  • Trauma
	  • Tumor

Lacrimal pump failure (6)	1. Facial nerve palsy • Combination of ectropion, punctal eversion, exposure keratopathy and pump failure

Q How do You Evaluate a Patient with Epiphora?

Functional Evaluation

1. **History**
   - Onset
   - Watery or mucoid discharge
   - Medical history (sinus disease, previous trauma, previous dacryocystitis)
   - Surgical or radiation history
2. **Slit lamp exam**
   - Lid position (entropian, ectropian)
   - Puncta (position, inflammatory changes)
   - Tear film
   - Cornea and conjunctiva
   - Dye disappearance test

3. **Syringing/irrigation with saline**
   - **Soft stop**
     - Diagnosis: **Complete canaliculi block (2)**
       - Reflex from upper canaliculi — common canaliculi block
       - Reflex from lower canaliculi — lower canaliculi block
   - **Hard stop**
     - If no saline enters nose/mucoid reflux into puncta:
       - Diagnosis: **Complete NLD block (4)**
     - If saline enters nose:
       - Possibilities: Hypersecretion (1), partial obstruction (3) or (5), lacrimal pump (6)
       - Proceed with Jones primary dye tests

4. **Jones primary dye test (largely of historical value)**
- **Positive (dye in nose):**
  - Diagnosis: **Hypersecretion (1)**
- **Negative:**
  - Possibilities: Partial obstruction (3) or (5), lacrimal pump failure (6)
  - Proceed with Jones secondary dye test

5. **Jones secondary dye test**
- **Positive (dye in nose after flushing):**
  - Diagnosis: **Partial obstruction NLD (5)**
- **Negative:**
  - Diagnosis: **Partial obstruction canaliculi (3), lacrimal pump failure (6)**

Q   How do You Perform a Dacryocystorhinostomy (DCR)?

"DCR is a **tear drainage** surgical procedure to **bypass** an NLD obstruction."
"Creating an anastomosis between the **lacrimal sac** and the **middle meatus.**"
"Through an artificial **bony ostium.**"

DCR

1. **Indications**
   - Persistent and symptomatic epiphora form NLD obstruction
   - Chronic and recurrent dacryocystitis
   - Mucocele
   - Congenital NLD obstruction

2. **Preoperative preparation**
   - Assess nose for deviated septum/polyp:
     - Consider ENT referral and X-ray to assess nasal septum
     - Consider dacryocystogram (to look for stone, tumor and anatomy)
   - Assess for bleeding tendencies:
     - Check BP and platelet levels
     - Stop warfarin/aspirin

3. **Intraoperative procedure**
   - GA (hypotensive anesthesia or LA — less bleeding postoperatively):
     - Consider reverse-Trendelenburg position
     - LA injection to skin (lignocaine, marcaine, adrenaline, wydase) 15 min before operation
     - Cocaine 4% nasal pack
   - Skin incised:
     - With #15 Bard Parker blade
     - 10 mm medial to medial canthus and 10–15 mm long incision
     - Blunt dissection of orbicularis oculi by blunt dissecting scissors down to periosteum
     - Divide anterior limb of medial canthal tendon
   - Periosteum incised:
     - With Rollet periosteal elevator (or #11 Bard Parker) medial to anterior lacrimal crest
     - Periosteum and lacrimal sac reflected with lacrimal retractor to expose operation site at lacrimal fossa

   - Osteotomy created:
     - With Traquair's periosteal elevator at anterior lacrimal crest
     - Osteotomy enlarged with Kerrison punch to create 10 mm hole nasal mucosa exposed
     - Bowman probe inserted into canaliculi to lacrimal sac to assess if common canalicular obstruction is present
   - Lacrimal sac incised:
     - With #12 Bard Parker blade creating vertical incision on medial wall of sac
     - Anterior and posterior flaps created with right angled scissors (Weib's scissor)
   - Nasal mucosa incised:
     - After injection with lignocaine and adrenaline (to decrease bleeding)
     - Posterior flap sutured to posterior lacrimal sac flap with 6/0 vicryl
     - Anterior flap sutured
   - Management of canalicular obstruction:
     - Canalicular obstruction >10 mm from punctum — lacrimal trephination to clear obstruction followed by intubation
     - Canalicular obstruction <10 mm from punctum — carunculectomy with insertion of Jones (pyrex) tube
   - Closure:
     - Reattach medial canthal tendon
     - Close skin with 7/0 silk
     - Pack nose with antibiotic soaked gauze
     - Silicon tube insertion (Bodkin intubation)

4. **Postoperative care**
   - Monitor carefully for bleeding (from anterior ethmoidal artery)
   - Tell patient not to blow nose
   - Skin suture removed by fifth day
   - Syringing at six months
   - Remove tube (if present) at six months

Notes
- What are the indications for intubation after DCR?
  - Associated canalicular obstruction
  - Repeat DCR
  - Sever bleeding during operation
  - Shrunken and scarred lacrimal sac found during operation

ENUCLEATION, EVISCERATION & OTHER ORBITAL SURGERIES

Overall yield: ✪✪   **Clinical exam:**   **Viva:** ✪✪   **Essay:**   **MCQ:** ✪

Q Opening Question: What are the Indications for Enucleation?

"Enucleation is the removal of the entire globe, including the sclera and cornea."

Indications

1. **Malignant tumors (e.g. retinoblastoma, choroidal melanoma)**
2. **Painful blind eye (e.g. advanced glaucoma)**
3. **Severe ocular trauma (prevention of sympathetic ophthalmia)**
4. **Blind eye with opaque media in which CA cannot be ruled out**
5. **Deformed phthisiscal eye in which CA cannot be ruled out**

Q How do You Perform an Enucleation?

Enucleation

1. **GA (or LA), clean, drape and speculum**
2. **Inject subconjunctival LA (lignocaine with adrenaline)**
   - 360° peritomy
   - Separate conjunctiva from Tenon's and Tenon's from sclera with blunt dissection scissors
3. **Identify MR with squint hook**
   - Suture MR with double armed 6/0 vicryl 3 mm behind insertion, and hold suture with artery forceps
   - Divide MR 1 mm behind insertion
   - Suture MR insertion with 4/O silk (suture to hold the globe)
   - Repeat for IR, LR, SR, then IO and SO
4. **Lift and abduct the globe to stretch ON**
   - Engage ON with curved artery forceps, by strumming ON

- Do not clamp/crush ON if enucleation performed for retinoblastoma
- Cut ON with right angled scissors placed above the forceps
5. **Pack socket with 2.5 mm wide ribbon gauze to secure hemostasis**
6. **Insert implant either within Tenon's capsule or behind posterior Tenon's**
7. **Close anterior Tenon's capsule layer with 4/0 vicryl**
   - Suture rectus muscles to fornix
   - Close conjunctiva with 6/0 vicryl
   - Place prosthesis conformer to maintain fornix

Q **What are the Indications for Evisceration?**

"Evisceration is the removal of the contents of the globe, leaving the sclera and ON."

Evisceration

1. **Indication**
   - Endophthalmitis (less orbital contamination, less risk of intracranial spread)

2. **Advantages over enucleation**
   - Less disruption of orbital anatomy
   - Better motility for prosthesis

- Technically simpler procedure
- Better for endophthalmitis (reduces risk of dissemination of infection)

3. **Disadvantages**
   - Risk of sympathetic ophthalmia not decreased
   - Not indicated for tumors

Q **How do You Perform an Evisceration?**

Evisceration

1. **GA (LA), clean, drape and speculum**
2. **Corneal incised**
   - With Beaver blade from 3 to 9 o'clock
   - Hold cornea with Jayles forceps and cut off entire cornea with corneal scissors
   - Retract sclera at 12-, 5- and 9-o'clock with Kilner's hooks
3. **Insert evisceration scoop between sclera and uvea and scoop out intraocular contents**
   - Send contents for culture
   - Remove uveal remnants with cellulose sponge

4. **Closure**
   - Pack scleral shell with adrenaline-soaked ribbon gauze for five min
   - Wash with 100% alcohol (destroy residual uveal tissue), followed by gentamicin
   - Pack with ribbon gauze again
   - Apply pressure bandage for 24–48 hours
5. **Allow sclera to granulate (healing by secondary intention)**

Q **Tell me about Orbital Implants.**

"Orbital implants are used to replace globe volume after enucleation or evisceration."

Orbital Implants

- **Ideal implant**
  - Replace volume
  - Enhance motility
  - Good cosmesis
  - Easy to insert, stable and promote healing
- **Material**
  - Inert (non-integrating):
    - Glass, silicon, plastic, methyl methacrylate
  - Bioreactive (integrating)·
  - Hydroxyapatite, porous polyethylene
  - 'Bio-eye': Hydroxyapatite coated with polyethylene with differential resorption rates:
    - Does not need wrap

- Anterior coat dissolves more slowly to allow conjunctival healing
- Posterior coat dissolves more quickly for bio-integration
- **Size**
  - 16 mm = 2 cm³ volume
  - 18 mm = 3 cm³ volume
- **Ball covered with donor sclera/autogenous fascia**
  - **For attachment of recti muscles**
- **Implanted within Tenon's capsule or behind post Tenon's capsule**
- May be drilled to create peg for ocular prosthesis

Postenucleation Socket Syndrome

1. **Infection**
2. **Contracture of fornices (conjunctival deficiency)**
3. **Implant-related**
   - Prominent upper lid sulcus (small implant)
   - Exposure of implant
   - Extrusion of implant
   - Giant papillary conjunctivitis
4. **Lid problems**
   - Anophthalmic ptosis
   - Anophthalmic ectropion
   - Lash margin entropion

- Volume deficiency:
  - Secondary orbital implants
  - Dermis fat grafts
- Conjunctival deficiency:
  - Buccal mucosal grafts
  - Autologous conjunctival grafts
- Lid malpositions:
  - Correct residual malposition after correction of volume and conjunctival deficiencies

Management of PESS

Directed at correcting underlying mechanisms in following order:

- Prosthesis modification:
  - Frequently able to correct most deficiencies — least invasive

Q   **What is Exenteration?**

"Exenteration is the removal of the globe and parts of the orbit."

Exenteration

1. **Types of exenteration**
   - Subtotal:
     - Periorbital tissue, eyelids and apex left behind
   - Total:
     - All intraorbital tissue removed
   - Extended:
     - All intraorbital tissue plus adjacent bony structures (wall and sinus) removed

2. **Indications**
   - Destructive orbital malignancies
   - Destructive intraocular tumors with extension into orbit
   - Malignant lacrimal gland tumors
   - Orbital sarcomas
   - Fulminating fungal infection

Uveitis, Systemic Diseases and Tumors

INTRODUCTION TO UVEITIS

Overall yield: ✷✷✷ **Clinical exam:** ✷✷ **Viva:** ✷✷✷ **Essay:** ✷✷ **MCQ:** ✷✷✷

Q Opening Question: What is Uveitis?

"Uveitis is an inflammation of the uveal tract...."
"Inflammation of the iris is referred to as iritis, the ciliary body referred to as cyclitis and the choroid referred to as choroiditis."
"It can be classified in a few ways...."

Classification of Uveitis

1. **Anatomical**
   - Anterior, intermediate, posterior and panuveitis

2. **Pathological**
   - Granulomatous vs nongranulomatous uveitis
   - **Clinical**
   - Infectious (e.g. bacterial, viral, fungal, parasitic)

- Noninfectious (e.g. known systemic associations, no known systemic associations)
- Masquerade (e.g. neoplastic, nonneoplastic)
"Common causes of uveitis can be classified based on the anatomical location of the uveitis."

Q What are the Common Causes of Uveitis?

Etiology of Uveitis (by Anatomical Classification According to the International Uveitis Study Group (IUSG))

1. **Anterior uveitis (iritis, iridocyclitis and anterior cyclitis)**
   - Idiopathic
   - HLA-B27 related uveitis (e.g. anklyosing spondylitis, Reiter's syndrome, inflammatory bowel disease and psoriatic arthritis)
   - Fuch's heterochromic iridocyclitis, Posner-Schlossman syndrome
   - Viral e.g. herpetic
   - Juvenile rheumatoid arthritis

2. **Intermediate uveitis (pars planitis, posterior cyclitis, hyalitis and basal retinochoroiditis)**
   - Pars planitis

3. **Posterior (focal, multifocal, or diffuse choroiditis, chorioretinitis, retinochoroiditis, neurouveitis)**
   - Infective
     - Viral e.g. Acute Retinal Necrosis (ARN) or Progressive Outer Retinal Necrosis (PORN)
     - Fungal
     - Parasitic e.g. toxoplasmosis, toxocara
   - Noninfective
     - Collagen vascular diseases e.g. SLE, PAN, Wegener's
     - Retinochoroidopathies
   - Masquerade

4. **Panuveitis (diffuse)**
   - See below

Exam tips:
- **There are many ways to answer this question. Decide on one and remember it.**

Q **What are the Causes of Granulomatous Uveitis?**

"The causes of granulomatous uveitis can be divided into infective, noninfective and masquerade syndromes of granulomatous uveitis."

- **Infective:**
  - TB
  - Syphilis
  - Leprosy
  - Toxoplasmosis
  - Lyme disease
  - Brucellosis
  - Viral

- **Noninfective:**
  - Vogt-Koyanagi-Harada syndrome (VKH)
  - Sympathetic ophthalmia
  - Sarcoidosis
  - Phacoantigenic uveitis
- Masquerade:
  - Lymphoma/leukaemias
  - Ocular metastases

Exam tips:
- **This is one of the most important LISTS to remember in uveitis.**
- **It is especially useful in the clinical examination. If you see "mutton fat" keratic precipitates, think of this list!**
- **Remember the causes in groups (TB, syphilis and leprosy) and (VKH and sympathetic ophthalmia).**

Q **How do You Manage a Patient with Uveitis?**

"The management involves a comprehensive history, physical examination, appropriate investigations and treatment."

Management of Uveitis

1. **History**
   - Symptoms of uveitis (redness, pain, photophobia, blurring of vision, etc.)
   - Systemic review
   - **Examination**
     - Ocular examination:
     - Anterior uveitis:
       - AC cells and flare, presence of hypopyon (severity), fibrin
       - Keratic precipitates (small, medium size, mutton fat)
       - Posterior synechiae and peripheral anterior synechiae, iris nodules
       - Complications (cataract, glaucoma, band keratopathy, phthsis bulbi)
     - Intermediate uveitis:
       - Snowflakes and snowbanks
       - Vitritis
   - Posterior uveitis:
     - Cystoid macular edema
     - Choroiditis, retinitis, vasculitis
     - Optic neuritis
   - Systemic examination (heart, skin, joints, etc.)

2. **Investigations**
   - Blood (directed by clinical evaluation):
     - FBC (eosinophilia for parasites), ESR
     - VDRL, FTA
     - Autoimmune markers (ANA, RF, anti-double stranded DNA, ENA, HLA B27)
     - Calcium, serum ACE levels (sarcoidosis)
     - Toxoplasma serology and other TORCH screen (toxoplasma, rubella, CMV, hepatitis B, HIV)
   - Urine:
     - 24-hour urine calcium (sarcoidosis)
     - Culture (Bechet's disease, Reiter's syndrome)

- Radiological:
  - CXR (TB, sarcoidosis, histoplasmosis), CT chest
  - Spine and sacroiliac joints X-ray (ankylosing spondylitis)
  - X-ray of other joints (rheumatoid arthritis, juvenile rheumatoid arthritis)
  - Skull X-ray for cerebral calcifications (toxoplasmosis)
- Skin tests:
  - Mantoux tests
    - Intradermal injection of tuberculin purified protein derivative
    - Inject five tuberculin units in 0.1 ml to produce a wheal of 6–10 mm size on forearm
    - Look for induration 48–72 hours later
    - Positive if induration > 10 mm, indicates previous infection with TB or immunization for TB
    - Anergy: May indicate immunosuppression (AIDS) or sarcoidosis
  - TB quantiferon:
    - "In-vitro", quantitative Mantoux test
    - Useful in areas with high levels of TB endemicity
    - Measures IFN production in response to Mantoux antigens in sample of patient's blood
    - Able to distinguish BCG immunization from TB infection
    - Cannot distinguish recent/active and past infection
- Pathergy test for Behcet's disease:
  - Increased dermal sensitivity to needle trauma (increase leukotactic response)
  - Only 10% of Behcet's patients respond
  - Intradermal needle puncture
  - Look for pustule 24–36 hours later
- Kveim test for sarcoidosis:
  - Similar to Mantoux test
  - Intradermal injection of sarcoid tissue (from spleen of another patient with sarcoidosis)
  - Look for sarcoid granuloma four weeks later

3. **Medications**
- Mydriatic and cycloplegic agents
- Immunodulating:
  - Corticosteroids (topical, periocular, systemic, intravitreal)
  - NSAIDS
  - Immunosuppressives (e.g. cyclosporin, methotrexate, azathioprine)
- Newer medications (biologic agents):
  - Etanercept, infliximab, IVIG, interferon alfa-2b

Exam tips:
- The skin tests for sarcoidosis and Behcet's disease are almost never used, but frequently asked in the examinations!

Notes
- "When do you need to investigate for a specific cause?"
  - Suggestive systemic features
  - Recurrent uveitis
  - Bilateral uveitis
  - Severe uveitis
  - Posterior uveitis
  - Young age of onset

"Panuveitis can be divided into granulomatous or nongranulomatous conditions."
"They can be either infective or noninfective in origin."

Panuveitis/Posterior Uveitis

1. **Granulomatous**
   - Infective:
     - TB, syphilis, leprosy and others
   - Noninfective:
     - Sympathetic ophthalmia (previous trauma or surgery in other eye) and VKH
     - Sarcoidosis and others
   - Masquerade

2. **Nongranulomatous**
   - Infective:
     - Endophthalmitis (severe hypopyon, previous surgery)

- Noninfective:
  - Behcet's disease (severe hypopyon, no surgery, mention other features)
  - Candida (immunosuppression)
  - Toxoplasmosis
  - Lymphoma
- Masquerade

> **Exam tips:**
> - The causes of panuveitis, posterior uveitis and vasculitis are nearly IDENTICAL.
> - The granulomatous vs nongranulomatous classification list is very handy here.

"There are three overlapping stages in phthsis bulbi...."

Phthsis Bulbi

- **Atrophic bulbi without shrinkage:**
  - Initially size and shape of globe maintained
  - Continuous loss of nutritional support
  - Lens becomes cataractous
  - Serous detachment and atrophy of retina
  - Anterior and posterior synechiae formation, leading to an increase in IOP
- **Atrophic bulbi with shrinkage:**
  - Ciliary body dysfunction leads to drop in IOP
  - AC collapse with corneal edema, pannus and vascularization

- Globe becomes smaller and square-shaped (maintained by four recti muscle)
- **Atrophic bulbi with disorganization (phthsis bulbi):**
  - Size of globe decreases from 24–26 mm to 16–19 mm
  - Disorganization of ocular contents
  - Dystrophic calcification of Bowman's layer, lens and retina
  - Sclera thickens
  - Bone replaces uveal tract

SYSTEMIC INFECTIOUS DISEASES AND THE EYE I

Overall yield: ✪✪✪✪ **Clinical exam: Viva:** ✪✪✪✪ **Essay:** ✪✪ **MCQ:** ✪✪✪✪✪

Q **Opening Question:** What are the Ocular Complications of AIDS?

"Ocular complications develop in **75%** of patients with AIDS."
"They can be divided into…."

Ocular Complications of AIDS

1. **AIDS: Disease related manifestations**
   - Posterior: Microangiopathy
     - 70% of patients with AIDS
     - Microaneurysms, hemorrhages, cotton wool spots
       - Lesions are:
         - Transient
         - Smaller and multifocal
         - Located in the posterior pole
   - Anterior
   - Ocular adnexa:
     - **Molluscum contagiosum**
   - Neuroophthalmic:
     - Optic neuritis and optic atrophy
     - CN palsies
     - Cortical blindness

2. **Opportunistic infections**
   - Viral
     - CMV retinitis (see below)
     - Herpes zoster:
       - **Progressive outer retinal necrosis (PORN)**
   - Parasitic
     - Toxoplasmosis (relatively uncommon)
     - Pneumocystis carinii choroiditis
   - Fungi
     - Cryptococcal choroiditis:
       - Presents with **optic neuritis** and meningitis
     - Candida retinitis
   - Bacteria:
     - TB
     - Syphilis

3. **Neoplasia**
   - Kaposi's sarcoma of eyelid, conjunctiva and orbit
   - Lymphoma
   - Squamous cell CA

4. **Treatment related**
   - Cidofovir, Rifabutin may cause uveitis

5. **Immune reconstitution uveitis**
   - Mediated by recovery of immune responses specific to residual cytomegalovirus antigen located in the eye
   - On commencement of HAART therapy

Exam tips:
- **Remember "AIDS" complications as Angiopathy, Infections Diseases and Sarcomas.**
- **Remember the "BIG 8" opportunistic infections.**

> **Notes**
> - "How do you differentiate AIDS microangiopathy from CMV retinitis?" In microangiopathy:
>   - Patient is usually asymptomatic
>   - CD4 levels are normal (200–500 cells/μl)

> **Notes**
> - "How do you distinguish PORN from CMV retinitis and acute retinal necrosis (ARN)?" Four characteristics of PORN:
>   - Absence of inflammation (unlike ARN)
>   - Early posterior pole involvement (unlike ARN)
>   - Multifocal (unlike CMV)
>   - Rapid progression (unlike CMV)

> **Notes**
> - "How do you differentiate toxoplasmosis in AIDS from the typical toxoplasmosis that occurs in immunocompetent patients?" In patients with AIDS, toxoplasmosis is:
>   - More severe
>   - Bilateral
>   - Multifocal
>   - Not necessarily confined to the posterior pole
>   - Not adjacent to old scars
>   - Associated with CNS involvement
>   - Requires treatment for life

Q **Tell me about CMV Retinitis.**

"CMV retinitis is an important ocular complication of AIDS."
"Developing in about 50% of patients in the past…."
"The clinical manifestations can be divided into central and peripheral retinitis."

CMV Retinitis

1. **Clinical features**
   - 50% of patients with AIDS (declining now with better treatment)
   - Classification:
     - Indolent/granular
     - Fulminant/hemorrhagic
   - Central
     - Dense, white, well-demarcated areas of retinal necrosis
     - Retinal hemorrhages along edge or within areas of necrosis
     - **"Cheese and ketchup"** appearance
     - Lack of inflammatory signs (like presumed ocular histoplasmosis syndrome)
   - Peripheral
     - More common than central type
     - Foveal sparing granular retinal necrosis

2. **Natural history**
   - **R**elentless progression (like a "bush fire")
   - **R**etinal detachment
   - **R**etinal atrophy
   - **R**esolution
   - **R**ecurrence

3. **Treatment**
  - Zone of involvement important and determines urgency of treatment:
    - Zone 1: Within 3,000µm of fovea/1,500µm of optic disc (vision-threatening)
    - Zone 2: Up to vortex vein entrances
    - Zone 3: Peripheral vortex vein entrances
  - All drugs inhibit **DNA polymerase**
  - Ganciclovir (IV, oral and intraocular):
    - 80% response
    - Induction phase with IV, followed by maintenance with oral (poor bioavailability), IV and/or intravitreal
    - Major complication is **bone marrow suppression**

- **Valganciclovir:**
  - **Oral prodrug of ganciclovir**
  - **Good bioavailability**
  - **Useful for oral prophylaxis but main limitation of cost (very expensive)**
- Foscarnet (IV, oral and intraocular):
  - Major complication is **nephrotoxicity**
- Cidofovir:
  - Main complications are **uveitis** and **nephrotoxicity**
  - Not for intravitreal use – causes severe permanent hypotony
- Response to treatment suggested by:
  - Decreasing size of lesions
  - Decreasing activity of lesions

> **Exam tips:**
> - One of the most important ocular complications of IADS. Remember the natural history is "5R"s.

Q **What are the Ocular Features of Syphilis?**

"Ocular involvement in syphilis is not common."
"Usually occurs in secondary and tertiary stages."

Ocular Syphilis

1. **Congenital syphilis**
  - **Keratouveitis (interstitial keratitis, may be bilateral)**
  - **Salt and pepper fundus**
2. **Primary syphilis**
  - Systemic: Chance on genitalia
  - Eye chancre (Conj chancre)
3. **Secondary**
  - Systemic: Skin rash, fever, weight loss, arthralgias
  - Orbit and eyelids:
    - Eyelid rash
    - Orbital periostitis
    - Dacryocystitis
    - Dacryoadenitis
    - Madarosis
  - Anterior segment:
    - Conjunctivitis
    - **Interstitial keratitis**
    - Episcleritis, scleritis
    - **Uveitis**
      - Iritis roseate (dilated iris capillaries)
      - Iritis papulosa (iris papules)
      - Iritis nodosa (iris nodules)

- Posterior segment:
  - Chorioretinitis
  - Neuroretinitis
  - Retinal vasculitis
- Neuroophthalmic:
  - **Optic neuritis and neuroretinitis**
  - CN palsies

4. **Tertiary**
  - Systemic:
    - Granulomas form when immune system unable to clear the organism
    - Gummas produce a **chronic inflammatory** state in the body with mass-effects upon the local anatomy
    - Main features: Neurosyphilis and cardiovascular syphilis
  - Anterior segment findings similar to secondary syphilis (intersitial keratitis, uveitis etc)
    - Lens subluxation
  - Neuroophthalmic:
    - **Pupils:**
      - Argyll Robertson pupil
      - Tonic pupils
      - Horner's syndrome
      - RAPD (optic atrophy)

- Others:
  - CN palsies
  - Ptosis
- Nystagmus
- VF defects

Exam tips:
- **Primary syphilis — conjunctiva, secondary syphilis = anterior and posterior segments and tertiary syphilis = neuroophthalmic lesions (i.e. involvement moves deeper with each stage).**

Q **What are the Ocular Features of TB?**

- Gumma of ocular structures
  "Ocular involvement in TB is rare, but TB is one of the commonest causes of uveitis in Asia."
  "It can occur at the anterior segment or posterior segment or can be a neuroophthalmic involvement or a result of complications from treatment."

Ocular TB

1. **Anterior segment**
   - Eyelids (blepharitis, meibomitis)
   - Lacrimal gland and system (dacryoadenitis, dacryocystitis)
   - Orbital periostitis, cellulitis
   - Follicular conjunctivitis
   - **Phlyctenulosis**
   - Conjunctiva nodules (tuberculomas)
   - **Interstitial keratitis**
   - Episcleritis/scleritis
   - **Uveitis** (granulomatous)

2. **Posterior segment**
   - Choroiditis (choroidal tubercles)
   - Retinitis
   - Vasculitis
   - Vitreous hemorrhage (**Eale's disease**)

3. **Neuroophthalmic**
   - Optic neuritis, optic atrophy
   - CN palsies
   - Internuclear ophthalmoplegia

4. **Treatment related**
   - **Ethambutol** and others (pages 249 and 414)

Exam tips:
- **Most of the lesions are immune-related.**

Q **What are the Ocular Features of Leprosy?**

"Ocular involvement in leprosy can be divided into...."

Ocular Leprosy

1. **Leprosy mycobacteria favor cooler parts of the body (e.g. skin). Ocular manifestations are thus primarily periocular or in the anterior segment**

2. **Eyelid and lacrimal gland**
   - Eyelid
     - **Madarosis**
     - Trichiasis, distichiasis, entropion, ectropion
     - Lepromatous nodules, thickening of skin

   - Lacrimal system
     - Dacryocystitis and nasolacrimal duct obstruction

3. **Cornea and sclera**
   - Interstitial keratitis
   - **Exposure keratopathy** (VII CN palsy)
   - **Neurotrophic keratopathy**
   - Band keratopathy

- Thickened corneal nerves
- Pannus and scarring
- Episcleritis, scleritis

4. **Intraocular**
   - **Granulomatous uveitis:**
     - Iris atrophy, iris pearls, nodular iris lepromas
   - **Pupils:**
     - Occlusio/seclusio pupillae

- Corectopia, polycoria
- Miosis (sympathetic nerves are preferentially involved)
- Anisocoria, secrease response to light
- Cataract and glaucoma

5. **Neuroophthalmic**
   - Optic neuritis
   - CN palsies

Exam tips:
- **Most of the signs involve the eyelids and the anterior segment.**

Notes
- "What are the possible mechanisms of pannus and scarring?" Combination of:
  - Lid lesions
  - Interstitial keratitis
  - Exposure keratopathy
  - Neurotrophic keratopathy
  - Secondary infective keratitis

Q **Tell me about Lyme's Disease.**

"Lyme's disease is caused by the bacteria ***Borrelia burgdorferi.***"
"Transmitted through the ***Ixodes sp.*** tick."
"There are three classical stages…."
"There are systemic and ocular symptoms in each stage."

Lyme's Disease

1. **Stage 1**
   - Systemic (localized disease):
     - **Erythema migrans rash**
     - Fever, headache, arthralgia, myalgia (flu like symptoms)
   - Ocular (**anterior** segment):
     - Follicular conjunctivitis
     - Periorbital edema

2. **Stage 2**
   - Systemic (disseminated disease):
     - **Heart (arrhythmia, myocarditis)**
     - CNS
     - Skin
     - Joints

   - Ocular (**posterior** segment):
     - **Granulomatous uveitis**
     - **Intermediate uveitis**
     - Retinal vasculitis
     - Choroiditis

3. **Stage 3**
   - Systemic (immune-related):
     - **Arthritis**
   - Ocular (**anterior** segment):
     - **Episcleritis**
     - **Interstitial keratitis**
     - Orbital myositis

Exam tips:
- Surprisingly, this uncommon condition is one of the favorite exam questions! Remember that ocular involvement goes from the anterior segment (Stage 1) to the posterior segment (Stage 2) and back to the anterior segment (Stage 3) again!

SYSTEMIC INFECTIOUS DISEASES AND THE EYE II

Overall yield: ✪ ✪   **Clinical exam:**   **Viva:** ✪ ✪   **Essay:** ✪   **MCQ:** ✪ ✪ ✪

Q | **Opening Question:** What are the Ocular Complications of Toxocariasis?

"Ocular complications of toxocariasis can be divided into three different presentations depending on the age of infection."

Syndrome	Age of presentation	Clinical features	Differential diagnoses
Chronic endophthalmitis	Child (2–9)	Leukocoria Panuveitis	Retinoblastoma (Endophytic type)
Posterior pole granuloma	Teenager (4–14)	Localized mass at posterior pole	Retinoblastoma (Exophytic type)
Peripheral granuloma	Adult (6–40)	Pseudoesotropia	Dragged disc Retinal detachment

Exam tips:
- Important differential diagnosis of dragged disc and leukocoria (page 400).

Q | What are the Causes of Dragged Disc?

"The commonest cause is due to advanced cicatricial ROP."

Dragged Disc

1. **Proliferative vascular diseases**
   - Cicatricial ROP
   - Proliferative DM retinopathy
   - Sickle cell retinopathy
   - Coat's disease

2. **Infectious**
   - Toxocariasis

3. **Developmental disorders**
   - FEVR (Familial exudative vitreoretinopathy)
   - Combined hamartoma of retina and RPE
   - Incontinentia pigmenti
   - Norrie's disease

Q **Tell me about Presumed Ocular Histoplasmosis Syndrome (POHS).**

"POHS is caused by fungal infection by *Histoplasma capsulatum*."
"The organism is acquired by inhalation and may spread by the blood stream to the choroid."
"Associated with HLA-B7."

Clinical Features of POHS

1. **Atrophic "histo" spots**
   - Yellow-white in color
   - Half disc diameter in size
   - Asymptomatic unless macula is involved

2. **Peripapillary atrophy**

3. **Subretinal neovascular membrane (SRNVM)**
   - Usually develops adjacent to "histo" spot

4. **No vitreous involvement**
   - One of few "white dot syndromes" **NOT** to have vitreous involvement

Exam tips:
- **Important differential diagnosis of "white dot syndromes" (page 353) and SRNVM (page 176).**

Notes
- "What are the other important causes of peripapillary atrophy?"
  - Myopic degeneration (page 179)
  - Vogt-Koyanagi-Harada syndrome (page 350)

Q **Tell me about Masquerade Syndromes.**

Masquerade Syndromes

1. **Nonneoplastic masquerade syndromes**
   - Ocular ischemic syndrome
   - Chronic retinal detachment
   - Endophthalmitis

2. **Neoplastic masquerade syndromes**
   - CNS/systemic lymphoma

   - Leukemia
   - Uveal lymphoid proliferations
   - Nonlymphoid malignancies (e.g. melanoma, retinoblastoma)
   - Metastases

TOXOPLASMOSIS AND THE EYE

Overall yield: ✦✦✦✦ **Clinical exam:** ✦✦✦ **Viva:** ✦✦✦ **Essay:** ✦ **MCQ:** ✦✦✦✦

Q Opening Question: Tell me about Toxoplasmosis.

"Toxoplasmosis is a common parasitic infection with systemic and ocular manifestations."
"It is caused by *Toxoplasma gondii*."
"The cat is the definite **host** and other organisms, including humans, are the intermediate hosts."
"Ocular manifestations can be divided into congenital, acute acquired and recurrent…."

Toxoplasmosis

1. **Life cycle**
   - Sporocyst:
     - Excreted in cat's feces
     - Human infection: Ingestion from soil
   - Bradyzoite:
     - Encysted in tissues (including retina)
     - Human infection: Ingestion from beef and other meat
   - Tachyzoite:
     - Active proliferative form, responsible for tissue destruction and inflammation
     - Human infection: Transplacental spread (from mother to fetus)

2. **Clinical manifestations**
   - Congenital toxoplasmosis (see below)
   - Acute acquired toxoplasmosis (not common)
     - Immunocompetent:
       - Fever
       - Lymphadenopathy
       - Rash
     - Immunosuppressed:
       - CNS and systemic manifestation
   - Recurrent (congenital or acquired) toxoplasmosis
     - Primary lesion is an **inner retinitis**

   - Anterior segment
     - Granulomatous **OR** nongranulomatous uveitis
   - Posterior segment (**ALL** structures in posterior segment are involved):
     - **Superficial necrotizing retinitis**:
       - Commonest form
       - Distinguishing features (see toxoplasmosis in AIDS for comparison, page 327):
       - Unilateral
       - Focal
       - Posterior pole
       - Adjacent to scar
       - Vitreous haze ("headlight in the fog")
       - Local vasculitis around lesion
   - Deep retinitis:
     - Yellow distinct lesion with no vitritis (deeper than superficial retinitis)
   - Outer retinitis:
     - Multifocal punctate white lesions
   - Choroid involvement:
     - Massive granuloma
   - Optic nerve involvement:
     - Papillitis secondary to retinitis and choroiditis next to **ON**
   - Vessel involvement:
     - Vasculitis and vascular occlusions

Exam tips:
- The life cycle can be remembered by sporocyst = soil, bradyzoite = beef, tachyzoite = transplacental spread.
- The majority of clinical features are in the posterior segment (all posterior segment structures involved i.e. retina, choroids, ON, vessels).

Q **What are the Features of Congenital Toxoplasmosis?**

"Congenital toxoplasmosis has systemic and ocular features."

Congenital Toxoplasmosis

1. **Transmitted through placenta via tachyzoites**
2. **Severity depends on duration of gestation at time of maternal infection**
3. **Systemic features**
   - CNS:
     - Epilepsy
     - Intracranial calcification
     - Hydrocephalus
   - Fever
   - Visceral organ involvement
     - Hepatosplenomegaly

4. **Ocular features**
   - **Bilateral chorioretinal scars:**
     - Usually situated at macula
     - May cause squint
     - Should be differentiated from Best macular dystrophy (which also causes bilateral macula scars)
   - Optic atrophy
   - Others:
     - Microphthalmos
     - Cornea scars
     - Iris scars
     - Cataract

Q **How do You Manage a Patient with Ocular Toxoplasmosis?**

"The management of ocular toxoplasmosis depends on the patient's immune status and severity of ocular involvement."
"In general, if the patient is not immunosuppressed, most ocular lesions do not need treatment…."
"The indications for treatment are…."

Management of Ocular Toxoplasmosis

1. **Natural history (note the number "3")**
   - Resolution
     - Three months
   - Recurrence
     - 50% recurrence rate within **3** years
     - Number of recurrence per person = **3**

2. **Indications for treatment**
   - Patient factors:
     - Immunosuppression (AIDS)
   - Severity of ocular involvement:
     - Location of lesion: Macula, papillomacular bundle or around the ON
     - Size of lesion: > 1 disc diameter
     - Severe inflammation: Severe vitritis, cystoid macular edema
     - Complications: Tractional RD, epiretinal membrane

3. **Treatment**
   - Manage uveitis and associated complications (e.g. RD)
   - Systemic therapy:
     - Clindamycin:
       - Major complication is pseudomembranous colitis
     - Sulphur drugs:
       - Sulphadiazine
       - Co-trimoxazole (septrin)
     - Pyrimethamine (folic acid antagonist):
       - Major complication is anemia (need to moniter blood counts and add oral folic acid supplements)
     - Spiramycin:
       - Indicated for pregnancy (spiramycin concentrated in the placenta)

- Systemic steroids:
  - Indicated for severe vitritis (avoid in AIDS)
- Atovaquone:
  - Cysticidal but no clinical superiority demonstrated so far

- Azithromycin
- Treatment regimes:
  - Typically given as 'triple-therapy': Pyrimethamine + sulphadiazine + steroids
  - May also be given as 'quadruple therapy': Triple therapy + clindamycin

Exam tips:
- A common mistake is to jump straight into the myriad of drugs available. Most do not need treatment.

 Clinical approach to toxoplasmosis scar

"On examination of this patient's fundus…."
"There is a solitary, round, pigmented, punched out retinal scar."
"Located temporal to the macula, measuring one disc diameter in size."

Look for
- *Vitritis overlying scar*
- *Satellite lesion*
- *Surrounding perivascular sheathing*
- *Disc hyperemia*

I'd like to
- *Perform SLE (granulomatous or nongranulomatous uveitis, cataract)*
- *Examine fellow eye*

Frequent question: Would you treat this patient?

ARTHRITIS AND THE EYE

Overall yield: ✪✪✪✪ **Clinical exam:** ✪✪ **Viva:** ✪✪✪✪ **Essay:** ✪ **MCQ:** ✪✪✪✪

Q Opening Question: What Arthritic Diseases are Associated with Uveitis?

"There are three groups of arthritic conditions commonly associated with uveitis."

Spectrum of Arthritic Diseases Associated with Uveitis

1. **Spondyloarthropathies/seronegative arthritis**
   - Ankylosing spondylitis
   - Reiter's syndrome
   - Psoriatic arthritis
   - Inflammatory bowel disease
2. **Rheumatoid arthritis/juvenile rheumatoid arthritis/seropositive arthritis**
3. **Others**
   - Systemic lupus and other connective tissue diseases
   - Behcet's disease

> **Exam tips:**
> - See also connective tissue disease and the eye (page 342).

Q What are Spondyloarthropathies?

"Spondyloarthropathies or seronegative arthritis are a group of arthritic conditions."
"With **systemic** clinical features that involves the **axial skeleton** and **extraarticular features**."
"And characteristic uveitis with intense fibrinous reaction."

Spondyloarthropathy/Ankylosing Spondylitis

1. **Systemic features**
   - Men (peak 20–40 years)
   - Blood tests:
     - Rheumatic factor negative (therefore called seronegative)
     - ANA usually negative
     - HLA-B27 usually positive
   - Family history common
   - Arthropathy:
     - Axial skeleton inflammation:
       - Spinal pain worse at night and with rest, better with activity (compare this with mechanical spinal disorders — pain worse with activity)
     - Sacroiliitis:
       - Buttock pain alternating from one side to another
     - Extraarticular features
2. **Uveitis (note: Six features)**
   - Acute
   - Anterior
   - Unilateral, alternating
   - Nongranulomatous
   - Response to steroids
   - Recurrent

Exam tips:
- **These features are useful to remember because they apply to ankylosing spondylitis and most of the other spondyloarthropathies!**

Q **What is HLA-B27?**

"HLA stands for human leukocyte antigen."
"HLA-B27 refers to a specific antigen."
"Commonly found in the population...."

Important Facts About HLA-B27

1. **HLA (Human leukocyte antigen)**
   - Iso/allo antigen found on surface of cells
   - Differentiate one individual from another
   - Basis for graft rejection and blood transfusion reaction
   - Genotype found on **chromosome 6,** region called MHC (major histocompatibility complex)

2. **Prevalence of HLA-B27**
   - General population: 8%
   - Acute anterior uveitis: 45%
   - Psoriatic arthritis, inflammatory bowel disease: 60%
   - Reiter's syndrome: 75%
   - Ankylosing spondylitis: 85%
   - Ankylosing spondylitis and anterior uveitis: 95%

3. **Relative risk of AS with HLA-B27 = 90**

4. **What are the indications for HLA testing?**
   - To determine the cause of acute, unilateral, anterior uveitis (e.g. not useful in chronic, bilateral, posterior uveitis)
   - To exclude other diseases
   - To predict prognosis for recurrence
   - To predict risk of spondyloarthropathy

Common HLA Associations

HLA	Diseases	Relative risk (Normal person = 1)
HLA-A29	Birdshot retinochoroidopathy	97
HLA-B27	Ankylosing spondylitis	90
	Other spondyloarthropathies	10
HLA-B5	Behcet's syndrome	—
HLA-B7	Presumed ocular histoplasmosis syndrome	—
HLA-DR4	Juvenile DM Vogt-Koyanagi-Harada syndrome	—

Q **Tell me about Reiter's Syndrome.**

"Reiter's syndrome is a spondyloarthropathy or seronegative arthritis."
"With the characteristic **TRIAD** of urethritis, conjunctivitis and arthritis."
"The systemic clinical features are...."

Reiter's Syndrome

1. **Systemic features**
   - Young men
   - Blood tests:
     - Rheumatic factor negative (seronegative)
     - ANA usually negative
     - HLA-B27 usually positive
   - **Urethritis** or dysentery:
     - Nonspecific
     - Sterile

- Arthropathy
  - Acute **arthritis** (knees or ankles)
  - Extraarticular features:
    - Painless mouth ulcers (compare this with Behcet's disease, page 350)
    - Skin rash (keratoderma blennorrhagica)
    - Penile erosions (circinate balanitis)
    - Cardiovascular problems

2. **Ocular**
   - **Conjunctivitis:**
     - Bilateral papillary conjunctivitis
     - Sequence of events: Urethritis, followed by conjunctivitis and arthritis
   - Keratitis
   - Uveitis:
     - Acute anterior uveitis

Q Tell me about Psoriatic Arthritis.

"Psoriatic arthritis is a seronegative arthritis."
"With characteristic skin rash and ocular features."

Psoriatic Arthritis

1. **Systemic features**
   - Both sexes
   - Blood tests:
     - Rheumatic factor negative (seronegative)
     - ANA usually negative
     - HLA-B27 usually positive
   - Skin rash:
     - Chronic scaling and plaques, "red with silvery scales"
     - Bilateral but asymmetrical
   - Arthritis:
     - **10%** of psoriasis:
       - Hand joints
     - Extraarticular features:
       - Nail changes

2. **Ocular**
   - **10%** of those with psoriatic arthritis (i.e. only **1%** of all psoriasis patients will have eye signs)
   - Conjunctivitis, keratitis, uveitis

Q Tell me about Inflammatory Bowel Disease.

"Inflammatory bowel disease (IBD) is a systemic condition, classically divided into Crohn's disease and ulcerative colitis."
"With characteristic gastrointestinal features and ocular features."

Inflammatory Bowel Disease

1. **Systemic features**
   - Gastrointestinal:
     - Crohn's disease:
       - Whole gastrointestinal tract, especially **small bowels**
       - **Segmental**, skip lesions
       - **Transmural**
       - Risk of **perforation**
     - Ulcerative colitis (compare this with Crohn's colitis):
       - Rectum and colon
       - Continuous lesions
       - Confined to mucosa
       - Risk of **CA colon**
   - Arthritis:
     - Typical spondyloarthropathy features
   - Others:
     - Hepatobiliary complications
     - Skin rash
     - Renal complications

2. **Ocular**
   - Primary:
     - Uveitis in 10% (more common in **ulcerative colitis** than Crohn's disease)
     - Conjunctivitis, keratitis, scleritis
   - Secondary:
     - **Hypovitaminosis** (page 413)

Q What are the Different Gastrointestinal Diseases that have Prominent Ocular Manifestations?

"Gastrointestinal diseases are associated with a variety of ocular manifestations."

Gastrointestinal Diseases and the Eye

1. **Corneal complications**
   - Primary biliary cirrhosis and Wilson's disease
   - Kayser-Fleischer ring
   - Corneal arcus

2. **Uveitis**
   - IBD (Crohn's disease and ulcerative colitis)
   - Reiter's
   - Whipple's disease
3. **Retina complications**
   - Familial polyposis coli
     - Congenital hypertrophy of RPE (CHRPE)

- Pancreatitis
  - Purtscher's retinopathy
- Liver diseases, chronic diarrhoea
  - Vitamin A deficiency and night blindness

Q **Tell me about Juvenile Rheumatoid Arthritis.**

"Juvenile rheumatoid arthritis (JRA) is a systemic condition in children."
"It is classically divided into three types...."
"With characteristic systemic and ocular features in each type...."

	Systemic (Still's disease)	Polyarticular (five or more joints)	Pauciarticular (four or fewer joints) Late onset type	Pauciarticular Early onset type
Frequency	20%	40% (20% RF positive, 20% RF negative)	20%	20%
Salient features	**Systemic** disease (fever, rash, hepatosplenomegaly) Uveitis rare	Resembles **RA** in adults, main problem is severe arthritis	Resembles **ankylosing spondylitis**	Highest **uveitis** rate Uncommon systemic or arthritic complications
Demographics	More common in boys Early to late childhood	More common in girls Early to late childhood	More common in boys Late childhood	More common in girls Early childhood
Arthritis	Any joints	Any joints, but small joints frequent (hand, fingers)	Sacroiliac and hip joints	Large joints (knee, ankle, elbow)
Uveitis	Rare	Uncommon	Common (10–20%)	Very common (20–40%)
Rheumatoid factor (RF) and HLA-B27	Negative RF Negative HLA-B27 Negative ANA	50% positive **RF** Negative HLA-B27 50% positive ANA	Negative RF 75% positive **HLA-B27** Negative ANA	Negative RF Negative HLA-B27 75% positive ANA
Frequency of ophthalmic follow-up required	Yearly	6–9 monthly	4 months	3 months

Complications

- Complications are *frequent* but usually minimally symptomatic, hence need for regular follow-up:
- Glaucoma

- Band keratopathy
- Cataract
- CME

Exam tips:
- See also arthritis and eye (above), skin and eye (page 415), renal diseases and eye (page 210), cardiovascular diseases and eye (page 200), and cancer and the eye (page 360).

Exam tips:
- Risk of uveitis = pauciarticular, early onset and ANA positive JRA.

CONNECTIVE TISSUE DISEASES AND THE EYE

Overall yield: ✪✪✪   **Clinical exam:** ✪✪   **Viva:** ✪✪✪   **Essay:** ✪✪   **MCQ:** ✪✪✪✪

Q Opening Question: What are the Ocular Features of Rheumatoid Arthritis (RA)?

"Rheumatoid arthritis (RA) is a chronic inflammatory disease of the joints."
"The ocular manifestations can be divided into those affecting the anterior segment, those affecting the posterior segment, and those due to treatment."

Ocular Manifestations of Rheumatoid Arthritis

1. **Cornea**
   - **Keratoconjunctivitis sicca** (plus xerostomia = Sjogren's syndrome)
   - **Peripheral keratitis** (note: Most important ocular manifestation, 4 types, 2 central, 2 peripheral):
     - Sclerosing keratitis
     - Acute stromal keratitis
     - Peripheral corneal thinning
     - Peripheral corneal melting
   - Filamentary keratitis
   - Microbial keratitis

2. **Sclera**
   - Episcleritis and RA nodules
   - **Scleritis**

3. **Posterior segment and beyond**
   - Venous stasis retinopathy
   - CN palsies
   - Orbital apex syndrome
   - Abnormal EOG
   - Cortical blindness

4. **Treatment complications**
   - **Steroids, gold, chloroquine**

> **Exam tips:**
> - RA affects mainly the anterior segment (cornea and sclera).

Q What are the Systemic Effects of Rheumatoid Arthritis (RA)?

"RA is a chronic multisystem inflammatory disease."
"Characterized by symmetrical arthritis, synovial inflammation, cartilage and bone destruction."

Systemic Manifestations of RA

1. **Diagnosis (American Rheumatological Association criteria: Needs four out of the seven points below for diagnosis. 1–4 must last > six weeks)**
   - Arthritis of three or more joints: Soft tissue swelling and fluid observed by physician
   - Arthritis of hand joints (wrist, metacarpal (MCP) or proximal interphalangeal (PIP) joints)
   - Symmetrical swelling of same joint area (wrist, MCP, PIP)
   - Morning stiffness lasting > one hour before improvement

- Rheumatoid nodules
- Serum RF
- Radiographic features of RA

2. **Manifestations**
   - Arthritis:
     - Symmetrical inflammatory polyarthropathy
     - Wrist, metacarpophalangeal (MCP), proximal interphalangeal (PIP) joints affected
     - Sparing of distal interphalangeal (DIP) joints
     - Swan-neck deformity (hyperextension of PIP)
     - Boutonniere's sign (flexion deformity of PIP)
   - Skin/subcutaneous:
     - RA nodules
     - Vasculitis
   - Cardiovascular and respiratory:
     - Pleurisy and pleural effusion
     - Fibrosing alveolitis
   - Neurological:
     - Atlantoaxial subluxation
     - Peripheral neuropathy and mononeuritis multiplex
     - Entrapment neuropathies
   - Hematological:
     - Anemia
     - Neutropenia (plus splenomegaly and leg ulcers = Felty's syndrome),
   - Renal:
     - Amyloidosis

3. **Treatment**
   - Drugs:
     - NSAIDS
     - Steroids
     - Immunosuppressants
   - Physiotherapy, occupational therapy
   - Surgery

Q **What are the Ocular Features of Systemic Lupus Erythematosus?**

"Systemic lupus erythematosus is a **multisystem autoimmune disease**."
"Commonly affecting young women."
"Common systems involved include skin, blood vessels and CNS."
"Ocular features are most commonly seen in the posterior segment."

Ocular Manifestations of Systemic Lupus Erythematosus

1. **Post segment (note: Clinical features are nearly IDENTICAL to that in hypertensive retinopathy)**
   - Retinal hemorrhages
   - Cotton wool spots (because arterioles preferentially affected)
   - Hard exudate
   - Arteriolar narrowing
   - Venous engorgement
   - BRVO/BRAO/CRVO/CRAO
   - Disc edema

2. **Anterior segment**
   - Cornea — punctuate epithelial keratitis, keratoconjunctivitis sicca, peripheral ulceration
   - Sclera — episcleritis/scleritis
   - Anterior uveitis

3. **Neurological**
   - Sensory:
     - **Optic neuritis, anterior ischemic optic neuropathy**
     - Pupil abnormalities
     - Homonymous hemianopia
     - Cortical blindness
   - Motor:
     - Ptosis
     - Nystagmus
     - III & IV CN palsy
     - Gaze palsy
     - Inter-nuclear ophthalmoplegia

4. **Treatment (similar to RA)**

Exam tips:
- **Systemic lupus erythematosus affects mainly the posterior segment (compared to RA).**

Q **What are the Systemic Effects of Systemic Lupus Erythematosus?**

"Systemic lupus erythematosus is a multisystem autoimmune disease."
"Characterized by involvement of skin, joints, cardiovascular and neurological systems."

Systemic Manifestations of Systemic Lupus Erythematosus

1. **Diagnosis (4 or more of 11 features)**
   - Malar rash
   - Discoid rash
   - Photosensitivity
   - Mucosal ulcers
   - Arthritis
   - Serositis
   - Renal involvement
   - Neurological involvement
   - Hematological involvement
   - Anti-DNA antibodies, anti-Sm antibody
   - ANA

Q **What are the Ocular Features of Wegener's Granulomatosis?**

"Wegener's granulomatosis is a multisystem inflammatory disease of unknown etiology."
"The ocular manifestations can be divided into orbital, anterior segment, posterior segment, neurological and treatment related."

Ocular Manifestations of Wegener's Granulomatosis

1. **Orbit**
   - **Orbital inflammatory disease (pseudotumor)**
   - Sinusitis leading to orbital abscess
   - NLD obstruction

2. **Anterior segment**
   - Conjunctivitis
   - Episcleritis/**scleritis (necrotizing)**
   - Keratitis — peripheral ulceration
   - Uveitis

3. **Posterior segment**
   - Vasculitis (CRAO, BRAO, cotton wool spots)
   - Hypertensive retinopathy

4. **Neurological**
   - Anterior ischemic optic neuropathy
   - CN palsies

5. **Treatment**
   - **Immunosuppression (cyclophosphamide)**

Exam tips:
- **Wegener's granulomatosis affects mainly the orbit.**

Q **What are the Systemic Effects of Wegener's Granulomatosis?**

"Wegener's granulomatosis is a multisystem inflammatory disease of unknown etiology."
"With primary involvement of lungs, vessels and kidneys."

Systemic Manifestations of Wegener's Granulomatosis

1. **Diagnosis (classic diagnostic TRIAD)**
   - Respiratory tract (necrotizing granuloma of lungs)
   - Vasculitis
   - Nephritis

2. **Investigations (to investigate the classic diagnostic TRIAD)**
   - Respiratory tract (CXR)
   - Vasculitis (serum C-ANCA levels)
   - Nephritis (urine exam)

Q **What are the Features of Polyarteritis Nodosa (PAN)?**

"PAN is a multisystem vasculitis of unknown etiology."
"It mainly involves medium size and small vessels."
"There are both systemic involvement and ocular involvement."
"The systemic features include…."
"The ocular manifestations can be divided into…."

Ocular Manifestations of PAN

1. **Anterior segment**
   - Episcleritis/**scleritis**
   - Keratitis — peripheral ulceration
   - **Interstitial keratitis** (one of the few systemic causes of interstitial keratitis)

2. **Posterior segment**
   - **Vasculitis** (CRAO, BRAO, cotton wool spots)
   - Hypertensive retinopathy

3. **Neurological**
   - Anterior ischemic optic neuropathy
   - CN palsies

4. **Treatment**

Systemic Manifestations of PAN

1. **General features**
   - Nephritis
   - Cardiovascular (myocardial infarct)
   - Bowel infarction
   - Skin (vasculitic lesions)
   - Arthritis
   - Neurological (peripheral neuropathy)

> **Exam tips:**
> - If the question is "What are the features…?", do not forget to mention the systemic features FIRST.
> - PAN affects mainly the blood vessels.

 Q **What are the Features of Systemic Sclerosis?**

"Systemic sclerosis is a multisystem disease of unknown etiology."
"It mainly involves the **skin** and **blood vessels.**"
"There are both systemic involvement and ocular involvement."
"The systemic features include…."
"The ocular manifestations can be divided into…."

Ocular Manifestations of Systemic Sclerosis

1. **Lids**
   - Lagophthalmos
   - Punctal ectropion and epiphora
   - Linear scleroderma

2. **Anterior segment**
   - **Keratoconjunctivitis sicca**

3. **Posterior segment**
   - Hypertensive retinopathy

Systemic Manifestations of Systemic Sclerosis

1. **General features**
   - Skin:
     - Sclerodermatous skin changes, "bird-like" facies
     - Raynaud's phenomenon
     - Calcinosis
   - Sclerodactyl
   - Nailfold infarcts
   - Telangiectasia
   - Bowel (esophageal fibrosis)
   - Nephritis
   - Cardiovascular (serositis)
   - Respiratory (fibrosis)

2. **CREST syndrome (a more benign form of systemic sclerosis)**
   - Calcinosis
   - Raynaud's phenomenon
   - Esophageal
   - Sclerodactyl
   - Telangiectasia

> **Exam tips:**
> - Systemic sclerosis affects mainly the eyelids and skin.

SPECIFIC UVEITIS SYNDROMES I

Overall yield: ✪✪✪ **Clinical exam:** ✪✪ **Viva:** ✪✪✪ **Essay:** ✪✪ **MCQ:** ✪✪✪

Q **Opening Question:** What are the Clinical Features of Sarcoidosis?

"Sarcoidosis is an idiopathic systemic condition."
"Characterized pathologically by presence of noncaseating granuloma."
"Affecting the lungs and other organs."

Sarcoidosis

1. **Pathology**
   - **Noncaseating granuloma**
2. **Systemic features**
   - Acute presentation:
     - Young adult
     - Lung:
       - Stage 1: Bilateral hilar lymphadenopathy
       - Stage 2: Bilateral hilar lymphadenopathy and reticulo nodular parenchymal infiltrates
       - Stage 3: Reticulo nodular parenchymal infiltrates alone
       - Stage 4: Progressive pulmonary fibrosis
     - Erythema nodosum rash
     - Parotid enlargement:
       - Plus VII CN palsy and anterior uveitis = **Heerfordt's** syndrome
     - Acute unilateral nongranulomatous anterior uveitis
   - Insidious onset:
     - Older adult
     - Nonspecific (weight loss, fever)
     - Lung, skin, joints, CNS, CVS, renal involvement, hepatosplenomegaly and lymphadenopathy
     - Chronic bilateral granulomatous panuveitis
3. **Ocular features**
   - 30% of patients
   - Orbit and lids:
     - Granuloma

   - Lupus pernio (sarcoid rash near eyelid margin)
   - Anterior segment:
     - **Acute unilateral nongranulomatous anterior uveitis OR chronic bilateral granulomatous panuveitis**
   - Posterior segment:
     - Vitritis (snowballs)
     - Retinitis
     - Vasculitis ("candle wax" appearance, BRVO, neovascularization)
     - ON involvement
4. **Investigation (STEPWISE APPROACH, from noninvasive to invasive)**
   - Step 1:
     - CXR
     - Serum angiotensin-converting enzyme (ACE) levels (monocytes secretes ACE in sarcoidosis)
     - Serum and urinary calcium levels
   - Step 2:
     - Chest CT or MRI
     - Gallium scan of head, neck and chest
     - Lung function tests
   - Step 3:
     - Lung and lymph node biopsy
     - Lacrimal gland and conjunctival biopsy
   - Step 4:
     - Bronchoalveolar lavage

Notes

- "What is a noncaseating granuloma?"
- Consists of:
- Epitheloid cells (derived from monocytes, macrophages)
- Giant cells (Langhans type):
  - Schaumann's body; cytoplasmic inclusion
  - Asteroid inclusion body (acidophilic, star-shaped)

Q **What is Fuch's Uveitis Syndrome? How is it Different from Posner-Schlossman Syndrome?**

"Fuch's uveitis is a common idiopathic uveitis with distinct clinical features."
"Posner-Schlossman syndrome is also an idiopathic uveitis characterized by recurrent attacks of glaucoma."
"There are several features which help distinguish the two conditions."
"The role of infectious agents, particularly rubella, toxoplasmosis, and CMV, in the pathogenesis of these forms of uveitis is currently under investigation."

	Fuch's uveitis	Posner-Schlossman syndrome
Age and sex	• Middle age to elderly • Females more common	• Young to middle age • Males
Presentation	• Asymptomatic, sometimes with blurring of vision	• Acute blurring of vision and halos • Acute pain
Keratic precipitates:	• Diffuse • Well-defined • Small, stellate-shaped • White-gray in color	• Inferior half of corneal endothelium • May be confluent • Larger • Colorless • May disappear with steroid treatment
IOP	• Mid-20s	• High 30–40s

Other features	• AC activity mild
	• Iris:
	  • Heterochromia iridis
	  • Iris atrophy (moth-eaten pattern at pupil border)
	  • Iris nodules
	  • No posterior or peripheral anterior synechiae
	  • Rubeosis (fine): Amsler's sign — acute hyphema following ocular decompression such as paracentesis
	• Cataract
	• Retina:
	  • Pigmentation/scarring (hence possible role for rubella/toxoplasmosis)
	  • No CME
	• Glaucoma (chronic POAG):
	  • Common (40%) and important cause of visual loss in FHI
	• Gonioscopy:
	  • Rubeosis
	  • Bleeding 180° opposite site of AC paracentesis (Amsler's sign)
		• Very similar to Fuch's uveitis
		• Less iris atrophy and heterochromia
		• Long term risk of glaucoma up to 40%

Clinical approach to Fuch's heterochromic uveitis

"On examination of this patient's anterior segment…."
"There are gray white keratic precipitates scattered diffusely throughout the endothelium."
"The keratic precipitates are well-defined, small, stellate-shaped and nonconfluent in nature."

Look for
- Cornea (should be clear)
- AC activity (mild)
- Iris:
  - Iris atrophy (moth eaten pattern at pupil border)
  - No posterior or peripheral anterior synechiae
  - Pupil is dilated but reactive
  - Rubeosis
- Cataract
- Fellow eye iris:
  - Affected eye's iris is hypochromia

I'll like to
- Check IOP
- Perform gonioscopy (rubeosis)

Exam tips:
- **Do not confuse Fuch's uveitis with Fuch's endothelial dystrophy (page 113).**
- **The comparison between Fuch's uveitis and Posner-Schlossman syndrome is clinically important because it is often difficult to tell the two apart in daily practice.**

Q **What are the Causes of Iris Heterochromia?**

"Iris hypochromia or iris hyperchromia can be either congenital or acquired."

	Congenital	Acquired
Hypochromia	• **Congenital Horner's syndrome** • Waardenburg's syndrome • Hirschsprung's disease • Facial hemiatrophy (Parry-Romberg syndrome)	• **Uveitis** (Fuch's, Posner-Schlossman, HZV, HSV, leprosy) • **Glaucoma** (pseudoexfoliation, pigmentary dispersion, post angle closure glaucoma) • Post trauma/surgery • Juvenile xanthogranuloma
Hyperchromia	• **Oculodermal/ocular melanosis** • Sector iris pigment epithelial harmatoma	• **Uveitis** (Fuch's) • **Glaucoma** (pigmentary dispersion) • **Iridocorneal endothelial syndrome (ICE)** • Diffuse pigmentation (siderosis, argyrosis, chalosis, hemosiderosis) • Iris tumors (nevus, melanomas)

SPECIFIC UVEITIS SYNDROMES II

Overall yield: ✴✴✴   **Clinical exam:** ✴   **Viva:** ✴✴   **Essay:** ✴✴   **MCQ:** ✴✴✴

Q Opening Question: What is Behcet's Disease?

"Behcet's disease is an idiopathic multisystem disorder."
"With characteristic, systemic clinical features and uveitis."

Behcet's Disease

1. **Pathology**
   - Associated with **HLA-B5**
   - Obliterative vasculitis with fibrinoid degeneration
   - **Type III** hypersensitivity

2. **Systemic features**
   - Young men of Japanese, Asian or Mediterranean origin
   - Diagnostic criteria (**five features**: Oral ulceration plus any two of the other four, International Study Group for Behcet's)
     - Oral ulceration:
       - Painful and recurrent
       - At least three times in last one year
       - 99% of cases
     - Genital ulceration

   - Skin lesions:
     - Erythema nodosum
     - Papular, pustular or nodular rash
   - Positive pathergy test (page 325)
   - Eye lesions
   - Other systemic features (**NOT** part of diagnostic criteria):
     - Arthritis
     - Thrombophlebitis
     - Gastrointestinal lesions
     - Cardiovascular involvement (myocardial infarct)
     - CNS involvement (stroke)

3. **Ocular features**
   - 70% of patients
   - Severe bilateral nongranulomatous panuveitis (iritis, retinitis, vitritis, **vasculitis**)

Q Tell me about Vogt-Koyanagi-Harada Syndrome.

"Vogt-Koyanagi-Harada syndrome is an idiopathic multisystem disorder."
"With characteristic systemic clinical features and uveitis."

Vogt-Koyanagi-Harada Syndrome

1. **Men of Japanese or Oriental origin**

2. **Systemic features**
   - **Triad** of:
     - Skin lesions, **triad** of:
       - Alopecia
       - Poliosis
       - Vitiligo

   - CNS lesions, **triad** of:
     - Encephalopathy
     - Meningeal irritation
     - CSF pleocytosis
   - Auditory symptoms, **triad** of:
     - Vertigo
     - Tinnitus
     - Deafness

3. **Uveitis**
- Bilateral granulomatous panuveitis
- Acute, **triad** of "**D**"s:
  - **D**etachment of retina (multifocal choroiditis and exudative RD)
  - **D**isc swelling
  - **D**alen-Fuchs nodules (inflammatory cells in RPE and Bruch's membrane)
- Chronic, **triad** of "**P**"s:
  - **P**igmentary changes and scarring ("pseudo" retinitis pigmentosa)
  - **P**eripapillary atrophy
  - **P**igment epithelial atrophy (sunset glow fundus)

4. **Imaging features**
- B-scan: Choroidal thickening
- FFA: Starry sky pattern, diffuse choroidal leakage, exudative RD
- ICG: Hypofluorescent dark areas

Diagnostic criteria formulated by Read *et al*. Revised diagnostic criteria or VKH disease: A Report of an International Committee on Nomenclature. *Am J Ophthalmol* 2001;131:647–652.

Diagnostic Criteria for Vogt-Koyanagi-Harada Disease

Complete Vogt-Koyanagi-Harada disease (criteria 1 to 5 must be present)
- No history of penetrating ocular trauma or surgery preceding the initial onset of uveitis
- No clinical or laboratory evidence suggestive of other ocular disease entities
- Bilateral ocular involvement (a or b must be met, depending on the stage of disease when the patient is examined)
  - Early manifestations of disease
- There must be evidence of a diffuse choroiditis (with or without anterior uveitis, vitreous inflammatory reaction, or optic disk hyperemia), which may manifest as one of the following:
  - Focal areas of subretinal fluid, or
  - Bullous serous retinal detachments
- With equivocal fundus findings; both of the following must be present as well
  - Focal areas of delay in choroidal perfusionv, multifocal areas of pinpoint leakage, large placoid areas of hyperfluorescence, pooling within subretinal fluid, and optic nerve staining (listed in order of sequential appearance) by fluorescein angiography, and
  - Diffuse choroidal thickening, without evidence of posterior scleritis by ultrasonography
- Late manifestations of disease
- History suggestive of prior presence of findings from 3a, and either both (2) and (3) below, or multiple signs from (3):
  - Ocular depigmentation (either of the following manifestations is sufficient):
  - Sunset glow fundus, or
  - Sugiura sign
- Other ocular signs:
  - Nummular chorioretinal depigmented scars, or
  - Retinal pigment epithelium clumping and/or migration, or
  - Recurrent or chronic anterior uveitis
- Neurological/auditory findings (may have resolved by time of examination)
  - Meningismus (malaise, fever, headache, nausea, abdominal pain, stiffness of the neck and back, or a combination of these factors;
    headache alone is not sufficient to meet definition of meningismus, however), or
  - Tinnitus, or
  - Cerebrospinal fluid pleocytosis
- Integumentary finding (*not* preceding onset of central nervous system or ocular disease)
  - Alopecia, or
  - Poliosis, or
  - Vitiligo

Incomplete Vogt-Koyanagi-Harada disease (criteria 1 to 3 and either 4 or 5 must be present):
- No history of penetrating ocular trauma or surgery preceding the initial onset of uveitis, and
- No clinical or laboratory evidence suggestive of other ocular disease entities, and
- Bilateral ocular involvement
- Neurologic/auditory findings; as defined for complete Vogt-Koyanagi-Harada disease above, or
- Integumentary findings; as defined for complete Vogt-Koyanagi-Harada disease above.

(Continued)

Probable Vogt-Koyanagi-Harada disease (isolated ocular disease; criteria 1 to 3 must be present):
- No history of penetrating ocular trauma or surgery preceding the initial onset of uveitis
- No clinical or laboratory evidence suggestive of other ocular disease entities
- Bilateral ocular involvement as defined for complete Vogt-Koyanagi-Harada disease above

Clinical approach to Vogt-Koyanagi-Harada's disease

"On examination of this patient's fundus, there are areas of atrophy and pigmentation seen."

Look for
- *Vitritis*
- *Disc hyperemia*
- *Peripapillary atrophy*
- *Multifocal areas of exudative RD*
- *Dalen-Fuchs nodules*
- *Pigmentary changes in periphery*
- *Sunset glow fundus*
- *Skin: Alopecia, vitiligo, poliosis, perilimbal vitiligo*

I'll like to
- *Check the anterior segment (granulomatous uveitis, cataract)*
- *Check IOP*
- *Examine fellow eye*
- *Ask for history of vertigo, tinnitus, deafness*
- *Examine patient neurologically*

Exam tips:
- **Remember the different "TRIADS."**
- **VKH may be subdivided into: Vogt-Koyanagi's syndrome (anterior uveitis and skin lesions) and Harada's syndrome (posterior uveitis and CNS lesions).**

Q **What are the Clinical Features of Sympathetic Ophthalmia? How does it Differ from VKH?**

"Sympathetic ophthalmia is a rare granulomatous panuveitis."
"With characteristic clinical features."

Sympathetic Ophthalmia

1. **Exciting eye: Penetrating injury or intraocular surgery**
2. **Sympathizing eye: Fellow eye**
3. **Clinical features**
   - Onset: Two weeks to one year after initial event
   - Earliest symptom: Decreased accommodation (ciliary body involvement)
   - Earliest sign: Retrolental cells
   - Bilateral granulomatous panuveitis

- Acute, **triad** of "D"s:
  - **D**etachment of retina (multifocal choroiditis and exudative RD)
  - **D**isc swelling
  - **D**alen-Fuch's nodules (inflammatory cells in RPE and Bruch's membrane)
- Chronic, **triad** of "P"s:
  - **P**igmentary changes and scarring ("pseudo" retinitis pigmentosa)
  - **P**eripapillary atrophy
  - **P**igment epithelial atrophy (sunset glow fundus)

	VKH	Sympathetic ophthalmia
Demographics	• 20–50 years • Asians and blacks	• Younger • No racial preference
History of trauma or surgery	• Uncommon	• Common
Clinical features	• Skin changes • CNS changes • Hearing changes	• Uncommon • Uncommon • Uncommon
Pathological features	• Involvement of choriocapillaris	• **Choriocapillaris spared** ("sympathize" with choriocapillaris)

Exam tips:
- **Usually compared closely with VKH because the ocular features are IDENTICAL.**

Q **What is Intermediate Uveitis?**

"Intermediate uveitis is an uncommon idiopathic uveitis."
"With characteristic clinical features."

Intermediate Uveitis

1. **Classification**
   - Primary
   - Secondary:
     - Sarcoidosis
     - Retinitis pigmentosa
     - Multiple sclerosis
     - TB, syphilis, Lyme's disease, toxocara

2. **Clinical features of idiopathic type**
   - Young adult
   - Bilateral involvement
   - Quiet anterior segment and no primary posterior pole involvement (note: Uveitis is "intermediate")
   - Vitritis with snowballs and snowbanking
   - Periphlebitis anterior to equator
   - Two spectrums:
     - Pars planitis: Snowbanking prominent
     - Cyclitis: No snowbanking
   - Complications:
     - Secondary anterior segment involvement (cataract)
     - Secondary posterior pole involvement (cystoid macula edema, RD)

"The white dot syndromes are a group of idiopathic posterior uveitis."
"They have overlapping clinical features."

	APMPPE	MEWDS	PIC	Multifocal choroiditis	Birdshot	Serpiginous
Age	• Young	• Young	• Young	• Young	• Middle age	• Middle age
Sex preference	• None	• Females	• Females	• Females	• Females	• None
Clinical features	• Bilateral • Subacute • **Flu-like illness** • Creamy lesions	• Unilateral • Acute • **Flu-like illness** • Tiny granular lesions • **Enlarged blind spot**	• **No vitritis/ anterior uveitis** • **Myopia** common • Small lesions	• **Severe vitritis/ anterior uveitis**	• Bilateral • Chronic • Indistinct lesions half disc diameter • Radiate from disc • **HLA-B29 (99%)**	• Bilateral • Chronic • Amoeboid "punched out" lesions • Radiate from disc

- APMPPE: Acute posterior multifocal placoid pigment epitheliopathy
- MEWDS: Multiple evanescent white dot syndrome
- PIC: Punctate inner choroidopathy
- Multifocal choroiditis: Multifocal choroiditis with panuveitis
- Birdshot: Birdshot retinochoroidopathy
- Serpiginous: Serpiginous choroidopathy

Exam tips:
- **One of the most difficult topics to remember in ophthalmology!**
- **The first step is to compare and contrast the syndromes in groups of two: APMPPE and MEWDS, PIC with multifocal choroiditis and birdshot with serpiginous. The first four occur in young adults, the last two in middle-aged adults.**
- **The next step is to identify the salient associations in each.**

ANTERIOR SEGMENT TUMORS

Overall yield: ✸✸✸ **Clinical exam:** ✸✸✸ **Viva:** ✸✸✸ **Essay:** ✸✸ **MCQ:** ✸✸✸

Q **Opening Question:** What are the Possible Diagnoses of a Pigmented Conjunctival Lesion?

"Possible differential diagnoses include...."

	Racial melanosis	Oculodermal melanosis	Nevus	PAM	Malignant melanoma
Age of onset and race	• Child • Pigmented races	• Young adult • Pigmented race	• Young adult • White	• Middle-aged • White	• Middle-aged • White
Laterality	• Bilateral	• Unilateral	• Unilateral	• Unilateral	• Unilateral
Clinical features	• **Limbal and interpalpebral region** • **Epithelial** • Static	• **Subepithelial (sclera or episclera)** • Adjacent dermal pigmentation (nevus of **Ota**)	• Bulbar conjunctiva • Sharply demarcated • **Inclusion cysts**	• Multifocal • Any part of conjunctiva • No cysts • **"Wax and wane"** in appearance	• Pigmented nodule • Can be non-pigmented • **Limbus** • Fixed to underlying • Spontaneous bleeding
Other associations	• None	• Dermal pigmentation on shoulder blades (nevus of **Ito**) • **Uveal melanoma** • **No** risk of conjunctival melanoma • Risk of **glaucoma**	• High risk of **conjunctival melanoma** (palpebral and fonix nevus, nevus straddling cornea, enlarging nevus)	• High risk of **conjunctival melanoma** (50% risk if biopsy shows atypia)	• Arise from PAM (50%), nevus (25%) and de novo (25%)

(Continued)

	Racial melanosis	Oculodermal melanosis	Nevus	PAM	Malignant melanoma
Treatment	• None	• Follow-up for melanoma • Manage **glaucoma**	• Local excision with bare sclera	• Local excisional biopsy and cryotherapy to sclera	• Wide margin local excision • Lamellar kerato-sclerectomy with lamellar keratoplasty • Cryotherapy • Topical MMC • Exenteration and chemotherapy

PAM: Primary acquired melanosis

Clinical approach to nevus of Ota

"There is an area of subepithelial melanosis...."
"Associated with pigmentation of the lids and face."
"In the distribution of the first and second divisions of the trigeminal nerve."

Look for
• *Proptosis (orbital melanoma)*
• *Iris pigmentation/melanosis/melanoma*
• *Lens subluxation (ciliary body melanoma)*
• *Trabeculectomy (glaucoma operation)*
• *Optic disc (cupping)*

I'd like to
• *Check IOP, gonioscopy (angle pigmentation)*
• *Examine the fundus for choroidal melanoma*
• *Examine patient's back for nevus of Ito*

Exam tips:
• **Fairly common clinical examination case.**

Q **What are the Differential Diagnoses of Iris Nodules?**

"The main causes can be divided into tumors and non-tumor lesions...."

Iris Nodule

1. **Tumors**
   • Benign:
     • Iris nevus
     • Iridocorneal endothelial syndrome (ICE)
     • Oculodermal melanosis (nevus of Ota)
   • Malignant:
     • Primary:
       · Maligant melanoma
       · Leiomyoma
       · Leukemia
     • Secondary

2. Non-tumor conditions

- Infection/inflammation:
  - Granulomatous uveitis (Koeppe and Busacca nodules)
  - Fungal endophthalmitis
- Trauma:
  - Inclusion cyst
  - Retained IOFB
- Developmental:
  - Neurofibromatosis (Lisch's nodule)

- What is the histology? Nevus cells
- Down's syndrome (Brushfield spots)
  - What is the histology? Areas of normal stroma surrounded by ring of hypoplasia
- Juvenile xanthogranuloma
  - What is the histology? Granulomatous lesion with lipid filled histiocytes and Touton giant cells

---

 Clinical approach to iris nodule

"This patient has a pigmented iris nodule at the 9 o'clock position."
"Measuring about 2 mm in size."

Look for

- _New vessels, pupil distortion, ectropian uvea, lens opacity (melanoma)_
- _Keratic precipitates and AC cells (Koeppe or Busccada nodules)_
- _Iris atrophy (ICE syndrome)_
- _Conjunctival subepithelial melanosis (nevus of Ota)_
- _Systemic features (neurofibromatosis, Down's syndrome)_

I'll like to

- _Check IOP (ICE syndrome, melanoma) and perform gonioscopy_
- _Ask for a history of trauma (traumatic inclusion cyst) and use of pilocarpine (iris cyst)_
- _Examine patient systemically (neurofibromatosis)_

Exam tips:
- **The suggestive features of malignant melanoma can be remembered by the mnemonic "RIPPLE."**

Notes
- "What are the suggestive features of malignancy?"
  - **R**ubeosis
  - **I**OP increase
  - **P**upil distortion
  - **Ph**otograph documentation of growth
  - **L**ens opacity
  - **E**ctropian uvea

Q Tell me about Tumors of the Ciliary Body.

"The most important ciliary body tumor is ciliary body melanoma."
"Other tumors can be divided into tumors arising from either the pigmented and nonpigmented epithelium."

Tumors of the Ciliary Body

1. **Ciliary body melanoma**
   - 15% of uveal melanomas
   - Anterior segment signs:
     - Dilated episcleral vessels ("sentinel vessels")
     - Cataract and subluxed lens
     - Uveitis
     - Glaucoma
   - Posterior segment signs:
     - Retinal detachment

2. **Tumors of ciliary epithelium**
   - Arising from pigmented epithelium:
     - Benign adenoma
     - Hyperplasia
   - Arising from nonpigmented epithelium:
     - Congenital
       - **Medulloepithelioma:**

   - Present in childhood
   - Clinical presentation: Ciliary body mass, raised IOP, subluxed lens and cataract
   - May be mistaken for retinoblastoma
   - Histology: Flexner-Wintersteiner and Homer Wright rosettes can be seen
     - Glioneuroma (rare)
   - Acquired:
     - Fuchs' adenoma (pseudoadenomatous hyperplasia) (rare)
     - Benign adenoma (rare)
     - Adenocarcinoma (rare)

3. **Others**
   - Leiomyoma
   - Hemangioma

Exam tips:
- **Remember only ciliary body melanoma and medulloepithelioma. The others are extremely rare.**

TOPIC 10

POSTERIOR SEGMENT TUMORS

Overall yield: ✸✸✸   **Clinical exam:** ✸   **Viva:** ✸✸✸✸   **Essay:** ✸✸   **MCQ:** ✸✸✸✸

Q   Opening Question: What are the Possible Diagnoses of a Choroidal Mass?

"Possible causes include tumors and non-tumor lesions."

Choroidal Mass

1. Tumors
- Choroidal melanoma
- Secondaries:
  - Bilateral, history of malignancy elsewhere
- Choroidal nevus:
  - Unilateral, flat, drusens located within lesion
- Choroidal hemangioma:
  - High internal reflectivity on B-scan
- Congenital hypertrophy of RPE:
  - Flat, lacunae located within lesion
- Melanocytoma of optic disc:
  - Jet black lesion at optic disc

2. Non-tumor lesions
- Choroidal and retinal detachment
- AMD with disciform scar:
  - Bilateral, drusens in both eyes, FFA diagnostic
- Exudative maculopathy:
  - FFA useful
- Posterior scleritis:
  - Anterior segment signs, systemic history, FFA useful

> **Exam tips:**
> - **See also retinoblastoma (page 395).**

Q   What are the Causes of Choroidal Folds?

"Possible causes include extrinsic compression, intramural lesions, ocular hypotony and idiopathic choroidal folds."

Choroidal Folds

Mechanisms	Etiology
Extrinsic compression	• Tumors (intraconal/extraconal) • Thyroid eye disease and pseudotumor • Retinal detachment surgery (scleral buckle)

(Continued)

Section 8: Uveitis, Systemic Diseases and Tumors   431

Mechanisms	Etiology
Intramural	• Choroidal tumors • Uveal effusion syndrome • Posterior scleritis • Optic nerve disorders (optic neuritis, tumors) • Chorioretinal scars
Intraocular (ocular hypotony)	• Post traumatic (rupture, cyclodialysis) • Post surgical (trabeculectomy, wound leak) • Uveitis
Idiopathic	• Usually in hypermetropic males with good VA • Spontaneous resolution

Q | **What are the Clinical Features of Choroidal Melanoma?**

"Choroidal melanoma is the most common primary intraocular malignant tumor in adults."
"They present with a variety of clinical features and are sometimes difficult to diagnose."

Clinical Features of Choroidal Melanoma

1. **Risk factors**
   - White race (rare in blacks and pigmented race)
   - Oculodermal melanosis (nevus of Ota)
   - Neurofibromatosis
   - Nevus

2. **Clinical features**
   - Age 50–60 years
   - Choroidal melanoma (**IDENTICAL** to pathological features, see below):
     - Pigmented or nonpigmented mass
     - Break through Bruch's membrane (mushroom-shaped)
     - Secondary exudative RD
     - Orange pigment within lesion (lipofuscin)
     - Choroidal folds
   - Anterior segment signs:
     - Uveitis (masquerade syndrome)

   - Cataract
   - Glaucoma
   - Systemic metastasis:
     - Liver (most common)
     - Lung (second most common)

3. **Investigation**
   - Diagnosis
     - B-scan
     - FFA
     - CT scan:
       - Extraocular extension
     - MRI:
       - Hyperintense to vitreous (T1 weighted film)
       - Hypointense to vitreous (T2 weighted film)
     - Phosphorus-32 uptake (differentiate from hemangioma)
     - Intraocular fine needle biopsy

Notes
- "What are the features of the nevus that suggest malignant transformation?"
  - Presence of lipofuscin within the nevus (instead of drusens)
  - Location near the optic disc
  - More than 2 mm thick
  - Associated with retinal complications (e.g. RD)

Notes
- "What are the mechanisms of glaucoma?"
  - Direct invasion of angles
  - Release of pigments clogging the trabecular meshwork
  - Rubeosis at the angles

Q What are the Pathological Features of Choroidal Melanoma?

"The pathology of choroidal melanoma can be described in terms of gross pathology and histopathology."

Pathology of Choroidal Melanoma

1. **Gross pathology**
   - Pigmented or nonpigmented mass
   - Breaks through Bruch's membrane (mushroom-shaped)
   - Secondary exudative RD
   - Orange pigment within lesion (lipofuscin)
   - Choroidal folds

2. **Histopathology**
   - Callender classification
     - Spindle A:
       - Cigar-shaped
       - Slender nuclei with basophilic line
       - No nucleolus
     - Spindle B:
       - Oval-shaped, larger
       - Oval nuclei
       - Prominent nucleolus
       - Syncytium
     - Epitheloid:
       - Large oval or round
         - Round nuclei
         - Prominent nucleolus
         - Polymorphism, varied pigmentation, mitotic figures
     - Mixed:
       - Combination
   - Modified Callender classification:
     - Spindle cell nevus = Spindle cell A (15-year mortality: < 5%)
     - Spindle cell melanoma = Spindle cell B (15-year mortality: 25%)
     - Epithelioid (15-year mortality: 75%)
     - Mixed (15-year mortality: 50%)
   - ISDNA classification (inverse of standard deviation of nucleoli area):
     - Newer classification using pleomorphism of cells as a guide
     - More objective quantification of risk

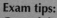

Exam tips:
- **One of the most common pathology questions in the exams. The gross pathology is IDENTICAL to the clinical features of the melanoma itself (see above).**

"The treatment is still being evaluated and should be individualized to the patient."
"The factors to consider are…."
"The options include…."

Treatment of Choroidal Melanoma

1. **Factors to consider**
   - VA of involved eye and fellow eye
   - Size, location and extent of tumor
   - Presence of metastasis
   - General health and age of patient

2. **General principles**
   - Large tumor (larger than 15 mm diameter and 5 mm thickness)
     - Enucleation
       - Indicated especially if:
         - Eye has poor visual prognosis
         - Tumor has extended to the anterior segment
         - No systemic metastasis is detected
         - Patient is of good general health
       - Pre-enucleation radiotherapy affords no additional benefit (COMS)
       - Bimodal incidence of death, initially at 2 years and later at 10 years
   - Small tumor (less than 10 mm diameter and 3 mm thickness)
     - Laser photocoagulation
       - Indicated especially if:
         - Eye has good visual potential
         - Tumor is situated away from the fovea
         - No systemic metastasis is detected
         - No subretinal fluid
     - Plaque radiotherapy may be considered
     - Close observation for growth before initiating treatment can be considered, especially if tumor is in less favorable location (macula, peripapillary) — small tumor arm of COMS showed slow progression without excess mortality with observation
   - Medium-sized tumor (between 10–15 mm diameter and 3–5 mm thickness)
     - Most **controversial**
     - Plaque radiotherapy vs enucleation (this is the primary objective of COMS):
       - Latest data suggests no difference in survival
       - Plaque radiotherapy saves eye **but** does not preserve vision

3. **Other treatment options**
   - Partial lamellar sclerectomy (for anterior tumors)
   - Exenteration
   - Chemotherapy
   - Radiotherapy

Exam tips:
- **Read the latest from COMS (Collaborative Ocular Melanoma Study) http://www.jhu.edu/wctb/coms/in.**

Notes
- "What is the Zimmerman hypothesis?"
  - Early peak in mortality due to increased metastasis after enucleation in the first two years of treatment

"Systemic malignancies can affect the eye in one of four ways...."

Systemic Malignancies and the Eye

1. **Spread to the eye**
   - Orbit (fairly common)
   - Iris (rare)
   - Choroid (most common):
     - 10 times more common than orbit
     - Primary tumor:
       - Breast CA in women (patient usually provides **previous** history of breast CA)
       - Lung CA in men (patient usually have **no** history of lung CA)
     - Clinical features:
       - Posterior pole (most common site)
       - Bilateral and multiple
       - Poorly defined borders
       - Not elevated or pigmented

2. **Spread to the CNS**
   - Papilledema and other neuroophthalmic features (page 262)

3. **PARANEOPLASTIC syndrome (Cancer Associated Retinopathy (CAR))**
   - Usually associated with lung CA (**small** cell CA)
   - Rapid loss of VA
   - Normal looking fundus (there may be slight narrowing of arterioles)
   - Severely reduced ERG
   - High serum levels of a particular 23 kD antibody (specific for a protein similar to recovering)

4. **Complications from TREATMENT**
   - Chemotherapy drugs

Q Tell me about the Combined Hamartoma of Retinal and RPE.

"The combined hamartoma of retinal and the RPE has distinct clinical features...."

Combined Hamartoma of Retinal and RPE

1. **Clinical features**
   - Males
   - Childhood
   - Hamartoma
     - Mossy gray-green lesion
     - Epiretinal membrane over hamartoma with subsequent fibrosis
     - Vessel tortuosity

2. **Associations**
   - Differential diagnoses for **retinoblastoma** (page 401)
   - Differential diagnoses for **dragged disc** (page 332)
   - Associated with **neurofibromatosis type II** (page 273)

Exam tips:
- **There are three significant ocular associations.**

IMMUNOSUPPRESSIVE THERAPY, STEROIDS AND ATROPINE

Overall yield: ✸✸✸ **Clinical exam:** **Viva:** ✸✸✸ **Essay:** ✸ **MCQ:** ✸✸

Q **Opening Question No. 1:** Tell me about the Types of Immunosuppressive Therapy.

"Immunosuppressive therapy can be classified into four different groups…."

Classification of Immunosuppressive Therapy

1. **Hormones**
   - **Steroids** (see below)
2. **Alkylating agents**
   - **Cyclophosphamide:**
     - Nitrogen mustard derivative
     - Reacts with guanine forming DNA cross-linkages — non cell cycle specific
     - Drug of choice for Wegener's granulomatosis, Mooren's ulcer and ocular cicatricial pemphigoid
3. **Antimetabolites — target DNA production and hence cell-cycle-specific**
   - **Folate** antagonists — methotrexate:
     - Folate analogue
     - Inhibits conversion of folate into tetrahydrofolate
   - **Purine** analogues — azathioprine:
     - Activited to 6-mercaptopurine
     - Incorporated into DNA causing false protein coding

   - Drug of choice for thyroid eye disease
   - **Pyrimidine** analogues — 5 fluorouracil (5FU):
     - See section on glaucoma (page 84)
   - Mycophenolic acid — mycophenolate mofetil:
     - Metabolized to mycophenolic acid
     - Inhibitor of inosine monophosphate dehydrogenase (involved in guanine synthesis)
4. **Natural products**
   - T-cell specific immunosuppressive agent — **cyclosporin:**
     - Fungal product
     - Modulates T-cell function
   - **Antibiotics** — mitomycin C (MMC):
     - See section on glaucoma (page 84)

"Immunosuppressive therapy is useful in ophthalmology in two broad categories...."

Indications of Immunosuppressive Therapy

1. **Inflammatory/immune diseases**
   - Cornea
     - Peripheral ulcerative keratitis:
       - Mooren's ulcer
       - Rheumatoid arthritis, systemic lupus, Wegener's granulomatosis, polyarteritis nodosa
     - Ocular surface diseases (ocular cicatricial pemphigoid, Stevens-Johnson syndrome)
   - Scleritis
   - Uveitis
     - Behcet's disease
     - Pars planitis
   - Vogt-Koyanagi-Harada
   - Sympathetic ophthalmia
   - Sarcoidosis
   - Orbit:
     - Thyroid eye disease
     - Inflammatory orbital disease (pseudotumor)
   - Retinitis/vasculitis
   - Optic neuritis

2. **Adjunctive to eye operations**
   - High risk penetrating keratoplasty
   - High risk glaucoma surgery

Q **What are the Complications of Immunosuppressive Therapy?**

"The complications can be divided into general complications and those specific to certain agents...."

Complications of Immunosuppressive Agents

1. **General**
   - Bone marrow suppression
   - Increased infection
   - Alopecia
   - Carcinogenesis (skin, lymphoma)

2. **Specific**
   - Cyclosporin and cyclophosphamide group:
     - Renal toxicity (cyclosporin)
     - Hemorrhagic cystitis (cyclophosphamide)
     - Hirsutism, gingivitis (cyclosporin)
   - Azathioprine and methotrexate group:
     - Hepatotoxicity (azathioprine, methotrexate, cyclosporin)
     - Gastrointestinal disturbance (azathioprine, methotrexate)
     - Azoospermia (azathioprine)
     - Rash/fever (azathioprine, methotrexate)

Q **Opening Question No. 3:** What are the Indications for Steroid Therapy in Ophthalmology?

"Steroid therapy is used in ophthalmology either via a topical, periocular or systemic route."
"Topical therapy are used for two broad categories of diseases...."

Indications of Steroid Therapy

1. **Topical**
   - **Inflammatory/immune diseases:**
     - Conjunctival diseases:
       - Atopic/allergic conjunctivitis
     - Cornea:
       - Marginal keratitis and other peripheral ulcerative keratitis
       - Specific keratitis (nummular keratitis, Thygeson's keratitis, interstitial keratitis, HSV stromal necrosis)
     - Ocular surface diseases (ocular cicatricial pemphigoid, Stevens-Johnson syndrome)
     - Scleritis
     - Uveitis
     - Glaucoma:
       - Acute angle closure glaucoma
   - **Adjunctive to eye operations**
     - Cataract and other intraocular surgeries (trabeculectomy, etc)

- Post-refractive surgery

2. **Periocular**
   - Cataract and other intraocular surgeries (trabeculectomy, etc)
   - Post-refractive surgery

3. **Systemic**
   - **Inflammatory/immune diseases:**
     - Cornea:
       - Peripheral ulcerative keratitis
       - Ocular surface diseases (ocular cicatricial pemphigoid, Stevens-Johnson syndrome)
       - Graft failure
     - Scleritis
     - Uveitis:
       - Behcet's disease
       - Pars planitis
       - Vogt-Koyanagi-Harada
       - Sympathetic ophthalmia
       - Sarcoidosis
     - Orbit:
       - Thyroid eye disease
       - Inflammatory orbital disease (pseudotumor)
     - Retinitis/vasculitis
     - Optic nerve:
       - Optic neuritis
       - Anterior ischemic optic neuropathy associated with giant cell arteritis
   - **Adjunctive to eye operations:**
     - High risk penetrating keratoplasty
     - High risk glaucoma surgery

4. **Intravitreal**
   - **Given as 4 mg dose (0.1 ml of 40 mg/ml suspension)**
   - **Inflammatory/immune diseases:**
     - Uveitis:
       - Behcet's disease
       - Pars planitis
       - Vogt-Koyanagi-Harada
       - Sympathetic ophthalmia
       - Sarcoidosis
   - **Adjunctive to eye operations:**
     - Highlight vitreous for anterior/posterior vitrectomy
   - Vascular diseases:
     - CME
     - CNV
     - CSME
     - Retinal vein occlusions

Exam tips:
- **Listen to the question, is it "steroid therapy" or "topical steroid therapy?"**
- **The indications for "systemic steroid therapy" are IDENTICAL to that for "immunosuppressive therapy."**

Q   What are the Complications of Steroids?

"The complications of steroid therapy can be divided into ocular and systemic complications."
"Topical therapy is usually associated with ocular complications while systemic therapy can be associated with both ocular and systemic complications...."

Complications of Steroid Therapy

1. **Ocular**
   - **Cataract** (posterior subcapsular type)
   - Raised IOP (see steroid responder, page 62)
   - Exacerbation of **infection** (bacterial keratitis, fungal keratitis, HSV)

2. **Systemic**
   - **C**ardiac complications (arrythmias, heart failure)
   - **U**lcer (gastric ulcer)
   - **S**uppression of hypothalamic — pituitary — adrenal axis (shock)
   - **H**ypertension, hirsutism, Hepatic (liver failure)
   - **I**schemic necrosis of femur and osteoporosis
   - **N**eutropenia and infection
   - **G**rowth problems in children
   - **S** for Psychosis

Exam tips:
- Listen to the question, is it "steroid therapy" or "topical steroid therapy?"
- There are three big ocular complications.
- The mnemonic for systemic complications is "CUSHINGS."

Notes
- "How do steroids cause cataract?"
  - Binding of steroids to lens proteins
  - Disulphide bond formation
  - Increased glucose concentration in lens
  - Increased cation permeability
  - Decreased G6PD activity

Notes
- "How do steroids cause glaucoma?"
  - Increased glycosaminoglycans in trabecular meshwork
  - Inhibition of phagocytic activity of meshwork cells
  - Inhibition of prostaglandins

Q **When is Atropine Needed in Ophthalmology?**

"Atropine is a cholinergic receptor blocker, specifically a muscarinic antagonist."
"It is used topically for diagnosis and treatment, as well as systemically…."

Atropine Indications

1. **Diagnostic**
   - Mydriasis for vitreoretinal surgery:
   - Prolonged duration, onset 30–40 min, duration 10–14D
   - Cycloplegic refraction:
     - Indicated for poor response to cyclopentolate or in cases of excessive accommodation

2. **Therapeutic**
   - Uveitis
   - Glaucoma:
     - Inflammatory glaucoma
     - Neovascular glaucoma
     - Malignant glaucoma

   - Cataract (posterior subcapsular type):
     - In situations when surgery is contraindicated or patient refused surgery
   - Amblyopia:
     - Penalization technique (give atropine to the good eye)

3. **Systemic use**
   - Inhibit oculo-cardiac reflex during orbital/squint surgery
   - Standby for tensilon test in myasthenia gravis (page 236)

Q What are the Complications of Atropine Use?

"Atropine is a cholinergic receptor blocker, specifically a muscarinic antagonist."
"It has both local and systemic complications."

Complications of Atropine

1. **Local**
   - Transient stinging effect
   - Conjunctival irritation, hyperemia, follicular conjunctivitis
   - Acute ACG
   - Visual blurring from mydriasis and cycloplegia
   - Amblyopia in children

2. **Systemic**
   - Flushing (red as a beetroot)
   - Dryness (dry as a bone)

   - Fever (hot as a hare)
   - Headache, dysarthria, ataxia, hallucination, amnesia (mad as a hatter)
   - Bladder distension, decreased gastrointestinal mobility (bloated as a barrow)
   - Tachycardia, dysarrhythmia
   - Hypotension, respiratory depression, coma and death

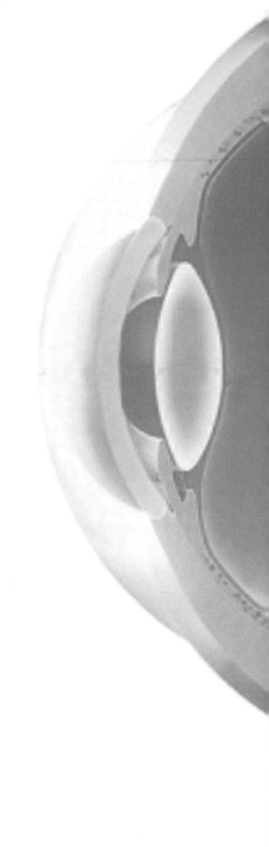

SQUINTS AND PEDIATRIC EYE DISEASES

ASSESSMENT OF STRABISMUS

Overall yield: ✸✸✸✸   **Clinical exam:**   **Viva:** ✸✸✸✸   **Essay:**   **MCQ:** ✸✸✸

Q Opening Question: What Clinical Tests are Used in the Assessment of Strabismus?

Assessment of Strabismus

1. **Light reflection tests:**
   - Hirshberg's test
   - Krimsky's test
   - Bruckner's test

2. **Cover tests:**
   - Cover and uncover test
   - Alternate cover test
   - Simultaneous prism cover test
   - Alternate prism cover test

3. **Dissimilar image tests:**
   - The Maddox wing
   - The Maddox rod
   - The Hess test/Lee's screen

4. **Binocular single vision tests:**
   - Base out prism test
   - Worth's four dot test
   - Bagolini striated glasses
   - Synoptophore
   - Stereopsis tests (Titmus test, TNO random dot tests)

Exam tips:
- **Alternate questions are "How do you perform the cover and uncover tests?" and "What is the Maddox rod?"**

Notes

Common scenarios in orthoptics examination:

1. Intermittent XT
2. Esotropia
3. Duane's syndrome
4. Fourth nerve palsy
5. Brown's syndrome
6. Monocular elevation deficit

Light Reflection Tests

1. **Hirshberg's test:**
   - Detects **gross heterotropias**
   - Based on Purkinje Sanson image no. 1
   - Look at symmetry of light reflex
   - Normal reflex:
     - Just nasal to center of pupil
   - Abnormal reflex:
     - Border of pupil (15° or 30 prism D)
     - In between border and limbus (30° or 60 prism D)
     - Limbus (45° or 90 prism D)
   - What are the possible differential diagnoses of an abnormal Hirshberg's test?
     - Strabismus (tropia)
     - Eccentric fixation
     - Large (positive) angle kappa — congenital or acquired (ROP)
     - Nonseeing eye

2. **Krimsky's test:**
   - Place prism in front of fixating eye until light reflex is symmetrical

3. **Bruckner's test:**
   - Use direct ophthalmolscope
   - Look at symmetry of red reflex
   - Brighter reflex comes from deviated eye

Exam tips:
- **Describe each test as simply as possible.**

Cover Tests

1. **Cover-uncover test:**
   - Cover component:
     - Detects **heterotropias**
     - Cover straight eye
     - Look at uncovered deviated eye (movement indicates tropia)
   - Uncover component:
     - Detects **heterophorias**
     - Uncover straight eye
     - Look at uncovered eye for deviation and refixation (movement indicates phoria in this eye)

2. **Alternate cover-uncover test:**
   - Detects **heterophorias**
   - Alternate cover and uncover both eyes

   - Look at uncovered eye for movement (movement indicates phoria in that eye)

3. **Simultaneous prism cover test:**
   - Measures **heterotropias**
   - Simultaneous cover of one eye and placing prism over the other until no movement

4. **Alternate prism cover test:**
   - Measures **total deviation (heterotropias and phorias)**
   - Prism over deviated eye and alternate cover each eye until no movement

Dissimilar Image Tests

1. **The Maddox wing:**
   - Measures **heterophorias**
   - Dissociates two eyes for near fixation:
     - Right eye sees white vertical arrow and red horizontal arrow
     - Left eye sees vertical and horizontal row of numbers
   - Patient asked which number arrow pointing at

2. **The Maddox rod:**
   - Measures **heterophorias**

- Dissociates two eyes for distance fixation
- Consists of series of fused high power cylinder red rods
- Coverts white spot of light into red line perpendicular to axis of rods
- Rods placed in front of deviated eye and patient asked to locate position of red line in relation to white spot of light:
  - If red line is temporal to light, indicates **esophoria (EP)**
  - If red line is nasal to light, indicates **exophoria (XP)**
- To estimate degree of squint, place prisms until red line is at center of white spot of light

3. **Hess test/Lee's screen:**
   - Principle: **Herring's law** of equal and simultaneous innervation of yoke muscle
   - Dissociates two eyes for distance fixation
   - Hess test: Dissociates two eyes with red and green filters
   - Lee's screen: Dissociates two eyes with mirror
   - Interpretation of Hess chart/Lee's screen:
     - Smaller field is from abnormal eye (eye with limited movement)

- Larger field is from normal eye (outward displacement indicates overaction in that direction)
- Equal size field indicates no deviation or equal deviation
- Narrow field indicates mechanical restriction of movements in opposing directions (blow out fracture)
- Sloping field indicates A or V pattern (**NOT** torsion)
- When do you perform a Hess test?
  - To differentiate ET from paretic squint (e.g. VI CN palsy)
  - Paretic squints
  - Thyroid eye disease
  - Myasthenia gravis (tensilon test)
  - Blow out fracture
- When is the Hess test contraindicated?
  - Patients who have monocular suppression
  - Patients who do not have normal retinal correspondence

BSV Tests

1. **The base out prism test:**
   - Place prism base out over eye
   - This displaces retinal image and initiates eye movement in direction of apex
   - Examiner looks for corrective movement of eye
   - No movement indicates scotoma/suppression in that eye
     - Four prism D base out prism will not induce corrective movement in eye with microtropia

2. **The Worth's four dot test:**
   - Test of BSV
   - Dissociates two eyes for distance fixation
   - Consists of box with 4 dots (1 red, 1 white and 2 green).
   - Patient wears glasses with red lens in right eye and green lens in left
   - Interpretation:
     - If 4 lights are seen, indicates **normal fusion**
     - If 4 lights are seen in presence of manifest squint, indicates **anomalous retinal correspondence (ARC)**
     - If 2 lights are seen, indicates **left suppression**

- If 3 lights are seen, indicates **right suppression**
- If 5 lights are seen, indicates **diplopia (uncompensated ET/XT)**

3. **Bagolini striated glasses:**
   - Test of BSV
   - Consists of glasses with fine striations orientated at 45° to each other
   - Converts point of light into a line perpendicular to striations (like Maddox rod) but principle is based on interference and diffraction of light (not refraction as in Maddox rod)
   - Patient wears glasses and sees point of light
   - Interpretation:
     - If lines cross at center, indicates **normal fusion**
     - If lines cross at center in presence of squint, indicates **ARC**
     - If one of the lines is missing, indicates **left or right suppression**
     - If lines do not cross at center (point of light), indicates **diplopia**

4. **The synoptophore:**
   - Test of BSV
   - Dissociates two eyes for **both near and distance** fixation
   - Instrument: two cylindrical tubes with pictures are inserted at end of each tube

> **Notes**
> - "What are the uses of the synoptophore?"
>   - Determine 3 grades of BSV
>   - Measure objective and subjective angle of deviation
>   - Measure angle kappa
>   - Measure primary and secondary deviation
>   - Assessment of retinal correspondence
>   - Measurement of IPD
>   - Assessment of anisokonia
>
> Therapeutic use (treatment of suppression, ARC, accommodative ET, intermittent tropias and phorias)

Q What are the Tests for Stereopsis?

"Stereopsis tests can be divided into...."

Stereopsis

1. **True 3-dimensional tests:**
   - Frisby plates:
     - Stereopsis test (600 — 15 seconds)
     - Consists of 3 clear plastic plates consisting of 4 squares with hidden circle in 1 of them
     - Plates are of varying thickness and tests can be varied by distance
     - Patient asked to pick square with circle in it

2. **Dissociated 2-dimensional tests:**
   - Titmus test:
     - Stereopsis test (3000 — 40 seconds)
     - Consists of three components: Fly, circle, animal
     - Needs polaroid glasses
   - TNO random dot:
     - Stereopsis test (1900 — 15 seconds)
     - Consists of 7 plates with various obvious and hidden shapes (squares, dots)
     - Needs red green glasses
     - No monocular clues (better than Titmus)
   - Lang test:
     - Stereopsis test (1200 — 200 seconds)
     - Consists of plates with various hidden objects (moon, sun)
     - No need for glasses (built-in cylindrical elements)
     - No monocular clues
   - Mentor BVAT:
     - Distance stereopsis test

TOPIC 2

BINOCULAR SINGLE VISION

Overall yield: ✪✪✪✪ **Clinical exam: Viva:** ✪✪✪✪ **Essay:** ✪ **MCQ:** ✪✪✪✪

Q Opening Question: Tell me about Fixation.

"Fixation is a **monocular** visual phenomenon."
"In which the image of an object is focused on the fovea."

Fixation

1. **Axes in fixation:**
   - **Optical axis** (**anatomical** axis) = line passing through center of cornea that bisects globe into two equal halves (OR = line passing through center of cornea and lens; OR = line that joins all Purkinje images)
   - **Pupillary axis** = line perpendicular to corneal center, which passes center of pupil
   - **Visual axis** = line from object of regard to fovea
   - **Angle kappa** = between VISUAL and PUPILLARY axis, subtended at anterior nodal point
     - Positive if Hirschberg light reflex is displaced nasally
     - Negative if displaced temporally
     - Normal: Up to 5° in adults/10° in infants
   - **Angle lambda** = between VISUAL and PUPILLARY axes, but subtended at pupil entrance
   - **Angle alpha** = between OPTICAL and PUPILLARY axes

2. **Abnormalities of fixation:**
   - If development in fixation is disturbed, two possible consequences
     - Nystagmus:
       - Appears at 3–4 months

- Eccentric fixation:
  - A monocular phenomenon, whereby an eye fixates upon a target with a nonfoveal area
  - Develops if there is an early-onset macular pathology and is also a very rare complication of strabismus
  - Compare with anomalous retinal correspondence (see below)

3. **Tests of fixation:**
   - Gross testing:
     - Occlude one eye and test fixation pattern of the other with target (e.g. cover-uncover test)
   - Visioscopy:
     - Performed with a direct ophthalmoscope, where examiner observes retinal position of projected target when viewed by fixating patient
   - Haidinger brushes:
     - Entoptic phenomenon appreciated only by a macular area with its center located at fovea
     - Patient sees rotating Maltese cross when stimulated with a rotating plane-polarized blue light. If eccentric fixation present, patient will be unable to localize "hub" of cross correctly

> **Exam tips:**
> - **BSV is an extremely difficult subject.**
> - **Definitions for BSV, fusion, retinal correspondence, the horoptor, Panum's space and stereopsis must be committed to memory. Use keywords for each.**

"Binocular single vision (BSV) is a binocular **acquired** phenomenon."
"Whereby **separate** and **similar** images seen by two eyes are perceived as one."
"The prerequisites of BSV are...."
"There are three grades of BSV."

BSV

1. **Prerequisites of BSV:**
   - Clear visual axis in both eyes, with normal function of visual pathways
   - Straight eyes — within 8 prism D horizontally (motor fusion)
   - Ability of cortex to integrate images (sensory fusion)

2. **Grades of BSV (Worth's three ascending levels):**
   - Simultaneous perception
   - Fusion
   - Stereopsis

"Simultaneous perception is the appreciation of two separate and **dissimilar** images being projected to the same position in space."
"Occurs in two sets of circumstances."

Simultaneous Perception

1. **Appreciation of dissimilar images (first grade of BSV):**
   - Two dissimilar images appear to be projected to same area
   - Involves fovea in one eye and peri-foveal area in the other (synoptophore — bird in cage)

2. **Appreciation of similar images too disparate to fuse leading to diplopia**

"This is a hypothetical "single eye" situated between the two eyes."
"An image which falls on the fovea in the two eyes is perceived to come from a straight ahead position."
"This direction is the subjective visual direction from the cyclopean eye."

"Fusion is a binocular phenomenon where **separate** images are perceived as one due to stimulation of **corresponding retinal areas** in the two eyes."
"This is associated with a **2-dimensional** localization of object in space."
"There are two types of fusion: Motor and sensory."

Fusion

1. **Motor fusion:**
   - A vergence movement designed to allow objects to stimulate corresponding retinal areas (reduce horizontal, vertical or torsional disparity of the retinal image)
   - Strength of motor fusion = fusional amplitude (in prism D)
   - Experiments have shown that vergence precision is not necessary for fusion and stereopsis. Up to 2.5 degree of vergence error can be tolerated

2. **Sensory fusion:**
   - The appreciation of two separate images located on the retina as a single unified percept
   - Strength of sensory fusion = fixation disparity
   - Similar foveal images of up to 14 minutes of ARC are fusible

Distant:	Convergence	15	Divergence	6	Vertical	2.5
Near:	Convergence	25	Divergence	15	Vertical	2.5

"Retinal correspondence is a phenomenon in which retinal areas…."

Retinal Correspondence

1. **Retinal correspondence**
   - Retinal areas in two eyes share a **common visual direction** and therefore project to same **position** in space and are connected to approximately the same area in **visual cortex**
2. **Normal retinal correspondence**
   - When these retinal areas bear identical relationship with fovea
3. **Anomalous retinal correspondence**
   - When they do not share same relationship with fovea

"Horoptor is an imaginary **surface** in space."
"All points of which will stimulate corresponding retinal points."
"All points will therefore be projected to same position in space."

Horoptor

1. **Each fixating point determines a specific horoptor.**
2. **All points located just off horoptor will stimulate non-corresponding retinal points, but images can still be perceived singly as long as they are located within Panum's space**
3. **Horoptor's surface is a torus, derived from experiments**
4. **Vieth-Muller circle is an imaginary circle derived from mathematical formulae, all points which will stimulate corresponding retinal points, with circle passing through optical centers of each eye**

"Panum's space is an imaginary **volume** in space surrounding the horoptor."
"Within which objects will be seen singly, although they may stimulate non-corresponding retinal areas."

Panum's Space

1. **Points falling outside of Panum's space are not fusible and will lead to physiological diplopia, which is then physiologically suppressed in nondominant eye**
2. **Panum's space widens out toward periphery:**
   - **To match the increasing coarseness of peripheral vision**
   - **To prevent bothersome peripheral diplopia**
   - **To help facilitate cyclofusion**
3. **Not a fixed space; it widens if the stimulus is:**
   - **Larger**
   - **Fuzzier**
   - **Slower moving**

"Stereopsis is the binocular perception of **depth**."
"Occurs when **separate** but **slightly dissimilar** objects are seen by two eyes as one."
"Stereopsis is caused by **horizontal retinal image disparity**."
"In contrast to fusion, there is 3-dimensional localization of the object in space."

Stereopsis

1. **Prerequisites**
   - Needs slight horizontal disparity (does not occur for vertical/torsional disparity)
   - Images must be fusible (i.e. within Panum's space), BUT not all fusible images give stereo:
   - Those pointing RIGHT on the horopter are not seen stereoscopically, as they project to corresponding retinal point with no horizontal disparity present!

- Retinal disparity must be large enough to prevent simple fusion, but not great enough for diplopia to occur
- Not possible beyond 700 m (insufficient image disparity)
- Cortically, must be able to have:
  - Binocular correlation (ability to determine that two similar images come from same object)
  - Disparity detection between these correlated images
2. Monocular clues to stereopsis
  - Apparent size (larger of two identical objects is nearer)
- Overlay (nearer object will cover further one)
- Aerial perspective (distant objects appear more indistinct and less color-saturated)
- Light shading
- Geometric perspective (parallel lines converge the further they are)
- Relative velocity
- Motion parallax (when observer's head is moved, closer object moves smaller amount in an opposite direction, while further objects move a larger amount in same direction)

Q What is Stereoacuity?

"Measure of the **threshold of horizontal disparity** required to perceive stereopsis."

Stereoacuity

1. **Smallest binocular disparity or parallax that can be detected**
2. **Dependent on three parameters: Interpupillary distance, object separation and object distance**
3. **Stereoacuity increases progressively as horoptor is approached, but reaches 0 at horoptor (where there is zero retinal image disparity)**
4. **Normal values:**
   - Centrally: 20–40 sec of ARC
   - Peripherally: 200 sec of ARC
   - Maximal at about 0.25° off dead-center in the foveola
   - Minimal beyond 15° eccentricity

Q What are the Differences between Fusion and Stereopsis?

"Both fusion and stereopsis are components of BSV...."

Comparison between Fusion and Stereopsis

	Fusion	Stereopsis
Image disparity	• Eliminates disparity of retinal images. The less the disparity, the more ideal the fusion	• Based on existence of retinal image disparity
Motor component stimuli	• Yes • Horizontal, vertical and torsional visual stimuli elicit a fusional response	• No • Only horizontal disparity will elicit stereopsis
Localization of object Range	• In 2-dimensional space • All ranges of distances	• In 3-dimensional space • Less effective as distance increases

BSV Abnormalities

1. **Compensatory mechanisms**
   - Physical adaptation:
     - Abnormal head posture
     - Conscious closure of one eye
   - Sensory adaptation:
     - Suppression (leads to amblyopia)
     - Anomalous retinal correspondence
     - Monofixation syndrome (initially a compensatory mechanism, later on becoming a BSV abnormality)

   - Blind spot syndrome
2. **BSV abnormalities**
   - Absent BSV (e.g. congenital ET)
   - Impaired BSV (e.g. monofixation syndrome)
   - Diplopia
   - Confusion

Q Tell me about Diplopia.

"Diplopia is an abnormality of BSV."
"Occurs when there is an **acquired** misalignment of visual axis (squint)."
"**Single** object stimulates **two non-corresponding retinal points**."
"Object is therefore perceived to come from two different locations in subjective visual space."

Diplopia

1. **Does not occur in congenital squints**
2. **Usually there is stimulation of fovea in one eye and a nonfoveal area in the other eye**
   - One of two areas must project to a point outside of Panum's space:
3. **Compensatory mechanism is peripheral suppression (nonfoveal area)**

4. **Classified as:**
   - Crossed diplopia (XT) (note: "cross" = "X")
   - Uncrossed diplopia (ET)

Q Tell me about Confusion.

"Confusion is an abnormality of BSV."
"Occurs when there is an **acquired** misalignment of visual axis (squint)."
"**Two** objects stimulate **corresponding retinal points**."
"Two objects are therefore perceived to come from single location in subjective visual space."

Confusion

1. **Less common than diplopia**
2. **Does not occur in congenital squints**

3. **Usually there is stimulation of both foveas by different objects in different locations**
4. **Compensatory mechanism is central suppression**

Exam tips:
- **Confusion = corresponding retinal points = central suppression!**

Q Tell me about Suppression.

"Suppression is a compensatory mechanism when there is an **interruption of BSV**."
"Visual sensation is prevented from reaching consciousness."
"Occurs when there is a misalignment of visual axis (squint)."
"Adaptation to **prevent** diplopia and confusion."

Suppression

1. Occurs mainly in children (congenital squints or early acquired squints)
2. Physiological suppression (prevents physiological diplopia) vs pathological suppression (squints)
3. Classified as:
   - Central (prevent confusion) vs peripheral (prevent diplopia)
   - Monocular (higher risk of amblyopia) vs alternating
   - Facultative (only when manifest squint is present) vs obligatory (all the time, higher risk of amblyopia)

Q Tell me about Monofixation Syndrome (Microtropia).

"Monofixation syndrome is an abnormality of BSV."
"Occurs when there is a **small angle squint**."
"The classical features include…."

Monofixation Syndrome

1. Scenarios
   - Primary (small angle ET most common squint, usually less than 8 prism D)
   - Secondary (treatment of ET with glasses or surgery, anisometropia, macular lesions)
2. Differential diagnosis of unilateral decrease in VA when no obvious squint is present
3. Variable features
   - Amblyopia is common
   - Central scotoma with peripheral fusion capability
   - Decreased stereopsis
   - May have ARC
   - May have central or eccentric fixation
4. Alternate prism cover test measurement will EXCEED simultaneous prism cover test
5. Treatment
   - Refractive correction of anisometropia
   - Occlusion to treat amblyopia
   - Poor prognosis for restoring binocular single vision

Exam tips:
- **Fairly rare syndrome, but fairly common exam question.**

AMBLYOPIA

Overall yield: ✸✸✸   **Clinical exam:**   **Viva:** ✸✸✸✸   **Essay:** ✸   **MCQ:** ✸✸✸✸

Q Opening Question: What is Amblyopia?

"Amblyopia is a unilateral or bilateral decrease in **visual acuity**."
"**Caused by** form vision deprivation or abnormal binocular interaction."
"**No organic** causes can be detected by the examination of the eye."
"In appropriate cases, is **reversible** by therapeutic measures."

Classification

1. **Strabismic amblyopia**
   - Most likely with constant tropias
   - Uncommon in intermittent XT
2. **Amblyopia related to refractive errors**
   - **Ametropic:**
     - Due to either bilateral hyperopia (> 4–5 D) or bilateral myopia (> 6–7 D)
     - More common in bilateral hyperopia
     - In bilateral amblyopia, high myopia less likely as near objects will still be in focus due to accommodation
   - **Anisometropic:**
     - Due to unequal refractive error between the two eyes:
       - Anisohyperopia — difference in hyperopia of > 1.5 D

   - Anisomyopia — difference in myopia of > 3 D
   - **Meridonal:**
     - Due to uncorrected astigmatism of > 1.5 D
3. **Stimulus-deprivation amblyopia**
   - Complete ptosis, corneal opacities, congenital cataracts, other media opacities
   - Iatrogenic origin (occlusion amblyopia)

Q What are the Pathophysiological Changes in Amblyopia seen in Animal or Experimental Models?

Pathophysiological Changes of Amblyopia

1. **Retina:**
   - Reduction in spatial resolving powers of retinal cells
   - Increased lateral inhibition between retinal cone cells
2. **Lateral geniculate nucleus — reduction in number of cells of all six layers**
3. **Visual cortex — reduction in number of cortical cells**

Clinical Features of Amblyopia

1. **Decreased VA commonly defined as loss of VA of two or more lines on Snellen chart**
   - VA paradoxically improves with neutral density filter
2. **Crowding phenomenon**
   - Represents an abnormality of contour interaction between point of fixation and adjacent objects
   - VA better for single optotypes than multiple optotypes (Sheridan Gardiner)
   - VA better on grating tests (FPL)
3. **Normal ocular exam and no RAPD**
4. **Eccentric fixation**
5. **Decreased contrast sensitivity and decreased brightness perception**
6. **Binocular suppression of amblyopic eye**
7. **Increased perception and reaction times**

"The management of amblyopia will depend on the **age** of patient, **cause** of amblyopia and **severity** of amblyopia."

"First, we need to exclude…"

Management of Amblyopia

1. **Exclude other organic causes of poor vision**
   - Refractive errors, cataract, tumors
2. **Remove obstacles to clear vision**
   - Refractive correction, cataract surgery
3. **Occlusion therapy (gold standard)**
   - Amount of occlusion depends on **age** of patient, **cause** of amblyopia and **severity** of amblyopia
   - Best achieved with adhesive patches
   - Practical guidelines:
     - Patching should be started as soon as amblyopia is detected
     - For part-time occlusion, duration of patching usually depends on age of child: 1 hour/day for each year of age
     - Full-time occlusion should not exceed **1 week per year of age**
     - Patching should be continued till VA reaches and maintains a plateau for 3–6 months
     - From full-time patching, decrease to half-time patching for a few months, then to several hours per day
     - If no progress is made for 3 consecutive months, patching may be considered a failure
     - Regular follow-up to ensure that vision remains stable
     - Maintenance patching may be required until 9 years of age when visual system is assumed to have "matured"

4. **Penalization**
   - Usually reserved for patching failure or noncompliance with patching
   - Pharmacologic:
     - 1% atropine placed in good eye to blur eye for near vision
   - Optical:
     - Degrades image in better eye to a degree such that amblyopic eye has a competitive advantage at a given fixation distance
     - Undercorrecting the refractive error in better eye
5. **Others — CAM visual stimulator, pleoptics (unproven alternatives to patching)**
6. **Prevention**
   - Education and awareness of primary care physician
   - Vision screening programs essential in any community
   - Red reflex of every baby should be checked at birth

Additional Management Principles

1. **Strabismic amblyopia**
   - Occlusion therapy should be instituted prior to surgery:
     - Fixation behavior will be harder to determine once eyes are surgically aligned

- Optimal acuity may maximize chances of restoring binocular vision
- Parent motivation toward patching might be increased by visual reminder of strabismus

2. **Amblyopia related to refractive errors**
   - Correct refractive error first before occlusion therapy

- Part-time occlusion preferable if binocular interaction present, amblyopia is mild and child is in school

3. **Stimulus deprivation amblyopia**
   - Remove barriers to vision preferably within first 6 weeks of life

Notes
- "What if there is no response after 3 months of patching?" Consider possible causes:
  - Wrong diagnosis
  - Noncompliance
  - Uncorrected refractive error
  - Failure to prescribe sufficient treatment
  - Irreversible amblyopia

ESOTROPIA

Overall yield: ✪✪✪ **Clinical exam:** ✪✪✪✪ **Viva:** ✪✪ **Essay:** ✪✪ **MCQ:** ✪✪✪✪

Q Opening Question: What are the Causes of Esotropia?

"Esotropia is a convergent misalignment of eyes."
"They can be divided according to age of onset…."

Causes of ET

1. **Infantile ET (<6 months)**
   - Essential or congenital ET
   - Early accommodative ET
   - Duane's syndrome Type 1
   - Mobius syndrome
   - VI CN palsy
   - Nystagmus blockage syndrome

2. **Acquired ET (>6 months)**
   - Comitant ET:
     - Accommodative ET
     - Sensory ET (disruption of BSV in children usually before 2 years of age e.g. congenital cataract)
   - Consecutive ET
   - Divergence insufficiency
   - Stress-induced ET
   - Cyclic ET
   - Incomitant ET:
     - VI CN palsy
     - Thyroid eye disease
     - Medial wall fracture
     - Mobius syndrome

Q Tell me about Essential/Congenital Esotropia.

"Essential or congenital ET is a common convergent squint."

Essential/Congenital ET

1. **Clinical features**
   - Presents at 6 months of birth
   - Family history common
   - Characteristic of ET:
     - Large angle (>30 prism D)
     - Stable
     - Angle at distance = near
   - Normal refractive error (therefore not accommodative ET)
   - Alternating fixation in primary position but cross fixation in side-gaze
   - Need to exclude VI CN palsy (cover one eye, elicit Doll's reflex)
   - Latent nystagmus, dissociated vertical deviation, IO overaction and asymmetrical OKN response may be present
   - Poor potential for BSV

2. **Management**
   - Correct amblyopia
   - Timing of surgery: 6 months to 2 years (usually before 1st birthday):
     - Angle of deviation stable over 2 visits, 3–4 weeks apart; no amblyopia; at least 2 cycloplegic refractions 3–4 weeks apart
     - "Why not before 6 months?"
       - There is a chance of spontaneous recovery before 6 months and angle is also smaller after 6 months
     - "Why not after 2 years then?"
       - Loses stereopsis after 2 years

- Type of surgery
  - Bilateral MR recession with IO overaction correction
  - Aim for 10 prism D of residual ET (allows good peripheral fusion although central BSV is still impaired)
- Subsequent management
  - Manage amblyopia (develops in 40% of congenital ET after surgery)

- Watch for:
  - Accommodative ET
  - Undercorrection (need further LR resection)
  - IO overaction and DVD

Q What are Accommodative Esotropias?

"Accommodative esotropias are common types of convergent squints."
"Due to an overaction of the accommodative reflex."
"There are three classical types."

Accommodative ET

1. **Classification**
   - Fully accommodative
   - Partially accommodative
   - Fully and partially accommodative with high AC/A ratio

2. **Clinical features**
   - Presents at 2.5 years
   - **5 cardinal features** common to all 3 types:
     - Usually intermittent in onset early on then becomes constant
     - Family history is common
     - May be precipitated by trauma or illness
     - Amblyopia is common
     - Diplopia is uncommon
   - Fully accommodative ET:
     - ET fully corrected with glasses
     - Deviation same near and distance
     - Normal AC/A ratio
     - Surgery not necessary. Reassure patient that the hypermetropia and ET will lessen as they grow older
   - Partially accommodative:
     - ET not fully corrected with glasses
     - Deviation same near and distance
     - Normal AC/A ratio
     - Surgery as soon as possible to correct the non-accommodative component. The patient will still require glasses post-surgery
   - Fully and partially accommodative ET with high AC/A ratio:
     - Deviation greater for near compared to distance
     - High AC/A ratio
     - Patient will require bifocals (in addition to surgery for partially accommodative ET)

3. **Management**
   - Correct refractive error (hypermetropia):
     - "Plus" bifocal component for nonrefractive accommodative ET
   - Miotic therapy (ecothiopate or pilocarpine):
     - Temporary measure for children who are noncompliant with glasses
     - Induces peripheral accommodation so that less accommodative effort is needed by patient
     - Side effects: Miosis, ciliary spasm, iris cysts, cataract, RD
   - Correct amblyopia
   - Surgery:
     - If ET is not fully corrected with spectacles
     - Determine the amount of surgical correction
       - Standard:
         - Target angle determined by residual distance ET that is not corrected with spectacles
         - Undercorrection rate high: 25–30%
       - Augmented:
         - Target angle determined by averaging near deviation with correction and near deviation without correction
         - 7% overcorrection rate for distance
       - Prism adaptation:
         - Target angle determined using prisms
         - Patient prescribed base-out prism for residual ET after being prescribed full hypermetropic correction. Prisms are increased at 2 weekly intervals until ET has stabilized

- Target angle determined by full prism-adapted angle
- 85% success rate, but time-consuming and costly
- Type of surgery:
  - Bilateral MR recession

- Recess-resect if amblyopia in one eye
- Other considerations:
  - Correct IO overaction
  - Correct V or A pattern

EXOTROPIA

Overall yield: ✪✪✪   **Clinical exam:** ✪✪✪   **Viva:** ✪✪   **Essay:** ✪✪   **MCQ:** ✪✪✪✪

Q Opening Question: What are the Causes of Exotropia?

"Exotropias are divergent misalignment of eyes."
"The commonest cause is intermittent XT."
"Other causes include...."

Causes of Exotropia

1. **Congenital**
   - Congenital XT: Present at birth, large and constant angle, frequently associated with neurological anomalies
   - Duane's syndrome Type 2
2. **Acquired**
   - Comitant XT:
     - Intermittent XT
     - Consecutive XT (after correction for ET)
   - Sensory XT (disruption of BSV in children usually after 2 years of age)
   - Convergence insufficiency
   - Incomitant XT:
     - III CN palsy
     - Myasthenia gravis
     - Thyroid eye disease
     - INO

Q Tell me about Intermittent Exotropias.

"Intermittent XT is a common divergent squint."
"It can be divided into 3 types based on severity of XT for near vs far."
"And into 3 phases...."

Intermittent XT

1. **Classification:**
   - Convergence insufficiency (worse for **near**, needs MR resection or recess-resect)
   - Divergence excess (worse for **distance**, needs LR recession):
     - Simulated excess (accommodative fusion controls deviation at near)
     - True excess (diagnosed by adding "plus" 3D lens at near to control for accommodation, or occluding one eye to relax the accommodation)
     - Basic (near and distance **same or within 10 Δ**, needs LR recession)
2. **Phases:**
   - Phase 1 (intermittent XP at distance)
   - Phase 2 (XT at distance, XP at near)
   - Phase 3 (XT at distance and near)
3. **Clinical features:**
   - Age of onset: 2 years
   - Precipitated by illness, bright light, day-dreaming, fatigue
   - Goes through 3 phases
   - Temporal retinal hemisuppression when eyes are deviated
   - Amblyopia not common
   - ARC and eccentric fixation may be present
4. **Management:**
   - Correct refractive errors (myopia)
   - Correct amblyopia
   - Orthoptic treatment:
     - Fusional exercise (pencil pushups, base-out prism)

- Diplopia awareness
- Surgery:
  - Indications **(4 classic indications)**
    - Increase angle of XT
    - Increase frequency of breakdown (i.e. progressing from Phase 1 to 2)
    - Decreasing stereopsis
    - Abnormal head posture
  - Determine the amount of surgical correction:
    - Basic and pseudo-divergence excess: Correct angle of deviation for distance
    - Divergence excess: Correct ½ (angle of deviation for distance + angle of deviation for near)
- Type of surgery:
  - Bilateral LR recession
  - If one eye amblyopic, recess LR and resect MR of amblyopic eye
  - If angle of deviation is large, 3 muscle surgery (bilateral LR recession + MR resection)
  - If there is a V-pattern XT:
    - Bilateral LR recession and IO weakening
    - Bilateral LR recession and upward transposition of LR (if there is no significant IO overaction)

Notes

"What are the causes of abnormal head posture?"

- **Ocular:**
  - Strabismus
  - Nystagmus
  - Ptosis
  - Refractive error

- **Non-ocular:**
  - Torticollis
  - Unilateral hearing loss
  - Habitual

VERTICAL SQUINTS AND OTHER MOTILITY SYNDROMES

Overall yield: ✪ ✪   Clinical exam: ✪ ✪ ✪ ✪   Viva: ✪ ✪   Essay: ✪   MCQ: ✪ ✪ ✪

Q Opening Question: What are the Types of Vertical Squints?

Vertical Squints

1. **SO and IO muscles**
   - SO palsy
   - SO overaction
   - IO palsy
   - IO overaction

2. **Multiple muscles**
   - Congenital fibrosis syndrome

   - Double elevator palsy
   - Dissociated vertical deviation (DVD)
   - A and V patterns

3. **Others (III CN palsy, thyroid eye disease, blowout fracture)**

Q Tell me about Inferior Oblique Overaction.

"IO overaction is a common vertical squint."
"50% of patients with essential or congenital ET have IO overaction."

Inferior Oblique Overaction

1. **Introduction**
   - Bilateral, but may be asymmetrical
   - Clinical scenarios:
     - With horizontal squints
     - Paresis of one or both SO
     - Primary (uncommon)
   - Significance of IO overaction:
     - Affects cosmesis
     - Disruption of BSV
     - Contributes to large angle ET

2. **Clinical features**
   - V pattern — difference of >15 prism D is considered significant
   - Upshoot of eye in adduction
   - Associated with SO underaction

3. **Surgery**
   - Grade +1:
     - IO recession 8–10 mm
   - Grade +2:
     - IO myomectomy
     - IO myotomy at insertion
   - Grade +3:
     - Extirpation of IO muscle
   - Grade +4:
     - Denervation
     - Anteriorization of IO tendon:
       · Marshall Parks point: 3 mm posterior to IR insertion +1 mm lateral
       · Equivalent to 12–15 mm of IO recession
       · Can correct for DVD as well

Notes

- "How do you differentiate IO overaction from DVD?" In IO overaction:
  - Elevation of eye in adduction only (in DVD, in primary position and abduction as well)
  - Hypotropia of fellow eye (in DVD, only hypertropia of affected eye)
  - Base-up prism over fellow eye will neutralize hypotropia (in DVD, only base down prism over affected eye will correct hypotropia)

Q **How do You Locate the IO Muscle During Surgery?**

Localization of IO During Surgery

- Isolate LR and IR
- IO is a pink tendon within white Tenon's capsule
- Tubular/worm-like structure
- Pull IO and feel tug at point of origin at orbital rim

Notes

- **Complications of IO surgery:**
  1. Injury to the macula
  2. Injury to the posterior ciliary artery
  3. Breach of the posterior tenon space → fat prolapse, adhesions
  4. Injury to the vortex veins

Q **What are the Advantages of an IO Myomectomy Compared to IO Recession?**

	Myomectomy	Recession
Advantages	• Easy visualization and technique • Skilled assistant not needed • Consistent result • Lower risk of undercorrection	• Graded • Reversible potentially • Anteriorization for DVD
Disadvantages	• Dilate pupils • Not reversible • Cannot be graded (all or none) • No benefit for DVD	• More difficult • Need skilled assistant • Results less consistent

Q **What is the Duane's Syndrome?**

"Duane's syndrome is an ocular motility disorder."
"The main clinical feature is retraction of the globe on attempted adduction."
"It can be classified into 3 types...."

Duane's Syndrome

1. **Classification**
   - Type 1:
     - 60%
   - Limitation in **abduction**
   - Can present as an ET

- Type 2:
  - 15%
  - Limitation in **adduction**
  - Can present as an XT
- Type 3:
  - 25%
  - Limitation in **both** adduction and abduction
  - Usually orthophoric

2. **Clinical features:**
   - **Females** more common
   - **Left** eye in 60%, bilateral in 20%
   - Retraction of globe on adduction (sine qua non)
     - Co-contraction of MR and LR
     - Associated with narrowing of palpebral fissure
     - "What is the underlying pathogenesis?" Pontine dysgenesis with III CN innervating both MR and LR.
   - Upshoot or downshoot (lease phenomenon, do not mistake for IO overaction!)

3. **Ocular and systemic associations:**
   - Ocular associations (8%):
     - Ptosis
     - Epibulbar dermoids (associated Goldenhar syndrome)

- Anisocoria
- Persistent hyaloid artery
- Myelinated nerve fibers
- Nystagmus
- Lid and iris colobomas
- Optic disc and foveal hypoplasia
- Systemic associations:
  - Agenesis of genitourinary system
  - Bone (vertebral column abnormalities, syndactyly, polydactyly)
  - CNS (epilepsy)
  - **Deafness** (sensory neural deafness is the most common association; 16% of all Duane's syndrome)
  - **Dermatological** (café au lait spot)
- **Wildervank** syndrome (Duane's syndrome, deafness and Klippel-Fiel anomaly of spine)

4. **Management:**
   - Correct amblyopia
   - Indications for surgery:
     - Abnormal head posture
     - Unacceptable upshoot or downshoot
     - Squint in primary position
   - Liberal MR recession (may add LR recession)

Exam tips:
- **Systemic associations can be remember as ABCD.**

Q What is Brown's Syndrome?

"Brown's syndrome is an ocular motility disorder."
"The main problem is pathology of the SO tendon."
"It can be either congenital or acquired…."

Brown's Syndrome

1. **Classification**
   - Congenital:
     - Bilateral in 10%
     - Pathology: Short SO tendon, tight trochlea, nodule on SO tendon
   - Acquired:
     - Trauma
     - Tenosynovitis (rheumatoid arthritis)
     - Marfan's syndrome
     - Acromegaly
     - Extraocular surgery (RD surgery)

2. **Clinical features**
   - Classical triad:
     - Defective elevation in adduction (most important)

- Less severe defective elevation in midline
- Normal elevation in abduction
- **Vertical gaze triad:**
  - No SO overaction (i.e. not IO palsy!)
  - V pattern
  - Hypotropia in primary position
- **Additional triad:**
  - Positive forced duction test
  - Downshoot in adduction
  - Widening of palpebral fissure on adduction

3. **Management**
   - Correct amblyopia
   - Spontaneous recovery common
   - Steroids (oral or injection into trochlear area)

- Indications for surgery:
  - Abnormal head posture
  - Squint (hypotropia) in primary position
- Diplopia in downgaze
- SO tenotomy, silicon expander or chicken suture

	Brown's syndrome	IO palsy
Deviation in primary position	• Slight	• Significant hypotropia
Muscle sequalae	• Contralateral SR overaction	• Ipsilateral SO overaction
A or V pattern	• V	• A
Compensatory head posture	• Slight	• Marked chin elevation
Forced duction test	• Positive	• Negative

Exam tips:
- **Sometimes hard to differentiate form IO palsy.**
- **The clinical features can be remembered in triads.**

Notes

- **Causes of V pattern strabismus:**
  1. Brown's syndrome
  2. IO overaction secondary to IV nerve palsy
  3. LR overaction
  4. SR underaction
  5. Craniofacial anomalies e.g. Crouzon syndrome

- **Causes of A pattern strabismus:**
  1. SO overaction
  2. LR underaction
  3. IR underaction

STRABISMUS SURGERY

Overall yield: ✪✪✪   **Clinical exam:**   **Viva:** ✪✪✪   **Essay:** ✪   **MCQ:** ✪✪✪

Q Opening Question: What are the Indications for Squint Surgeries?

"In general, the indications for squint surgeries are...."

Indications for Squint Surgeries

1. **Anatomical (largely a "cosmetic" indication):**
   - Correct misalignment (large angle, increase frequency of breakdown if intermittent)

2. **Functional:**
   - Restore BSV (if child is young enough)
   - Correct abnormal head posture
   - Treat diplopia and confusion

Q What are the Principles of Squint Surgeries?

"The principles of squint surgeries are...."

Principles of Squint Surgeries

1. **Recess or resect? Recession is more forgiving**
2. **MR or LR? If deviation at near > at distance, consider operation on MR. If distance > near, consider LR**
3. **What are the indications of recess = resect operation on 1 eye?**
   - Constant squint in 1 eye

   - Amblyopia in 1 eye
   - Previous surgery in 1 eye
4. **How much to correct?**
   - Recess 1 mm = 4 prism D
   - Vertical muscle surgery 1 mm = 3 prism D
   - Resect 1 mm = 2 prism D
   - Recession of MR more effective than LR

Q How do You Perform a Recession (Resection) Operation?

"In a simple case of an XT with deviation worse at distance, I would perform a bilateral LR recession."

Recession Operation

1. **GA**
2. **U shaped fornix-based conjunctival peritomy**
3. **Isolate LR:**
   - Dissect Tenon's capsule on either side of LR muscle with Weskott scissors
   - Isolate LR muscle with squint hook
   - Clear off fascial sheath and ligaments with sponge
   - Spread muscle using Stevens hook

4. **Stitch two ends of muscle with 6/0 vicryl:**
   - One partial and 2 full-thickness bites dividing muscle into 3 parts
   - Clamp suture ends with Bulldog
   - For resection, measured distance to resect from insertion
5. **Cut muscle just anterior to stitches (for resection, cut muscle at the desired site)**
6. **Measure distance of recession**

7. **Resuturing of LR:**
   - Diathermize point of insertion to create ridge
   - Stitch each end of muscle to sclera or stitch to insertion stump using a hangback technique
   - For resection, stitch end to insertion stump

8. **Close conjunctiva with 8/0 vicryl**

Notes

- **Strabismus surgery with forniceal incision**
  - Advantages:
    1. Cosmetically superior
    2. Less discomfort
    3. No trauma to limbal area (stem cells, tear film disturbances etc)
    4. Obeys anatomical planes, hence less bleeding and scarring.
  - Disadvantages:
    1. Adequate exposure difficult — needs good assistant
    2. Suitable only for younger patients (usually less than 45 years of age) as Tenon's layer is atrophic in older patients

---

Q **What are the Indications for Adjustable Squint Surgeries?**

"In general, it is indicated in adult squints when a precise outcome is needed...."

Adjustable Squint Surgeries

1. **Indications:**
   - Adult squints:
     - Best for **rectus** muscles
     - Best with **recession** (principle: Recess more than necessary and adjust postoperatively)
   - Vertical squints
   - Thyroid eye disease
   - Blow out fractures
   - VI CN palsy
   - Reoperations

2. **Contraindications:**
   - Childhood squints
   - Patient unwilling to cooperate after operation
   - Oblique dysfunctions and DVD
   - Concomitant nystagmus

Q **What are the Complications of Squint Surgeries?**

"The complications can be divided into intraoperative, early and late postoperative complications...."
"The most dangerous intraoperative complications are scleral perforation and malignant hyperthermia."

Complications of Squint Surgeries

1. **Intraoperative ("M")**
   - Malignant hyperthermia (see below)
   - Lost muscle:
     - **MR** most common muscle lost
     - Muscle retracts into Tenon's capsule and usually ends up at apex
   - Slipped muscle:
     - Slip within muscle capsule
     - Prevented by adequate suture placement
     - Management similar to lost muscle
   - Scleral perforation:
     - Thinnest part of sclera (<0.3 mm just posterior to insertion)
     - Potential sequelae: RD, endophthalmitis, vitreous hemorrhage
     - Usually end up with chorioretinal scar
     - Management:
       - Stop operation and examine fundus
       - Consider cryotherapy at site of scar
       - Refer to retinal surgeon

- Others:
  - Oculo-cardiac reflex
  - Hemorrhage

2. **Early postoperative ("A")**
   - Alignment:
     - Most common complication
     - Under- or over-correction
     - Late misalignment caused by scarring, poor fusion, poor vision, altered accommodation
   - Anterior segment ischemia:
     - Operate on 3 or more recti
   - Adherence syndrome:
     - Tenon's capsule is violated
   - Allergic reaction
   - Infection:
     - Mild conjunctivitis

- Preseptal cellulites/orbital cellulites
- Endophthalmitis (missed perforation)

3. **Late postoperative ("D")**
   - Diplopia:
     - Can be early or late
     - Scenarios:
       - In children, diplopia resolves because of new suppression scotoma or of fusion
       - In adults, diplopia usually persists if squint is acquired after 10 years of age
     - Management:
       - Prisms
       - Diplopia awareness
       - Reoperation (adjustable surgery)
   - Droopy lids (ptosis)
   - Dellen and conjunctival cysts

Exam tips:
- The complications can be remembered using the mnemonic "MAD."
- Intraoperative complications begin with "M" (muscle and malignant hyperthermia).
- Early postoperative complications begin with "A" (anterior segment ischemia, alignment, etc).
- Late postoperative complications begin with "D" (diplopia, droopy lids, etc).

Notes
- "How do you manage a lost muscle?"
  - Stop operation (do not dig around frantically)
  - Microscopic exploration (look for suture ends within Tenon's capsule)
  - Irrigate with saline and adrenaline (Tenon's usually appears more white)
  - Watch for oculocardiac reflex when structures are pulled
  - If muscle cannot be found, abandon search
  - Postoperatively, can try CT scan localization
  - May consider reoperation/muscle transposition surgery

Q **How do You Manage Malignant Hyperthermia?**

"Malignant hyperthermia is a medical emergency and requires immediate recognition and management."

Malignant Hyperthermia

1. **Mechanism of action:**
   - Acute metabolic condition characterized by extreme heat production
   - Inhalation anesthetics (e.g. halothane) and muscle relaxants (succinlycholine) trigger following chain of events:
     - Increase free intracellular calcium
   - Excess calcium binding to skeletal muscles initiates and maintains contraction
   - Muscle contraction leads to anaerobic metabolism, metabolic acidosis, lactate accumulation, heat production and cell breakdown

2. **Clinical features:**
   - More common in children
   - Isolated case or family history (AD inheritance)
   - Early signs:
     - Tachycardia is earliest sign
     - Unstable BP
     - Tachypnea
     - Cyanosis
     - Dark urine
     - Trismus
     - Elevated carbon dioxide levels
     - Electrolyte imbalance
     - Renal failure
     - Cardiac failure and arrest
     - Disseminated intravascular coagulation

3. **Management:**
   - Stop triggering agents and finish surgery
   - Hyperventilate with 100% oxygen
   - Muscle relaxant (dantrolene)
   - Prevent hyperthermia:
     - IV iced saline
     - Iced lavage of stomach, bladder, rectum
     - Surface cool with ice blanket
   - Treat complications:
     - Sodium bicarbonate (metabolic acidosis)
     - Diuretics (renal failure)
     - Insulin (hyperkalemia)
     - Cardiac agents (cardiac arrhythmias)

Exam tips:
- One of the few life-threatening conditions in ophthalmology you need to know.

Q Tell me about Botulinum Toxin.

"Botulinum toxin or Botox is a toxin used for chemodenervation."
"The mechanism is believed to be...."
"The indications in ophthalmology include either squint or lid disorders...."

Botulinum Toxin

1. **Mechanism of action:**
   - Purified botulinum toxin A from *Clostridium botulinum*
   - Permanent blockage of **acetylcholine release** from nerve terminals
   - Injection with electromyographic guidance
   - After injection, Botox bound and internalized within 24–48 hours
   - Paralysis of muscle within **48–72** hours
   - Recovery by sprouting of **new** nerve terminals; paralysis recovers in 2 (squint) to 3 months (lid)

2. **Indications:**
   - Squint:
     - VI CN palsy (weakening of antagonistic MR to prevent contracture)
     - Small angle squints
     - Postoperative residual squint
   - Assess possibility of postoperative diplopia before squint operation in adults
   - When surgery is contraindicated
   - Part of transposition operation
   - Cyclic ET
   - Lid disorders:
     - Essential blepharospasm
     - Hemifacial spasm

3. **Complications:**
   - Intraoperative:
     - Scleral perforation
     - Retrobulbar hemorrhage
   - Postoperative:
     - Temporary ptosis (common)
     - Vertical squints
     - Diplopia
     - Mydriasis

TOPIC 8

RETINOBLASTOMA

Overall yield: ✪✪✪✪✪ **Clinical exam:** **Viva:** ✪✪✪✪✪ **Essay:** ✪✪✪✪ **MCQ:** ✪✪✪✪

Q Opening Question No. 1: Tell me about Retinoblastoma (RB).

"RB is a tumor of the primitive retinal cells."

Epidemiology

1. **RB is the most common primary, malignant, intraocular tumor of childhood**

2. **Eighth most common childhood cancer**

3. **Second most common intraocular tumor (after choroidal melanoma)**

4. **Incidence is 1 in 20,000 births (range 1 in 14,000 to 1 in 34,000)**

5. **No gender or racial variation**

Q Opening Question No. 2: Tell me about the Genetics of Retinoblastoma.

"Retinoblastoma gene is a tumor suppressor gene, which is located on…."
"RB can be divided into hereditary vs nonhereditary RB."

Genetics of Retinoblastoma

1. **RB gene (RB1)**
   - Maps to **chromosome 13 q14** (13 associated with bad luck)
   - Produces RB protein (pRB) that binds various cellular proteins to suppress cell growth
   - RB1 is a **recessive** oncogene at cellular level
   - Mutations of RB1 alleles result in cancer only in developing retina; other cell types die by apoptosis in absence of RB1
   - Primitive retinal cells disappear within first few years of life so RB is seldom seen after 3 or 4 years of age

2. **Knudson's 2 hit hypothesis**
   - Both alleles must be knocked out for tumor to develop

3. **Hereditary RB**
   - The patient inherits one mutant allele from parents and one normal allele which undergoes subsequent new mutation after conception

   (one of Knudson's 2 hits occur **prior** to conception)
   - **40**% of RB is hereditary type of RB
   - The risk of the Knudson's second hit/new mutation is extremely high (therefore RB is inherited as **AD trait** with 90% penetrance)
   - There is risk of bilateral RB (as all cells have inherited one mutant allele)
   - There is risk of non-ocular malignancies elsewhere (as all cells have one mutant allele)
   - Age of presentation: 1 year

4. **Nonhereditary RB**
   - Both alleles are normal after fertilization, but two or more subsequent spontaneous mutations inactivate both alleles (both of Knudson's 2 hits occur **after** conception)
   - **60**% of RB is nonhereditary type of RB
   - No risk of bilateral RB
   - No risk of nonocular malignancies elsewhere
   - Age of presentation: 2 years

Distinguish Between

Hereditary (inherited RB gene) vs nonfamilial	Bilateral vs Unilateral	Familial (positive family history) vs nonfamilial
Hereditary (40%) Nonhereditary (60%)	Bilateral (30%) Unilateral (70%): • 10–15% of unilateral cases are still hereditary RB • Therefore absence of bilateral RB does not rule out hereditary RB	Familial (6%) Nonfamilial (94%): • 25–30% of nonfamilial cases are still hereditary RB (the rate of new mutation is high) • Therefore a negative family history does not rule out hereditary RB

Exam tips:
- The FIRST of a few important topics in RB.
- Be clear about percentages (see table below).
- Distinguish between hereditary vs nonhereditary, familial vs nonfamilial and unilateral vs bilateral RB. It is conceptually easiest to talk about hereditary vs nonhereditary RB.

Q How do You Counsel Parents with a Child with RB?

"Risk of RB depends on presence or absence of family history and whether tumor is unilateral or bilateral."
"If there is a positive family history, the risk to the next child is 40%."
"If there is no family history, but the tumor is bilateral, the risk to the next child is 6%."
"If there is no family history and the tumor is unilateral, the risk to the next child is only 1%."

Genetic Counseling

	Chance of the following people having a baby with RB:		
	Parent	Affected child (patient)	Normal sibling
Family history	• 40%	• 40%	• 7%
No family history			
• Bilateral	• 6%	• 40%	• 1%
• Unilateral	• 1%	• 8%	• 1%

Q Opening Question No. 3: What is the Pathology of Retinoblastoma?

"RB is a tumor of the primitive retinal cells."
"Pathological it has distinct gross and microscopic features."

Pathology

1. **Originates from neuroretina (primitive cone cells)**

2. **Gross pathology**
   - **Endophytic** tumor:
     - Projects into vitreous cavity
     - White or pink
     - Cottage cheese appearance
   - Dystrophic calcification
   - Presents with endophthalmitis picture
   - **Exophytic** tumor:
     - Grows into subretinal space
     - Presents with total retinal detachment
   - **Diffuse** infiltrative tumor:

- Age of presentation: 6 years
- Presents with uveitis, glaucoma

3. Histopathology
- RB cells (**5 features**):
  - Twice the size of lymphocytes with round or oval nuclei
  - Hyperchromatic nuclei with little cytoplasm

- High mitotic activity
- Necrosis
- Calcification
- Arrangement (Homer Wright, Flexner Wintersteiner rosettes and fleurettes)

Type of arrangements	Differentiation	Features
Homer Wright	• **Neurobastic** differentiation	• Single row of columnar cells surrounding a central lumen • Central lumen is tangle of neural filaments • Can be seen in neuroblastoma and medulloblastoma
Flexner Wintersteiner	• **Early retinal** differentiation	• Single row of columnar cells surrounding a central lumen with a refractile lining • Cilia projects into lumen • Central lumen is subretinal space • Refractile lining is external limiting membrane • Can be seen in retinocytoma and pinealoblastoma
Fleurettes	• **Photoreceptor** differentiation	• Two rows of curvilinear cells • Inner cluster represents rod and cone inner segments • Outer cluster represents outer segment

Exam tips:
- **The SECOND of important topics in RB.**
- **The 5 histological features of RB should be contrasted with the 5 features of retinocytoma (see below).**

Q **What is a Retinocytoma?**

"Retinocytoma can be considered a benign variant of RB."
"Pathological and genetically it shares many characteristics of RD."

Retinocytoma
1. **Originates from neuroretina**
2. **Same genetic implications**
3. **Histopathology**
   - Retinocytoma (**5 features**):
     - Round or oval nuclei with even chromatin distribution

- More cytoplasm
- Low or no mitotic activity
- No necrosis
- Calcification not common
- Arrangement (Flexner Wintersteiner rosettes and fleurettes)

Exam tips:
- **A fairly common follow-up question to the pathology or genetics of RB.**

"The aims of management of RB are…."
"This depends on a team approach involving…."

Indications for Enucleation for RB

1. **Large unilateral tumor**
   - Large unilateral RB occupying more than 1/2 of globe
   - Large unilateral RB with no visual potential

2. **Associated complications**
   - Massive vitreous seeds

- Total retinal detachment
- Iris neovascularization
- Ciliary body involvement

3. **Failure of other treatment**

Exam tips:
- **Extremely difficult question. Answer with broad principles.**
- **Do not get into details too quickly.**

Q Tell me about Chemotherapy for Retinoblastoma.

"The indications for chemotherapy in RB are…."
"The current drugs under investigations include…."

Chemotherapy for RB

1. **Indications**
   - Curative:
     - Chemoreduction for small- and medium-size tumors
     - Vitreous/subretinal seeds (isolated local therapy is not good enough)
   - Palliative:
     - Tumor cells crossed lamina cribrosa/extraocular extension
     - Orbital recurrences
     - Metastasis

2. **Drugs used**
   - VEC (vincristine, etoposide, carboplatin)
   - VTC (tenoposide instead of etoposide)
   - Cyclosporin

3. **Cycles**
   - Four cycles:
     - Small to medium-size tumors, 4–10 disc diameters, <4mm thick
   - Seven to nine:
     - Larger tumors, vitreous seeds, RD, bone marrow or orbital involvement

4. **Response to chemotherapy**
   - 80% remission at 3 years
   - RB tumors frequently become "multi-drug resistant" and regrow after initial response
   - Related to expression of **P-glycoprotein (P170)** (note: This is a relatively "hot" topic!)
     - Increased P170 correlated with therapeutic failure in other tumors (neuroblastoma, rhabdomyosarcoma, leukemia, myeloma, lymphoma)
   - Favorable response to chemotherapy:
     - Considerable shrinkage after 2 cycles
     - Reduced vascularization or avascular tumor
     - Calcification (cottage-cheese appearance)
     - Disappearance or significant clearance of vitreous seeds
     - Resolution of extensive RD
   - Unfavorable response to chemotherapy:
     - Little shrinkage or calcification
     - Remains vascular or translucent (fish-flesh appearance)
     - Unchanged vitreous seeds

Exam tips:
- **Relatively "hot" topic for RB.**
- **See *Ophthalmology* 1997; 104: 2101–2111.**

Tell me about Second Cancers in Retinoblastoma.

"Second cancers are leading causes of death in patients with the hereditary type of RB."
"The incidence is…."
"The common tumors include…."
"The different modalities available include…."
"Factors to consider are…."

Management of Retinoblastoma

1. **Aims of management**
   - First goal to save life
   - Second goal to save eye
   - Third goal to maximize vision

2. **Team approach**
   - Ophthalmologist
   - Pediatric oncologist and radiation oncologist
   - Geneticist
   - Ocular prosthetist
   - Medical social worker and RB support group

3. **Treatment methods**
   - Enucleation
   - External beam radiotherapy
   - Chemotherapy (e.g. chemoreduction, systemic chemotherapy, subconjunctival chemoreduction, intrathecal cytosine arabinoside)
   - Focal therapy (e.g. laser, cryotherapy, radioactive plaque, thermotherapy)
   - Orbital exenteration

4. **Trends**
   - In the past, **enucleation** was standard treatment for small tumors within globe and external beam radiotherapy was standard for large tumors extending out of globe
   - Trend towards more **conservative** treatment for small to medium-size tumors
   - Increasing use of **chemotherapy** followed by **focal** therapy for small tumors and **plaque radiotherapy** for medium-size tumors

5. **Factors to consider**
   - Tumor size and location
   - Bilateral or unilateral disease
   - Visual potential of affected eye
   - Visual potential of unaffected eye
   - Associated ocular problems (e.g. RD, vitreous hemorrhage, iris neovascularization, secondary glaucoma)
   - Age and general health of child
   - Personal preferences of parents

6. **Follow-up**
   - Patients with treated RB and siblings at risk need to be followed up indefinitely
   - After initial treatment, re-examine patient 3–6 weeks later:
     - Active tumor on treatment requires follow-up every 3 weeks
     - If tumor is obliterated, follow-up 6–12 weeks later
   - 3-monthly until 2 years post-treatment, then 6 monthly until 6 years of age, then yearly for life

7. **Risk of new or recurrent retinoblastoma**
   - Risk of new RB decreases rapidly after 4 years of age to negligible risk after 7 years of age
   - Risk of recurrence of treated RB negligible after 2 years of completed treatment (unrelated to patient's age)

8. **Prognosis**
   - Location (**most important factor**):
     - **95**% 5-year survival if intraocular tumor
     - **5**% 5-year survival with extraocular extension/optic nerve involvement
   - Tumor size and grade
   - Iris rubeosis
   - Bilateral tumors (risk of second malignancy)
   - Age of patient (older is worse)

Notes

- **Presenting features of retinoblastoma:**
  - Leukocoria (60%)
  - Strabismus (20%)
  - Secondary glaucoma
  - Masquerade syndrome/iris nodules

(Continued)

(Continued)

- Orbital inflammation
- Routine examination of a patient at risk of RB
- Late presentation: Orbital invasion, metastases

Q | What are the Current Indications for Enucleation of Retinoblastoma?

"Enucleation remains the treatment of choice for large tumors."
"And in eyes with little or no potential vision."

Second Cancers in RB Patients

1. **Incidence**
   - Hereditary RB: **6%** over lifetime
   - Hereditary RB with external beam radiotherapy: Incidence **1% per year** in field of radiation (i.e. 30% in 30 years, 50% in 50 years)
   - Average age of diagnosis: **13 years** (note: Remember that RB gene is on chromosome **13**!)

2. **Type of tumors**
   - **Osteogenic sarcoma** is the most common cancer

- Pineoblastoma, ectopic intracanial RB (trilateral RB) is common up to 2 years after diagnosis of RB
- Beyond 2 years after diagnosis of RB:
  - Bony and soft tissue sarcomas (Ewing's tumor, chondrosarcoma, rhabdomyosarcoma)
  - Skin tumors (malignant melanoma, sebaceous cell CA, squamous cell CA)
  - Neuroblastoma, medulloblastoma, leukemia

Q | What is the Reese-Ellsworth Classification?

"Refers to a classification which relates to **VISUAL** prognosis (not mortality)."
"Based on size, number, location of tumor and vitreous involvement."

Reese-Ellsworth Classification

- Group I (very favorable, cure rate 95%):
  - Less than 4 DD
  - Solitary or multiple
  - Behind equator
  - No vitreous seeding
- Group II (favorable, 87%):
  - 4–10 DD
  - Solitary or multiple
  - Behind equator

- Group III (doubtful, 67%):
  - Larger than 10 DD
  - Anterior to equator
- Group IV (unfavorable, 50%):
  - Multiple, some larger than 10 DD
  - At ora
- Group V (very unfavorable, 34%):
  - Massive tumors involving 1/2 of retina
  - Vitreous seeding

Notes

International classification of RB (predicts those likely to be cured without need for enucleation or EBRT):

Group A: Small intraretinal tumors (≤3 mm) away from foveola (>3 mm) and disc (>1.5 mm)

Group B: All remaining discrete tumors confined to the retina

Group C: Discrete local (≤ 1/4 of retina) disease with minimal subretinal or vitreous seeding

Group D: Diffuse disease with significant vitreous or subretinal seeding

Group E: Presence of any one or more of these poor prognosis features:

- Tumor touching lens
- Tumor anterior to anterior vitreous face, involving ciliary body or anterior segment

(Continued)

- Diffuse infiltrating RB
- Neovascular glaucoma
- Opaque media from hemorrhage
- Tumor necrosis with aseptic orbital cellulitis
- Phthisis bulbi

Q **How do You Manage a Child with Leukocoria?**

"In a child with leukocoria, the most important diagnosis to exclude is retinoblastoma."
"However, the other common diagnoses for leukocoria are…."
"The management involves a complete history, ocular and systemic examination and appropriate investigations."

Leukocoria

1. **Causes of leukocoria**
   - Retinoblastoma
   - Other common causes:
     - Persistent hyperplastic primary vitreous (PHPV) (30% of cases)
     - Coat's disease (15%)
     - Toxocara (15%)
     - Congenital cataract
   - Vascular diseases:
     - ROP
     - Incontinentia pigmenti
   - Congenital/developmental anomalies:
     - Large coloboma
     - Retinal dysplasia
     - Juvenile retinoschisis
     - Norrie's disease
     - Combined hamartoma of retina and RPE
   - Other tumors:
     - Medulloepithelioma
     - Retinal astrocytoma

2. **History**
   - Age of presentation:
     - Birth (PHPV)
     - 1–3 years (RB)
     - Preschool (Coat's disease, toxocara)
   - Sex:
     - Male (Coat's disease, juvenile retinoschisis, Norrie's disease)
     - Female (incontinentia pigmenti)
   - Pregnancy history:
     - Gestational age (ROP)
     - Maternal health (TORCH syndromes)

   - Birth history:
     - Weight (ROP)
     - Trauma (congenital cataract, retinal detachment, vitreous hemorrhage)
     - Oxygen exposure (ROP)
   - Family history:
     - None (PHPV, Coat's disease, toxocara)
     - AD (RB)
     - SLR (juvenile retinoschisis, Norrie's disease)
     - AD/SLD (incontinentia pigmenti)

3. **Examination**
   - Unilateral (RB, PHPV, Coat's disease, toxocara and cataract)
   - Bilateral (RB, ROP, cataract, Norrie's disease, incontinentia pigmenti)
   - Normal size eye and no cataract (RB)
   - Microophthalmia or concomitant cataract (PHPV)
   - Other ocular abnormalities (Norrie's disease)

4. **Investigation**
   - Ultrasound:
     - Acoustically solid tumor with high internal reflectivity (RB)
     - Calcification (RB)
   - CT scans:
     - Calcification (RB)
     - Optic nerve, orbital and CNS involvement (RB)
   - MRI:
     - Detect pinealoblastoma (RB)
     - Optic nerve involvement (RB)

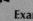

Exam tips:
- **Relatively common essay question.**
- **Remember NOT to focus solely on retinoblastoma.**

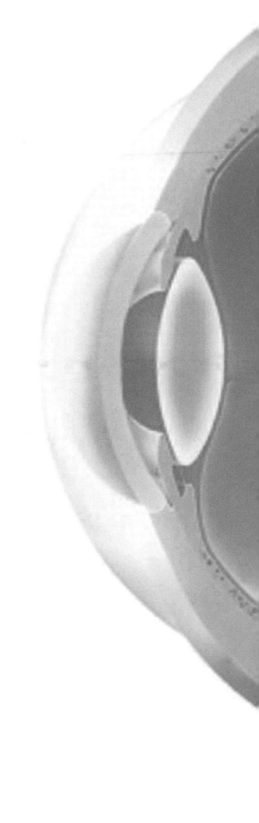

MISCELLANEOUS EXAMINATION PROBLEMS

TOPIC 1

OCULAR TRAUMA

Overall yield: ✪✪✪✪✪ **Clinical exam:** ✪✪ **Viva:** ✪✪✪✪ **Essay:** ✪✪✪✪ **MCQ:** ✪✪✪✪

Q **Opening Question:** What are the Possible Manifestations of Blunt Ocular Trauma?

"The ocular manifestations can be divided into orbit, anterior and posterior segment and neurological."

Blunt Ocular Trauma

1. **Orbital fracture**

2. **Anterior segment:**
   - Hyphema
   - Iris and angles:
     - Traumatic mydriasis, miosis
     - Angle recession, iridodialysis, cyclodialysis
   - Lens:
     - Traumatic cataract (Vossius ring)
     - Lens subluxation/dislocation

3. **Posterior segment:**
   - Vitreous hemorrhage
   - Commotio retinae
   - Vitreous base avulsion

- Retinal breaks and detachment:
  - Retinal dialysis
  - U-shaped tears and operculated retinal holes in the periphery
  - Giant retinal tear
  - Macular hole
- Choroidal rupture:
  - SRNVM
- Scleral rupture
- Optic nerve avulsion

4. **Neurological:**
   - Traumatic optic neuropathy
   - SO palsy

Exam tips:
- Because this problem is so "common" in daily clinical practice, candidates are frequently not adequately prepared for this question in examinations!

Q What are the Signs of Penetrating Ocular Trauma?

Signs of Penetrating Ocular Trauma

1. **Suggestive signs:**
   - Deep lid laceration
   - Conjunctiva:
     - Hemorrhage, laceration
     - Chemosis
   - Iris and AC:
     - Iridocorneal adhesion
     - Iris defect
     - Shallow AC
     - Hypotony

- Localized cataract
- Retinal tear/hemorrhage

2. **Diagnostic:**
   - Laceration with positive Siedal's test
   - Exposed uvea, vitreous and retina at wound
   - Visualization of IOFB
   - XR diagnosis of IOFB

"Management must be individualized…."

"The principles of management are to manage life-threatening injuries first, then assess severity of the eye injury, exclude IOFB and infection, restore globe integrity, and manage secondary injuries…."

Principles of Management of Penetrating Injury

1. **Manage life-threatening injuries first**

2. **Assess severity and extent of penetrating injury**

3. **Tetanus vaccine**

4. **Exclude IOFB:**
   - Suggestive features:
     - History (projectile foreign body, hammering related activities)
     - Examination: Visible entry wound, iris defect
   - Dilated fundal examination
   - XR orbit
   - B-scan
   - Consider CT scan

5. **If IOFB is present:**
   - Removal of IOFB indicated if injury is acute (e.g. within 24–48 hours):
   - If patient presents much later (e.g. 7 days), removal is indicated if:
     - Endophthalmitis is present
     - IOFB is toxic (e.g. copper, iron material)
     - IOFB is organic
     - Associated vitreous hemorrhage
     - IOFB is impacted onto retina
     - Secondary surgery is being considered (e.g. RD surgery)
   - Otherwise, can consider leaving IOFB *in situ*

6. **Exclude infection:**
   - No obvious signs of infection
     - Clean wound → prophylactic antibiotics (topical)
     - Dirty wound → prophylactic antibiotics (topical and systemic)
   - Endophthalmitis → therapeutic antibiotics (intravitreal, topical and systemic)

7. **Restore globe integrity:**
   - Principles:
     - Surgical closure of wound
     - Minimal distortion of globe anatomy
   - Procedure:
     - Eye shield to protect the eye before surgery

- Non-depolarizing anesthesia
- Eyelids retracted with Jeffrey's speculum (less pressure on globes) or lid sutures
- Swab for gram stain and cultures
- Clean eye with chlorhexidine (rather than iodine)
- Assess extent of injury
- AC paracentesis, re-form AC with viscoelastic, reposit prolapsing uveal tissue if still viable
- If wound limited to the cornea:
  - Close wound with 10–0 nylon
  - Sutures should be longer and more widely spaced near the limbus
  - Central corneal sutures are shorter and more closely spaced
  - Sutures should be deep (~3/4 of corneal thickness)
  - Water-tight closure essential (as wound may leak when corneal edema resolves)
- If wound involves both cornea and sclera:
  - Conjunctival peritomy to determine posterior limits of scleral wound (may need to disinsert extraocular muscles)
  - Appose limbus first with 8/0 or 10/0 nylon
  - Suture corneal wound (see above)
  - Scleral wound sutured with 8/0 nylon
  - Conjunctiva sutured with 8/0 vicryl
- Assess for Siedel's — ensure wounds are not leaking
- Subconjunctival and intracameral antibiotics
- KIV bandage contact lens
- Eye shield to protect eye
- Post-surgery:
  - Monitor closely for signs of infection
  - If no signs of infection, steroids can be started cautiously

8. **Assess secondary injuries and complications and manage accordingly**

Notes
- Ocular trauma score derived from:
  - Initial VA
  - Globe rupture
  - Endophthalmitis
  - Perforating injury
  - Retinal detachment
  - RAPD

Notes
- Parameters used to classify ocular trauma developed by the Ocular Trauma Classification Group *(Am J Ophthalmol* 1998;125:565–56):
  - Type of injury
  - Grade of injury (visual acuity)
  - Pupil (presence of RAPD)
  - Zone of injury (location)

Q   How would You Manage a Patient with a Penetrating Injury?

"Management of a patient with IOFB must be individualized...."
"The principles of management are to assess time of injury, site and nature of IOFB, exclude other complications and decide on whether the IOFB needs to be removed...."

Principles of Management of Penetrating Injury

1. **Factors to consider:**
   - **Time** of injury:
     - Acute or late presentation
   - Assess **site** of IOFB:
     - Anterior or posterior segment
     - Free-floating in vitreous or incarcerated with tissues
   - Assess **nature** of IOFB:
     - Organic or nonorganic
     - Inert or toxic

2. **Exclude infection and secondary injuries**
   - Cataract will cause poor view of posterior segment
   - RD

3. **Removal of IOFB indicated if injury acute (e.g. 24–48 hours):**
   - If patient presents much later (e.g. 7 days), removal is indicated if:
     - Endophthalmitis is present
     - IOFB is toxic (e.g. copper, iron material)

   - IOFB is organic
   - Associated vitreous hemorrhage
   - IOFB is impacted onto retina
   - Secondary surgery is being considered (e.g. RD surgery)

4. **Type of surgery:**
   - Small, free-floating metallic IOFB in vitreous → removal with intraocular magnet
   - Large nonmetallic IOFB incarcerated in retina → vitrectomy, lensectomy and intraocular forceps:
     - A small rare earth magnet can be used to mobilize foreign body from retinal surface

Clinical approach to ocular trauma

"This patient had ocular injury three months ago. Please examine him."
"There are periorbital and lid scars seen…."

Look for
- Corneal injury — laceration scars, suture wounds, siderosis bulbi, blood staining
- AC depth — uneven (lens subluxation)
- Iris — iridodialysis, traumatic mydriasis
- Lens — phacodonesis, cataract
- Vitreous in AC

I'd like to
- Check IOP and perform a gonioscopy (angle recession, cyclodialysis)
- Examine the pupils for RAPD (traumatic optic neuropathy)
- Examine the fundus:
  - Macular hole
  - Retinal breaks, detachment and dialysis
  - Choroidal rupture
  - Optic atrophy
- Check extraocular movements (SO palsy)

COLOR VISION

Overall yield: ✪✪✪✪ **Clinical exam:** **Viva:** ✪✪✪✪ **Essay:** ✪ **MCQ:** ✪✪✪

Q Opening Question: What is Color Vision?

"Color vision is the ability to **perceive** and **differentiate** colors."
"It is the sensory response to stimulation of **cones** by light of wavelength **400–700 nm.**"
"The physiological basis is the **relative absorption** of different wavelengths by the three cones."
"Color itself can be described in terms of its **hue, saturation** and **brightness**...."

Color Vision

1. **Definition:**
   - Sensory response to stimulation of cones by light of wavelength 400–700 nm
   - Relative absorption of different wavelengths by cone outer segment visual pigments

2. **Two basic theories:**
   - **Trichromatic theory** = selective wavelength absorption
     - Three types of photolabile visual pigments:
       - Short wavelength: Absorbed by "blue" cones
       - Middle wavelength: Absorbed by "green" cones
       - Long wavelength: Absorbed by "red" cones

   - **Opponent color theory** = stimulation and inhibition of different "receptive fields"
     - "Receptive fields" of color sensitive cells have regions that compare intensity of:
       - Red vs green
       - Blue vs yellow

3. **Description of color:**
   - Hue ("color"): Refers to wavelength
   - Saturation: Refers to depth of color, purity or richness of color
   - Brightness: Refers to intensity or radiant flux

Exam tips:
- **Extremely common question in the *viva*.**

Q What is Color Blindness?

"Color blindness can be divided into congenital vs acquired...."

1. **Color blindness**
   - Congenital:
     - 8% of all males and 0.5% all females
     - **SLR** inheritance
     - **Red-green** abnormality
     - Patients are not "aware" of wrong color
     - Bilateral and symmetrical between 2 eyes
   - Acquired:
     - Males and females equally affected
     - No inheritance pattern
     - **Yellow-blue** abnormality
     - Patients use incorrect color names or report that color appearance of familial objects (e.g. apple) has changed
     - Unilateral or asymmetrical between two eyes

2. **Classification:**
   - Clinical: Based on **color matching:**
     - Trichromats: Require all 3 primary colors to match an arbitrary color (possess 3 normal cones)
     - Dichromats: Require only 2 colors (loss of 1 type of cone)
     - Monochromats: Cannot match any color (loss of 2 or 3 types of cones)
   - Anomalous trichromats: Require 3 colors, but in abnormal proportions
   - Pathological: Based on loss or abnormality of **cone pigments:**
     - Loss of red sensitive cone: Protan defect
     - Loss of green sensitive cone: Deutan defect
     - Loss of blue/yellow sensitive cone: Tritan defect

Q   **What is Achromatopsia?**

"Achromatopsia is a congenital color blindness with absence of color discrimination."
"It can be divided into blue cone monochromatism of rod monochromatism…."

Achromatopsia

1. **Types:**
   - Blue cone monochromatism:
     - Only blue sensitive cones present. Loss of both red and green cones. Because only one cone is present, there is no effective cone function
     - SLR
   - Rod monochromatism:
     - Loss of 3 cones (e.g. true achromatopsia/true color blindness)
     - AR
     - Sees with shades of gray

2. **Diagnosis:**
   - Present with congenital nystagmus, poor VA and photoaversion
   - ERG:
     - Absence of cone responses
     - Rod ERG normal
   - Dark adaptation test:
     - No cone plateau
     - No cone rod break

Q   **Tell me about Color Vision Tests.**

"They can be divided into **quantitative** or **qualitative** tests…."

Color Vision Tests

1. **Quantitative (both sensitive and specific)**
   - **Farnsworth-Munsell 100 hue test:**
     - Based on matching hues/color
     - Consists of 84 colored discs
     - Discs arranged in sequence (increasing levels of hue)
     - Test is then scored
     - Difference in hues between adjacent tablets is 1–4 nm
     - Accurate in classifying color deficiency
     - Very sensitive
     - Time consuming and tiring
   - **Nagel's anomaloscope:**
     - Based on matching luminance or brightness
     - Good for congenital red-green color defects
     - Sensitive

2. **Qualitative (more sensitive, but less specific):**
   - **Farnsworth 15 panel**
     - More rapid and convenient to use than 100 hue test
     - 15 colored tablets
     - Hues more saturated than 100 hue test
     - Tablets arranged in sequence
     - Errors plotted very quickly on a simple circular diagram to define nature of color deficiency
     - Not very sensitive
     - Useful in judging practical significance of color deficiency
     - Desaturated versions available to recognize more subtle degrees of color deficiency
     - Discriminates well between congenital and acquired defects
       - Congenital defects:
         - Very precise protan/deutan pattern
       - Acquired defects:
         - Irregular pattern or errors
         - Shows tritan errors very clearly
   - **Pseudoisochromatic color plate test:**
     - Examples: Ishihara/AO Hardy Rand Rittler

- Gross estimate of acquired color loss and central visual dysfunction

- Quick, available, useful
- Test congenital red-green defects

"The Ishihara plates is a type of qualitative color vision test...."

Ishihara Plates

1. **Test in well-illuminated room**
2. **Held 75 cm from subject and perpendicular to line of sight**
3. **Literate patients use plates 1–17**
   - Answer given within 3 seconds
4. **Illiterate patients use plate 18–24**
   - Lines traced with a brush within 10 seconds
5. **Results:**
   - 13 plates correct: Normal color vision
   - < 9 plates correct: Deficient color vision

- Only reads "12": Total color blindness
- Reads first 7 plates (except "12") incorrectly and unable to read the rest: Red-green deficiency
- Reads "26" as 6 and "42" as 2: Protan defect
- Reads "26" as 2 and "42" as 4: Deutan defect
- Unable to read all plates, including "12" (despite good VA): Suspect functional color blindness

LASERS IN OPHTHALMOLOGY

Overall yield: ✸ ✸ ✸   **Clinical exam:**   **Viva:** ✸ ✸ ✸   **Essay:** ✸   **MCQ:** ✸ ✸ ✸

Q Opening Question: What is a Laser? What are the Basic Components of a Laser System?

"Laser stands for…."

Lasers

1. Definition:

- Laser = **L**ight **A**mplification by **S**timulated **E**mission of **R**adiation
- Laser light is:
  - Monochromatic (same wavelength)
  - Coherent (in phase)
  - Polarized (in one plane)
  - Collimated (in one direction and nonspreading)
  - High energy

2. Basic components:

- Power source:
  - Generate energy
- Active medium:
  - Special properties to emit photons
- Chamber:
  - Stores active medium
  - Mirrors at opposite ends to reflect energy back and forth (optical feedback)
  - One of the mirror partially transmits energy

> **Exam tips:**
> - **See relevant sections in glaucoma (page 77) and retina (pages 178 and 190).**

Q What are the Lasers available in Ophthalmology?

"Lasers can be classified either by their clinical effects or by the active medium…."

Laser Classification

1. Clinical effects

- Photocoagulation (thermal effect):
  - Temperature raised to 80°C
  - Coagulation of **proteins**
  - Clinical effect: Burn tissue
  - Example: Argon laser, Nd:YAG laser in "continuous mode"

- Photodisruption:
  - Temperature raised to 15,000°C
  - **Interatomic** forces are destroyed (electrons stripped from atoms)
  - Plasma formation (fourth state of matter, physical properties of gas, electrical properties of metal)
  - Clinical effect: Cut tissue

- Example: Nd:YAG laser in "Q switched or mode locked"
- Photoablation:
  - No release of heat
  - **Interatomic** forces are destroyed (carbon-carbon bonds are broken)
  - Clinical effect: Etch tissue
  - Example: Excimer

2. **Active medium**
   - Gas lasers:
     - Argon, krypton, carbon dioxide
   - Solid state (crystals) lasers:
     - Nd:YAG, holmium: YAG
   - Liquid lasers:
     - Dye lasers
   - Others:
     - Diode, excimer

VITAMINS, ALCOHOL, DRUGS AND SKIN

Overall yield: ✹✹   **Clinical exam:**   **Viva:** ✹✹   **Essay:** ✹   **MCQ:** ✹✹✹

Q Opening Question: What are the Associations between Vitamin and the Eye?

"Vitamin **deficiency** or **excess** causes eye diseases."
"Vitamins can also be used for **treatment.**"

Vitamins and the Eye

1. **Deficiency:**
   - Vitamin A (see below)
   - Vitamin B:
     - Optic neuropathy
     - Angular blepharoconjunctivitis (B2)
     - Gyrate atrophy (B6) (page 220)
     - Flame-shaped hemorrhage (B12)
   - Vitamin C:
     - Subconjunctival hemorrhage
   - Vitamin D:
     - Associated with proptosis

2. **Excess:**
   - Vitamin A:
     - Benign intracranial hypertension (page 262)

   - Vitamin D:
     - Band keratopathy (metastatic calcification)

3. **Treatment:**
   - Vitamin A (abetalipoproteinemia in Bassen Kornzweig syndrome) (page 215)
   - Vitamin B6 (gyrate atrophy, homocystinuria)
   - Vitamin C (chemical injury)
   - Vitamin E (abetalipoproteinemia in Bassen Kornzweig syndrome, ROP)
   - Vitamin K (coagulation problem)

Q Tell me about Vitamin A Deficiency.

"Vitamin A deficiency is one of the common causes of blindness in the world."

1. **Role of vitamin A:**
   - Precursor of photosensitive visual pigment
   - Outer segment turnover
   - Maintain conjunctival mucosa and corneal stroma

2. **Clinical features/WHO classification:**
   - XN: Night blindness
   - X1
   - X1A: Conjunctiva xerosis
   - X1B: Bitot's spots

   - X2: Corneal xerosis
   - X3
     - X3A: Corneal ulceration/keratomalacia < 1/3 corneal surface
     - X3B: Corneal ulceration/keratomalacia > 1/3 corneal surface
   - XS: Corneal scarring
   - XF: Xerophthalmic fundus

Exam tips:
- Vitamins affect both the front (conjunctiva/cornea) and the back (retina) of the eye.
- See also vitamin A cycle (page 145).

Q **What Systemic Drugs Have Established Ocular Toxicities?**

Classification	Site	Syndrome	Drugs
Anterior segment	• Conjunctiva	• Steven Johnson's syndrome	• Sulphonamides
	• Cornea	• Vortex keratopathy (page 117)	• Amiodarone • Chloroquine • Chlorpromazine • Tamoxifen • Indomethacin
		• Band keratopathy	• Vitamin D
	• Angles	• Glaucoma	• Steroids
	• Lens	• Cataract	• Steroids • Amiodarone • Chlorpromazine • Gold • Busulphan
Posterior segment	• Retina	• Retinotoxicity	• Chloroquine (see below)
	• Optic nerve	• Optic neuropathy (page 248)	• Ethambutol, boniazid, streptomycin • Alcohol • Chloroquine • Chloramphenicol • Digitalis • Tamoxifen • Chemotherapeutic agents
Neurological		• BIH Benign intracranial hypertension (page 262)	• Steroid • Tetracycline • Nalidixic acid • Vitamin A

Q **What are the Patterns of Retinal Toxicity with Systemic Drugs?**

Retinal Toxicity

1. **RPE/photoreceptor dysfunction**
   - Chloroquine, hydroxychloroquine
   - Phenothiazines
   - Deferoxamine (treatment of thalassemia)

2. **Vascular**
   - Quinine
   - Oral contraceptive

3. **Macular edema**
   - Nicotinic acid (treatment of hyperlipidemia)
   - Oral contraceptive

4. **Crystalline retinopathy**
   - Tamoxifen
   - Canthaxanthine (used to enhance sun-tanning)
   - Methoxyflurane (anesthetic agent)

5. **Color vision**
   - Digoxin

Effects of Alcohol

1. **Indirect effects on the eye:**
   - Risk factor for cardiovascular disease and ocular ischemia (see page 200)
   - Risk factor for ocular trauma
   - Drug interactions

2. **Direct effects on the eye:**
   - Toxic optic neuropathy (page 248)
   - Fetal alcohol syndrome

Skin Disorders and the Eye

1. **Acneiform disorders:**
   - Acne rosacea

2. **Bullous dermatoses:**
   - Ocular pemphigus, ocular pemphigoid
   - Steven Johnson's disease

3. **Congenital skin disorders:**
   - Albinism
   - Incontinentia pigmenti
   - Xeroderma pigmentosum
   - Congenital ichthyosis

4. **Connective tissue disorders:**
   - Systemic lupus
     - Butterfly rash, discoid lupus, photosensitivity, alopecia, telangiectasia
   - Scleroderma
     - Sclerodactyly, telangiectasia, Raynaud's phenomenon, digital ulcers
   - Rheumatoid arthritis
     - Rheumatoid nodules, vasculitic skin lesions, generalized rash of Still's disease
   - Sarcoidosis
     - Erythema nodosum, lupus pernio, sarcoid granulomas
   - Wegener's granulomatosis
     - Purpura, hemorrhagic vesicles, gingival hyperplasia

5. **Dermatitis:**
   - Atopic dermatitis

6. **Infections:**
   - Herpes simplex, herpes zoster, AIDS

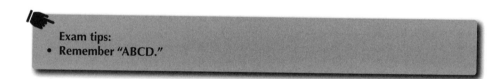

Exam tips:
- Remember "ABCD."

"Atopic dermatitis is a chronic inflammatory dermatitis with skin and ocular manifestations."

Atopic Dermatitis

1. **Skin findings:**
   - Acute: Exudation, vesicles, crusting
   - Chronic: Lichenification, pigmentation

2. **Ocular findings:**
   - Blepharitis, conjunctivitis
   - Vernal or atopic keratoconjunctivitis
   - Keratoconus
   - Cataract (anterior lamellar cataract)
   - RD (increased risk of RD after cataract surgery)

EPIDEMIOLOGY, PUBLIC HEALTH AND RESEARCH METHODS

Overall yield: ✪   **Clinical exam:**   **Viva:** ✪   **Essay:** ✪   **MCQ:** ✪

Q **Opening Question:** How would You Test a New Drug X in the Treatment of Glaucoma?

Steps in RCT

1. **Background research into clinical problem:**
   - Do you need a new drug?
   - What are the current therapies and how effective are they? (e.g. efficacy, side effects)
   - What are the characteristics of the ideal drug (long-term efficacy, side effects, costs, etc)

2. **Define study population:**
   - Restricted population or generalized population?
   - Early glaucoma or advanced glaucoma?
   - New cases or those on previous follow-up?
   - Include patients with concomitant diseases (e.g. DM)?

3. **Randomization:**
   - New drug vs placebo?
   - New drug vs established drugs?
   - Cross-over study design (drug and placebo are exchanged in course of RCT)?

4. **Masking:**
   - Single (participants), double (participants and investigators) or triple (participants, investigators and reviewers) masking?
   - Unmasking protocol (when do you stop?)

5. **Outcome:**
   - VA?
   - Lower IOP?
   - Optic disc and VF changes?
   - Complications?

6. **Exit protocol:**
   - Failure definitions (when do you consider whether a drug has worked or not worked?)
   - If it does not work, then what? How long do you wait?
   - If it works better than old therapy, how much is the effect?

7. **Statistics:**
   - Sample size and power issues
   - Randomization protocol
   - Statistical significance

8. **Other issues:**
   - Ethics

Exam tips:
- Candidates will be expected to know something about research methods and randomized clinical trials (RCT).

Prevention Strategies

1. **Primary prevention — prevent disease, usually before occurrence of symptoms**
   - Screening for DR and glaucoma
2. **Secondary prevention — prevent progression of disease, before occurrence of complications**
   - Lower IOP in glaucoma
3. **Tertiary prevention (controversial) — prevent effects of complications on morbidity (and mortality)**
   - PRP for PDR

Screening

1. **Definition:**
   - Presumptive identification of unrecognized disease by application of tests which can be applied rapidly
   - Screening for asymptomatic people
   - Raises ethical and societal issues (who to screen? At what costs?)
2. **Goals of screening:**
   - Primary prevention if possible; usually this cannot be achieved
   - Secondary prevention by improving outcome of disease by early detection and treatment
3. **Criteria for screening of a disease:**
   - Important public health problem (high prevalence, high rate of morbidity).
   - Natural history understood (asymptomatic latent phase must be present)
   - Acceptable, effective and available treatment
   - Early detection has effect on treatment outcome and natural history
   - Acceptable, reliable (repeatable) and valid (high sensitivity and specificity) screening test at reasonable cost

Disease	Public health problem	Natural history and treatment	Screening test
Glaucoma	• 50–60 million • 5–6 million blind • Can measure glaucoma • Can treat risk factor (IOP)	• Definition of glaucoma? • Natural history not well understood • Natural history of ocular hypertension (risk of glaucoma is 1%/year) • Need for treatment? • Better outcome with early treatment? • Medical vs surgical?	• Screening tests? • All screening test low sensitivity and specificity • Screening tests acceptable? • Costs of screening?

(Continued)

(*Continued*)

Disease	Public health problem	Natural history and treatment	Screening test

Diabetic retinopathy	• Most common cause of blindness in 30–50 years (working population):
	• 2% of population in U.S. (50 million patients)
	• 30% NPDR
	• 13% vision threatening DR (6 million patients/12 million eyes need treatment)
	• 24% million laser sessions or 500,000 per week
	• Cost US$4.8 billion/year
		• Natural history fairly clear
		• Well-defined asymptomatic stage
		• High risk factors identified:
		  • Duration of DM
		  • Control of DM
		  • HPT
		  • Smoking is not risk factor
		• Early treatment beneficial
		• Cost savings for society
			• What screening tests?
			  1. DR photography — dilated vs nondilated
			  2. Direct fundoscopy — dilated vs nondilated
			  3. FFA
			• Who should screen?
			  1. Ophthalmologists
			  2. Internists
			  3. Family physicians
			  4. Optometrists
			• How often to screen?
			• Training of family physicians?

Amblyopia	• Usually not reflected in prevalence of blindness statistics • No good prevalence data on amblyopia • 2% of population (estimate in white population) • 15% of unilateral blindness	• Definition of amblyopia? • Different types of amblyopia • Long term effectiveness of amblyopia treatment not proven • Optimal length of occlusion? • No value in treatment after age 6 years • Early treatment beneficial (proven)	• Screening may be important because treatment ineffective • School children too old? • No captive population for preschool children • Vision screening tests difficult in children under 3
Cataract	• 15 million people blind from cataract	• Surgery is effective • Cost-effectiveness of surgery?	• ICCE vs ECCE? • Cataract camps? • One eye vs two?
Trachoma	• 5 million people blind	• Natural history fairly clear • Well-defined disease • Early treatment beneficial • Treatment cheap	

Exam tips:
• **Only certain issues are highlighted here. Refer to textbooks for details.**

LAST MINUTE PHYSIOLOGY

Overall yield: ✹ ✹ ✹ **Clinical exam:** **Viva:** ✹ ✹ ✹ **Essay:** **MCQ:** ✹ ✹

Q Opening Question: What is Visual Acuity? What is Snellen VA?

"Visual acuity is the measurement of **spatial resolution** of the eye."

Visual Acuity

1. **Minimum VISIBLE VA**
   - Determines presence or absence of target
   - Threshold: 1 second of ARC

2. **Minimum RESOLVABLE VA (ordinary VA)**
   - Determines presence of identifying/ distinguishing feature in visible target
   - Threshold: 30 sec to 1 min of ARC
   - Snellen VA:
     - Measures minimum resolvable visual acuity
     - In normal observer, the minimum resolvable angle is 30 sec to 1 min of ARC
     - Snellen chart has letters that subtend 5 min of ARC, each part (stroke) of the letter subtends 1 min of ARC

   - Letters are made of different sizes and designated by distance at which letter subtends 5 min of ARC, e.g. letters on 20/20 line subtend 5 min of ARC when viewed at 20 feet
   - Patient asked to recognize progressively smaller letters or forms

3. **Minimum DISCRIMINABLE (hyperacuity)**
   - Spatial distinctions can be made at lower than ordinary VA
   - Determines positions of 2 or more visible features relative to each other
   - Threshold: 2–10 sec of ARC

Q What is Contrast Sensitivity?

"Contrast sensitivity is the ability to detect slight **changes** in luminance/brightness."

Contrast Sensitivity

1. **Contrast is a variation of brightness of an object:**
   - Dependent on **difference** in maximum brightness and minimum brightness
   - A 100% contrast target is a target composed of letters printed with perfectly black ink (i.e. totally nonreflecting) on perfectly white paper (100% reflecting)

2. **Snellen chart is a measure of VA under approximately 100% contrast condition**

3. **Clinical measurement: Present targets of various spatial frequencies and various peak contrast**

"Visual adaptation is phenomenon in which exposure of eye to light results in...."

- Increased spatial acuity
- Increased temporal acuity

- Decreased sensitivity
- And exposure to darkness results in reverse of above

"Dark adaptation is the measure of rod and cone **sensitivity** in darkness after exposure to light."
"Ability of visual system (both rod and cone mechanisms) to recover sensitivity following exposure to light."

EXPLANATION OF TERMS

Overall yield:

☆ = Rarely asked in any parts of the exams. Study only if you have enough time.
☆☆ = Uncommon question in some areas of the exams. Study to do well.
☆☆☆ = Common basic core knowledge. Expected to know principals of topic fairly well.
☆☆☆☆ = Important and common. Expected to know topic with a fair amount of details included.
☆☆☆☆☆ = Extremely important and common. Condition is usually sight threatening. Expected to have in-depth knowledge of topic. Poor answer in this topic will likely lead to failure in that question.

Clinical exam:

☆ = Rare clinical condition of no significance. Expected to have heard of condition.
☆☆ = Uncommon clinical condition. Expected to describe clinical signs.
☆☆☆ = Common clinical condition. Expected to come to diagnosis or differential diagnoses.
☆☆☆☆ = Important and common condition. Expected to diagnose condition with ease.
☆☆☆☆☆ = Extremely important and common. Expected to diagnose condition, exclude other conditions, ask appropriate questions and initiate discussion.

Viva:

☆ = Rarely asked.
☆☆ = Uncommon question.
☆☆☆ = Basic core viva knowledge. Expected to know principles around the topic.
☆☆☆☆ = Important and common. Expected to know topic reasonably well with a fair amount of details.
☆☆☆☆☆ = Extremely important and common. Expected to know topic inside out. Poor answer in this topic will likely lead to failure of that question.

Essay:

☆ = Rarely asked.
☆☆ = Uncommon question.
☆☆☆ = Basic core knowledge. Expected to know principles about the topic.
☆☆☆☆ = Important and common. Expected to write full-length essay on topic.
☆☆☆☆☆ = Extremely important and common. Expected to write with enough details to get a good score.

MCQ:

☆ = Rare.
☆☆ = Uncommon.
☆☆☆ = Common.
☆☆☆☆ = Very common.
☆☆☆☆☆ = Extremely common. High-yield facts for MCQ.

COMMON ABBREVIATIONS

AC	Anterior chamber
ACE	Angiotensin-converting enzyme
ACG	Angle closure glaucoma
AD	Autosomal dominant
AMD	Age-related macular degeneration
ANA	Anti-nuclear antibody
AR	Autosomal recessive
ARC	Anomalous retinal correspondence
B scan	B-mode ultrasonography
BIO	Binocular indirect ophthalmolscopy
BP	Blood pressure
BRAO	Branch retinal artery occlusion
BRVO	Branch retinal vein occlusion
CA	Carcinoma
CBC	Complete blood count
CDR	Cup-disc ratio
CME	Cystoid macular edema
CMV	Cytomegalovirus
CN	Cranial nerve
CNS	Central nervous system
CRA	Central retinal artery
CRAO	Central retinal artery occlusion
CRV	Central retinal vein
CRVO	Central retinal vein occlusion
CSF	Cerebrospinal fluid
CT scan	Computer tomographic scan
CVA	Cerebrovascular accident
CXR	Chest X-ray

DM	Diabetes mellitus
DR	Diabetic retinopathy
DRS	Diabetic retinopathy study
DVD	Dissociated vertical deviation
DXT	Deep radiotherapy
ECCE	Extracapsular cataract extraction
ECG	Electrocardiogram
EOM	Extraocular movements
EP	Esophoria
ERG	Electroretinogram
ERM	Epiretinal membrane
ESR	Erythrocyte sedimentation rate
ET	Esotropia
ETDRS	Early treatment for diabetic retinopathy study
FFA	Fundal fluorescein angiography
FTA	Fluorescein treponemal antibody test for syphilis
GA	General anesthesia
HM	Hand movement
HPT	Hypertension
HSV	Herpes simplex virus
HVF	Humphrey visual field
HZV	Herpes zoster virus
ICCE	Intracapsular cataract extraction
IDDM	Insulin dependent diabetes mellitus
INO	Inter-nuclear ophthalmoplegia
IO	Inferior oblique
IOFB	Intraocular foreign body
IOL	Intraocular lens implant
IOP	Intraocular pressure
IR	Inferior rectus
IV	Intravenous
LA	Local anesthesia
LPS	Levator palpebrae superioris
LR	Lateral rectus
MG	Myasthenia gravis
MLF	Medial longitudinal fasiculus
MR	Medial rectus
MRI	Magnetic resonance imaging
MS	Multiple sclerosis

NIDDM	Non-insulin dependent diabetes mellitus
NLD	Nasolacrimal duct
NPDR	Non-proliferative diabetic retinopathy
NPL	No perception of light
NV	New vessels
NVD	New vessels at the disc
NVE	New vessels elsewhere
OAG	Open angle glaucoma
OCT	Optical coherence comography
OKN	Optokinetic
ON	Optic nerve
PACG	Primary angle closure glaucoma
PC	Posterior chamber
PCO	Posterior capsule opacification
PCR	Posterior capsule rupture
PDR	Proliferative diabetic retinopathy
PI	Peripheral iridotomy
PKP	Penetrating keratoplasty
PMMA	Polymethylmethacrylate
POAG	Primary open angle glaucoma
POHS	Presumed ocular histoplasmosis syndrome
PPRF	Parapontine reticular formation
PRP	Panretinal photocoagulation
PVD	Posterior vitreous detachment
RA	Rheumatoid arthritis
RAPD	Relative afferent papillary defect
RB	Retinoblastoma
RD	Retinal detachment
RF	Rheumatoid factor
ROP	Retinopathy of prematurity
RP	Retinitis pigmentosa
RPE	Retinal pigment epithelium
SLE	Slit lamp examination
SLR	Sex linked recessive
SO	Superior oblique
SR	Superior rectus
SRF	Subretinal fluid
SRNVM	Subretinal neovascular membrane
SXR	Skull X-ray

TB	Tuberculosis
TRD	Tractional retinal detachment
VA	Visual acuity
VDRL	Venereal disease research laboratory test for syphilis
VEGF	Vascular endothelial growth factor
VEP	Visual evoked potential
VF	Visual field
VH	Vitreous hemorrhage
VKH	Vogt Koyanagi Harada syndrome
VOR	Vestibulocular reflex
XP	Exophoria
XR	X-ray
XT	Exotropia

INDEX

vitrectomy 13, 36–38, 42, 87, 103, 152, 183, 185, 188, 191–194, 219, 221, 222, 227–229, 231, 247, 251, 439, 485

diplopia
examination 453
pathophysiological basis 454

dissociated vertical deviation 459, 465

Doll's eye reflex 338

Down's syndrome 7–9, 11, 12, 139, 140, 217, 429

dragged optic disc 401, 435

dropped nucleus 35, 37, 191

drug toxicity 234

Drusens 181, 200, 209–211, 242, 431, 432
age-related macular degeneration 209
optic disc 9, 31, 49, 55, 56, 69, 71, 73–75, 79, 82, 85, 87, 143, 148, 178, 197, 210, 222, 234, 247, 253, 257, 258, 263, 295, 301, 303, 309, 317, 332, 335, 342, 343, 397, 428, 431, 432, 467, 497

Duane's syndrome 112, 269, 270, 276, 278, 279, 282, 295, 445, 459, 463, 466, 467

dysthyroid eye disease. See thyroid eye disease

E

ectropian 11, 122, 364

electrooculogram 205, 206

electrophysiology 205
electroretinogram 205
electrooculogram 205, 206
visual evoked potential 205, 207, 341

electroretinogram 205

empty sellar syndrome 316

empty socket syndrome 387

endophthalmitis 25, 35, 36, 38, 39, 67, 89, 100, 102, 105, 121, 153, 189, 191, 192, 213, 214, 219, 386, 394, 401, 402, 429, 471, 474, 484, 485

entoptic phenomenon 198, 339, 449

entropian 122

enucleation 118, 255, 385–387, 434, 476–478

epidemiology
eye disease 52, 107, 125, 126, 214, 269, 271, 272, 278, 285, 302, 358, 367, 370–372, 431, 437–439, 443, 447, 459, 463, 465, 470, 493

epiphora 381, 382, 416

epiretinal membrane 178, 191, 218, 219, 220, 235, 339, 404, 435

esotropia 459, 460
accommodative 459
cause 459
congenital 459

evisceration 385, 386

exenteration 377, 379, 387, 428, 434, 477

exotropia 463
cause 463
intermittent 463

extracapsular cataract extraction. See cataract surgery

extraocular movement
examination 372

eyelid
anatomy 347

F

facial nerve palsy 354, 355, 363, 364, 381

Farnsworth-Munsell test
for color vision 488

filtering shunts in glaucoma surgery 105

five-fluorouracil (5-FU). See anti-metabolite in glaucoma surgery

fixation 59, 152, 358, 449, 456

fleck retina syndrome 261

Flexner Wintersteiner rosettes
retinoblastoma 11, 12, 65, 254, 255, 262, 385, 401, 402, 430, 431, 435, 473, 474, 476–479

fovea. See macula

Foville's syndrome 277, 278, 365

Frey's syndrome 276

Frisby plates
test for binocular single vision 448

Fuch's adenoma
ciliary body 4, 28, 40, 41, 47, 48, 51, 56, 62, 63, 78, 86, 90, 96, 97, 104, 178, 186, 189, 330–332, 391, 394, 423, 428, 430, 476, 478

Fuch's endothelial dystrophy 29, 72, 118, 119, 137, 138, 141, 149, 419

Fuch's uveitis 126, 418, 419

fundal fluorescein angiography 199
age-related macular degeneration 209
central serous retinopathy 200, 221, 339, 343
diabetic retinopathy 32, 33, 39, 49, 81, 191, 218, 219, 223–225, 227–229, 249, 499

fundus albipunctata 262

fundus flavimaculatus 261, 265

fungal keratitis 122–124, 155, 439

fusion 447, 449–452, 460, 463, 471

G

galactosemia 7, 8, 11, 12

ganglion cells of the retina 175

gastrointestinal disease 409

giant cells 359, 418, 429, 430

suprachoroidal hemorrhage 35–37, 40, 83, 85, 102, 187, 192
sympathetic ophthalmia 96, 385, 386, 392, 394, 423, 424, 438, 439
synchisis scintillans 180
synoptophore
 test for binocular single vision 450
syphilis 133, 147, 153, 258, 260, 271, 293, 294, 296, 303, 304, 363, 392, 394, 395, 397, 398, 424, 430
systemic lupus erythematosis 122
systemic sclerosis 416

T

tensilon test 283, 284, 440, 447
Terrien's marginal degeneration 129–131, 157
thyroid eye disease 52, 269, 271, 272, 278, 285, 302, 358, 367, 370, 371, 372, 431, 437, 438, 439, 447, 459, 463, 465, 470
 clinical approach 370
 management 368
 ocular sign 8, 9, 294, 319, 322, 335, 367
 pathology 135–137, 182, 183, 210, 250, 271, 278, 368, 369, 375, 376, 378, 380, 417, 421, 433, 449, 467, 474, 475
Titmus test
 test for binocular single vision 445
TNO random dot tests
 test for binocular single vision 445
tonometry 53, 75, 199
toxocariasis 401
toxoplasmosis 11, 12, 210, 262, 391–396, 403–405, 418, 502
trabecular meshwork 47–49, 51, 52, 67, 84, 109, 432, 440
trabeculectomy
 clinical approach 84
trabeculodialysis 67
trabeculotomy
 congenital glaucoma 11, 41, 65–68, 111, 141, 155, 217
tractional retinal detachment. See retinal detachment
trauma
 blunt 85, 86, 177, 299, 382, 385, 483
 chemical 4, 5, 113–115, 118, 122, 155, 157, 169, 180, 191, 250, 263, 353, 368, 369, 493
 penetrating 21, 85, 114, 122, 127, 131, 151, 166, 423, 438, 439, 483–485
traumatic optic neuropathy 297, 300, 301, 335, 336, 483, 486
tuberculosis 398

tuberous sclerosis 331, 342
tumor
 brain 319
 choroidal 222, 432
 ciliary body 4, 28, 40, 41, 47, 48, 51, 56, 62, 63, 78, 86, 90, 96, 97, 104, 178, 186, 189, 330–332, 391, 394, 423, 428, 430, 476, 478
 conjunctiva 67, 101, 103, 113, 114, 131, 188, 250, 347, 354, 355, 359, 361, 376, 381, 385, 395, 398, 427, 470, 483, 484, 493, 494
 iris 419
 lacrimal gland 122, 363, 368, 371, 372, 377, 378–380, 387, 398, 417
 lid 357–361
 optic nerve 300
 orbital 19, 28, 122, 223, 233, 252, 270, 302, 324, 325, 329, 330, 335, 345, 347, 348, 350, 352, 367–372, 375–379, 385–387, 397–399, 413, 415, 428, 433, 438–440, 466, 471, 476–479, 483

U

ulcerative colitis 409, 410
Usher's syndrome 259, 260
uveitis. See also specific type 391–394
 common causes 391
 investigation 392

V

Van Herick's method
 anterior chamber depth assessment 63
varix
 orbital 376, 377
Vieth-Muller circle 451
viscoelastics 16, 17, 19, 20, 32, 37, 40
visual acuity 12, 75, 214, 220, 455, 485, 501
 assessment in children 11
visual adaptation 502
visual cortex 205, 291, 309, 321–323, 451, 455
visual evoked potential 205, 207, 341
visual field 57–60, 309
 bitemporal hemianopia 309, 310, 313, 315
 changes in glaucoma 55
 examination in neuroophthalmology 57
 humphrey visual field 58, 59
visual hallucination 309–311, 315, 322, 338, 339
vitamins
 deficiency and excess 493
 Vitamin A 122, 174–176, 318, 410, 493, 494